NURSING PHOTOBOOK™

Aiding Ambulatory Patients

NURSING85 BOOKS™
SPRINGHOUSE CORPORATION
SPRINGHOUSE, PENNSYLVANIA

NURSING85 BOOKS™

NURSING PHOTOBOOK™ SERIES
Providing Respiratory Care
Managing I.V. Therapy
Dealing with Emergencies
Giving Medications
Assessing Your Patients
Using Monitors
Providing Early Mobility
Giving Cardiac Care
Performing GI Procedures
Implementing Urologic Procedures
Controlling Infection
Ensuring Intensive Care
Coping with Neurologic Disorders
Caring for Surgical Patients
Working with Orthopedic Patients
Nursing Pediatric Patients
Helping Geriatric Patients
Attending Ob/Gyn Patients
Aiding Ambulatory Patients
Carrying Out Special Procedures

NEW NURSING SKILLBOOK™ SERIES
Giving Emergency Care Competently
Monitoring Fluid and Electrolytes Precisely
Assessing Vital Functions Accurately
Coping with Neurologic Problems Proficiently
Reading EKGs Correctly
Combatting Cardiovascular Diseases Skillfully
Nursing Critically Ill Patients Confidently
Dealing with Death and Dying
Managing Diabetics Properly
Giving Cardiovascular Drugs Safely

NURSE'S REFERENCE LIBRARY®
Diseases
Diagnostics
Drugs
Assessment
Procedures
Definitions
Practices
Emergencies

NURSING NOW™ SERIES
Shock
Hypertension
Drug Interactions
Cardiac Crises
Respiratory Emergencies
Pain

NURSE'S CLINICAL LIBRARY™
Cardiovascular Disorders
Respiratory Disorders
Endocrine Disorders
Neurologic Disorders
Renal and Urologic Disorders
Gastrointestinal Disorders
Neoplastic Disorders
Immune Disorders
Infectious Disorders

***Nursing85* DRUG HANDBOOK™**

NURSING PHOTOBOOK™ Series

PROGRAM DIRECTOR
Jean Robinson

CLINICAL DIRECTOR
Barbara McVan, RN

ART DIRECTOR
Lisa A. Gilde

EDITORIAL MANAGER
Patricia R. Urosevich

**Springhouse Corporation
Book Division**

CHAIRMAN
Eugene W. Jackson

PRESIDENT
Daniel L. Cheney

VICE-PRESIDENT AND DIRECTOR
Timothy B. King

VICE-PRESIDENT, BOOK OPERATIONS
Thomas A. Temple

VICE-PRESIDENT, PRODUCTION AND
PURCHASING
Bacil Guiley

Staff for this volume

BOOK EDITORS
Patricia K. Lawson
Patricia R. Urosevich

CLINICAL EDITOR
Paulette J. Strauch, RN

ASSOCIATE EDITORS
Dario F. Bernardini
Paul Vigna, Jr.

PHOTOGRAPHER
Paul A. Cohen

ASSOCIATE DESIGNERS
Scott M. Stephens
Carol Stickles

ASSISTANT PHOTOGRAPHER
Thom Staudenmayer

EDITORIAL/GRAPHIC COORDINATOR
Doreen K. Stowers

CLINICAL/GRAPHIC COORDINATOR
Evelyn M. James

COPY EDITORS
Barbara Hodgson
David R. Moreau

EDITORIAL STAFF ASSISTANT
Cynthia A. O'Connell

PHOTOGRAPHY ASSISTANT
Frank Margeson

ART PRODUCTION MANAGER
Robert Perry

ARTISTS
Donald G. Knauss   Joan Walsh
George Retseck   Ron Yablon
Louise Stamper

RESEARCHER
Vonda Heller

TYPOGRAPHY MANAGER
David C. Kosten

TYPOGRAPHY ASSISTANTS
Janice Haber   Diane Paluba
Ethel Halle   Nancy Wirs

PRODUCTION MANAGERS
Wilbur D. Davidson
Robert L. Dean, Jr.

PRODUCTION ASSISTANT
Terry Cooney

ILLUSTRATORS
Michael Adams   Bud Yingling
Robert Jackson

SERIES GRAPHIC DESIGNER
John C. Isely

COVER PHOTO
Photographic Illustrations

**Clinical consultant
for this volume**

Ellen Marszalek, RN, BSN, MS, CNP
Administrator, Ambulatory Care
University of Michigan
Ann Arbor

Amended reprint, 1985

© 1983, 1982 by Springhouse Corporation,
1111 Bethlehem Pike, Springhouse, Pa. 19477
All rights reserved. Reproduction in whole or part by
any means whatsoever without written permission of
the publisher is prohibited by law.
Printed in the United States of America.

PB-030185

Library of Congress Cataloging in Publication Data

Main entry under title:

Aiding ambulatory patients.

　(Nursing photobook)
　"Nursing82 books."
　Bibliography: p.
　Includes index.
　1. Nursing.　2. Ambulatory medical care.
　I. Springhouse Corporation　II. Series.
RT120.09A36　1982　610.73'4　82-21253
ISBN 0-916730-49-2

Contents

Introduction

Giving care in the community

Managing head and neck problems

Managing skin, muscle, and bone problems

Managing thoracic problems

Managing abdominal/pelvic problems

Managing other problems

Contributors

At the time of original publication, these contributors held the following positions:

Marion B. Dolan is executive director of Heritage Home Health Hospice in Bristol, New Hampshire. A diploma graduate of St. Mary's Hospital School of Nursing in Brooklyn, New York, she is studying health administration and planning at the University of New Hampshire in Durham. She is president-elect of the New Hampshire National League for Nursing.

Holly McGinn is a staff and visiting nurse for the Visiting Nurse Association of Eastern Montgomery County in Abington, Pennsylvania. She received her nursing diploma from the School of Nursing, Temple University Hospital in Philadelphia.

Ellen Marszalek, also an advisor for this book, is a certified nurse practitioner and administrator of ambulatory care at the University of Michigan in Ann Arbor. Ms. Marszalek earned a BSN degree from Worcester (Mass.) State College and an MS degree in public health from Clark University in Worcester. She is past president of the American Academy of Ambulatory Nursing Administration.

Sister Barbara A. Molloy is assistant professor of nursing at the New Hampshire Technical Institute in Concord. She earned an associate degree at the New Hampshire Technical Institute and a BSN degree at the University of New Hampshire in Durham. Sister Barbara is vice-president of the New Hampshire National League for Nursing.

Barbara J. Morgan, professor of nursing at the New Hampshire Technical Institute in Concord, holds a BSN degree from Hunter College in New York City and an MS degree from Boston University. She is a member and former president of the New Hampshire National League for Nursing, the president of the board of the Central New Hampshire Home Health Agency, and a member of Sigma Theta Tau.

Debra Sullivan Roberge, an instructor at the New Hampshire Technical Institute in Concord, received a BSN degree from the University of New Hampshire in Durham.

Therese C. Vogel is an instructor in the Department of Family Nursing at the Oregon Health Sciences Center, University of Portland. She graduated with a BSN degree from the University of Virginia School of Nursing in Charlottesville and earned an MN degree from the University of Pittsburgh School of Nursing.

Introduction

The role of the ambulatory-care nurse has changed drastically in the past few decades. And it continues to change. Gone are the days when your responsibilities were confined to administering oral medications, giving bed baths, and reinforcing dressings.

Today you use sophisticated equipment, initiate and manage comprehensive screening programs, provide preventive and primary health care, and teach patients about health maintenance.

But that's not all. As you care for your patient's physical problems, you consider his emotional, financial, family, and psychosocial problems as well. You work with him toward the mutual goal of problem management. And by doing so you put him in charge of his care.

If you're properly prepared, patient-centered intervention and autonomy go hand in hand. To help you meet the challenges of ambulatory-care nursing, we've written this PHOTOBOOK. In it, you'll find valuable information on the wide range of problems you encounter every day.

We start by reviewing the problem-oriented approach. Doing so is important, because you'll want to develop a care plan you—or any member of the health-care team—can rely on. We give you helpful suggestions for incorporating the problem-oriented approach in your patient assessment, treatment, and ongoing evaluation. We've also included documentation forms to use as guides.

You'll probably be using assessment and diagnostic equipment in your day-to-day patient care. We've gathered the most up-to-date equipment information we could find. For example, we tell you how to assess hearing using an audiometer, how to monitor heart activity using a portable microprocessor electrocardiograph, and how to evaluate a pacemaker using your telephone.

Dealing with emergencies? You'll find clearly written, step-by-step procedures for managing an avulsed eye, removing a barbed fishhook, and treating a snakebite. To help your patient maintain good health, you'll find tips on teaching him how to prevent low back pain, take a blood pressure reading, and check for testicular problems.

But as we've said, not all your patient's problems are physical. This is why we give you guidelines on dealing with psychosocial problems. We tell you how to recognize drug or alcohol abusers and how to help your patient cope with a sexually transmitted disease, such as genital herpes.

When you study these pages, you'll find AIDING AMBULATORY PATIENTS a book you can depend on. It'll help you expand the scope and depth of your accountabilities and autonomy.

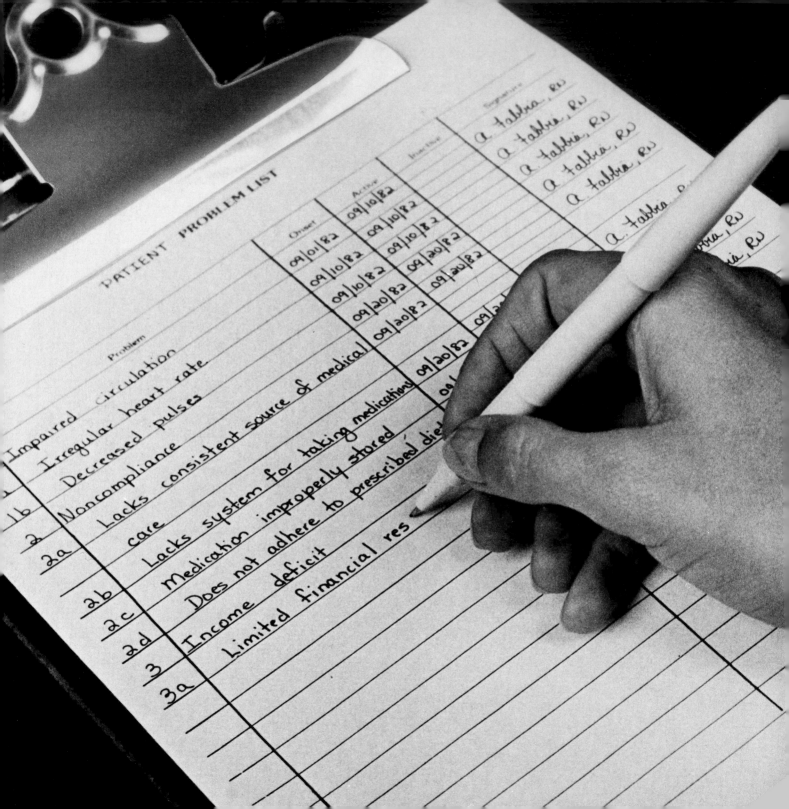

PATIENT PROBLEM LIST

	Problem	Onset	Active	Inactive	Signature
1	Impaired Circulation	09/01/82	09/10/82		a. Tabba, RN
1b	Irregular heart rate	09/10/82	09/10/82		a. Tabba, RN
	Decreased pulses	09/10/82	09/20/82		a. Tabba, RN
2	Noncompliance	09/20/82	09/20/82		a. Tabba, RN
2a	Lacks consistent source of medical care			09/20/82	a. Tabba, RN
2b	Lacks system for taking medications			09/	a. Tabba, RN
2c	Medication improperly stored				
2d	Does not adhere to prescribed diet				
3	Income deficit				
3a	Limited financial res				

Giving Care in the Community

Ambulatory care

Problem-oriented assessment

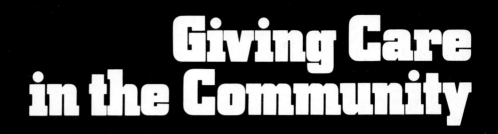

Ambulatory care

You're probably familiar with many aspects of ambulatory nursing. But do you know how ambulatory care and hospital nursing differ? In the next few pages, you'll learn about:
• typical ambulatory-care settings
• major ambulatory-care nursing responsibilities, such as health teaching, health promotion, case finding, and follow-up care
• specific ambulatory-care nursing areas, including occupational health nursing, school nursing, clinic nursing, and community health nursing.

For the concise introduction to ambulatory care you need, read the following pages.

Reviewing ambulatory nursing
As an ambulatory-care nurse, you provide family-centered nursing care in the community, rather than in an inpatient hospital setting. In doing so, you emphasize maintenance of health and optimal functioning. You approach the patient holistically, considering the physical, psychological, social, economic, and environmental components of a health problem.

Ambulatory-care nursing challenges you to work swiftly and competently. You routinely assess and identify your patient's problem and give immediate, skilled care. You're prepared to deal with almost any problem, from a sore throat to a cardiac disorder. You can also give prompt emergency care, when necessary.

You know which conditions you can care for and which you need to refer. You have up-to-date community resource information at your fingertips to make appropriate referrals. Then, in guiding your patient through the health-care system, you act as his advocate.

In addition to providing nursing care, you plan and carry out health promotion activities, such as health screening to identify health risks, and community health education to reduce health risks. Health teaching is a major ambulatory-care responsibility.

Also, because of your access to patients in the community, you're in a good position to identify environmental and social factors contributing to poor health. You don't just focus on the patient—you view him in the context of his family and community. You encourage family members to participate in patient care and to actively support the patient.

Nursing responsibilities
Now that we've outlined the scope of your work, let's review your major nursing responsibilities. You'll find that most of your work falls into one or more of the following categories:
• *Primary care:* assessing the patient, identifying problems

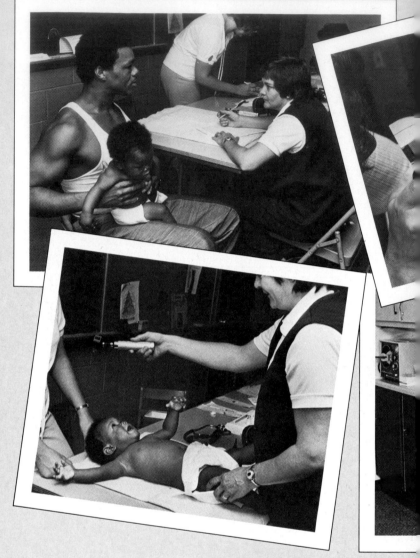

on initial contact, and following up with immediate care or referral. Includes triage, history taking, physical assessment, necessary treatment, health counseling, and referral.
• *Therapeutic care:* giving direct patient care and assessing the effects of intervention. Includes eye irrigation, wound cleansing, dressing changes, and other procedures you perform, as well as monitoring of results.
• *Health-care maintenance:* preserving a state of wellness through monitoring patient health status and providing general health education. Includes

teaching normal body function, daily hygiene, and physical fitness, as well as conducting follow-up assessment and making referrals.
• *Preventive care:* teaching and implementing preventive health care. Includes initiating screening programs, developing educational programs, and reinforcing teaching through follow-up monitoring.
• *Patient education:* teaching the patient and his family about his specific problem and about self-care measures. Includes demonstrating equipment, teaching self-administered procedures, giving care guidelines,

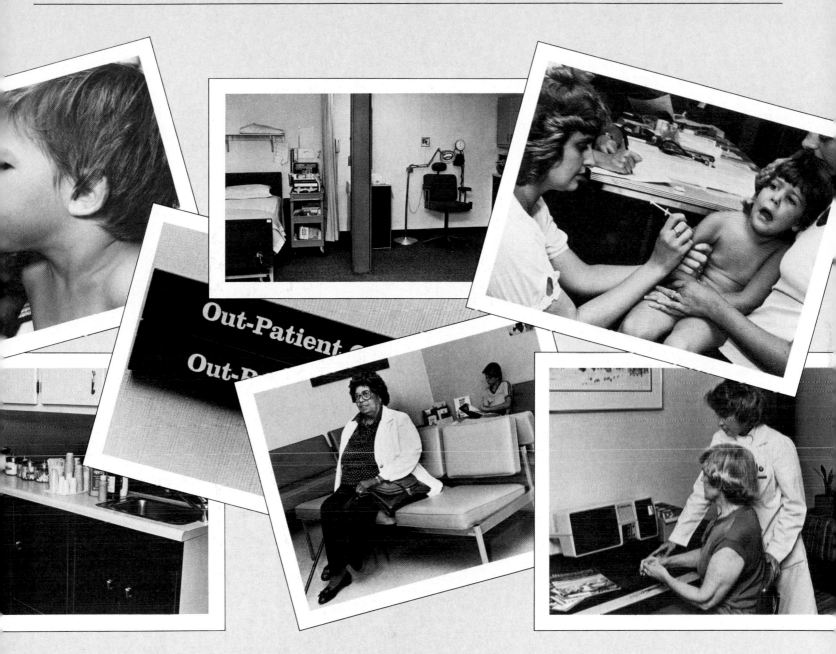

and reinforcing teaching through follow-up monitoring.
• *Patient counseling:* providing emotional support and professional guidance (to patient and family) for dealing with the patient's health status or disease state. Includes giving support during procedures and counseling patients with serious acute conditions as well as terminally ill patients and their families.
• *Coordinating care:* providing services during patient admission to and discharge from an ambulatory setting. Includes documenting, coordinating appointments, and directing the patient to another care provider,

if necessary.

Ambulatory settings
Traditionally, ambulatory care was administered through public health agencies, hospital outpatient departments, private doctors' offices, schools, and industries. But increasingly, it's administered through programs geared to specific settings (for example, a neighborhood clinic), special populations (for example, migrant workers and the elderly), and specific health problems (for example, drug abuse and mental health). In addition, new patterns are emerging in health-care

delivery, including health maintenance organizations (HMOs) and independent nursing practices.
   Ambulatory-care settings include:
• hospital ambulatory-care centers
• multiservice medical centers
• neighborhood health centers
• specialized clinics, such as for family planning and mental health
• health departments
• community health nursing agencies
• homes
• schools
• industries

• home health-care agencies
• private nursing practices
• HMOs
• nontraditional settings, such as senior citizens' centers.
   Not only are new programs emerging, but ambulatory care is increasing. Why? One obvious reason is the already high and continually rising cost of inpatient hospital care. Many treatments and procedures can be performed less expensively on an outpatient basis. Also, as explained above, ambulatory care offers advantages in terms of providing preventive care, community-centered care, and patient teaching.

Ambulatory care

Ambulatory nursing: Four examples

For a number of reasons, you may find useful a run-down of four major ambulatory-care nursing areas: clinic nursing, community health nursing, school nursing, and occupational health nursing.

For example, suppose you're working as an occupational health nurse. If so, a review of your responsibilities may help you organize your nursing priorities.

Or, perhaps you're considering working in another ambulatory-care capacity; for example, as a school nurse. In this case, you might find a list of the school nurse's responsibilities helpful in making your decision.

For the detailed information you need, read the text that follows.

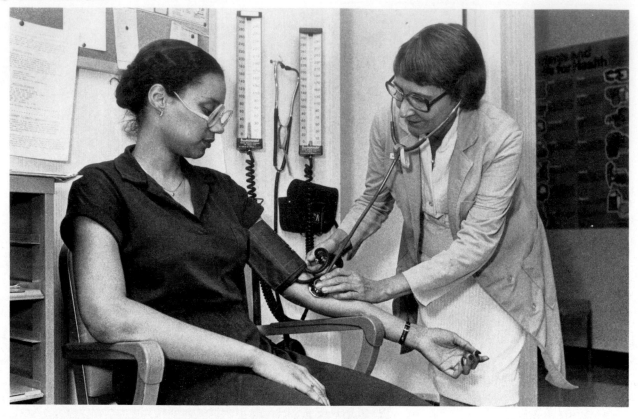

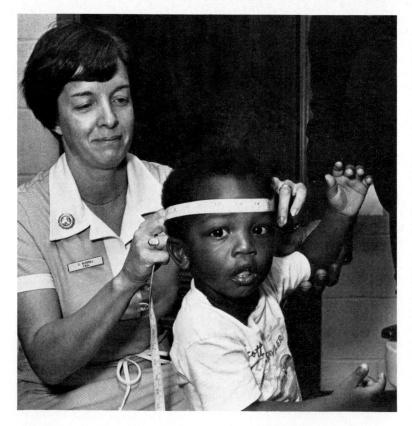

Community health nursing

Are you a community health nurse? Then you take a step *beyond* the clinic nurse; you reach out to the community to identify persons needing help (or those *likely* to need help).

You probably work through an official health agency, a voluntary health agency, a private nonprofit home health agency, or a proprietary home health agency. You're responsible for identifying population subgroups requiring health services and for directing resources toward the families within these groups. Usually, you're responsible for a case load in a specific geographic area, although you're not limited to this area.

Your goals include health promotion, illness prevention, early detection and treatment of disease, health education for self-care, control of communicable disease, and promotion of a healthful environment. Like all ambulatory-care nurses, you give special consideration to environmental, social, and personal factors affecting your patients' health.

You practice primary prevention by taking specific measures to prevent ill-ness; secondary prevention through early case finding, diagnosis, and treat-

Clinic nursing

As a clinic nurse, you could be working in a variety of settings. Depending on clinic staffing patterns and your experience and education level, you could function independently, under an established protocol. Of course, the procedures you perform depend on your clinic's requirements. Following are some of your general functions:
• giving primary care (assessment, shown at left, and treatment or referral)
• administering ordered tests and providing patient teaching about tests
• assisting the doctor with procedures or performing procedures under protocol
• providing patient teaching for self-care and prevention of complications
• documenting patient care thoroughly
• providing follow-up evaluation and care
• referring patients to the appropriate community resources
• communicating with outside agencies
• conducting special programs in health education
• providing support for patients and families
• making sure the clinic is adequately supplied.

ment or referral; and tertiary prevention through patient rehabilitation.
    Your specific responsibilities may include:
• assessing and diagnosing patient problems and formulating and implementing a care plan.
• making home visits to provide nursing care, to monitor and screen patients, and to perform patient and family teaching.
• making follow-up visits to patients with identified needs.
• referring patients to appropriate community resources.
• serving as a client advocate and as an agent for change in improving community health.
• serving as a liaison with community health and social agencies.
• providing direct care in public health clinics (such as well-baby clinics, shown at left, and tuberculosis clinics).
• planning and implementing community health education.
• analyzing the community for risk factors.
• participating in epidemiologic investigations.
• providing disaster nursing services.

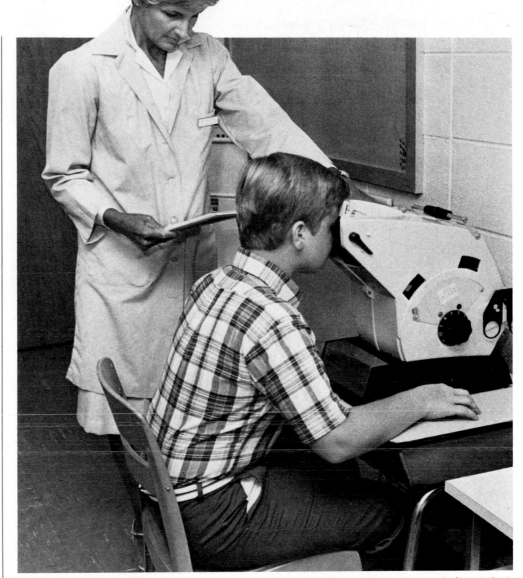

School nursing

If you're a school nurse, your position in the community is a vital one. You're responsible for maintaining the health of the school population by providing health services, offering health education, and promoting a healthy environment. You screen children for early detection of health problems, promote control of communicable disease, and prevent illness by teaching good health habits at an early age.
    Your specific duties probably include:
• conducting health screening; for example, of vision (shown above), hearing, and mental health.
• giving emergency care for illness and injury that occur in school.
• implementing programs for protection and promotion of student health, including immunization programs.
• coordinating school and community health programs.

• monitoring the return to school of a student who has been ill.
• identifying, evaluating, and coordinating health services for handicapped children.
• evaluating, referring, and following up student physical, emotional, and social problems.
• counseling students and parents concerning medical problems.
• documenting health care accurately.
• compiling health statistics, as necessary.
• developing a health curriculum.
• assessing and caring for school personnel, as necessary.
• working with school personnel to maintain an environment conducive to student health.
• interpreting school health and safety policies to parents, students, and school personnel.
• serving as consultant to school system personnel on health matters, as necessary.

Ambulatory care

Ambulatory nursing: Four examples continued

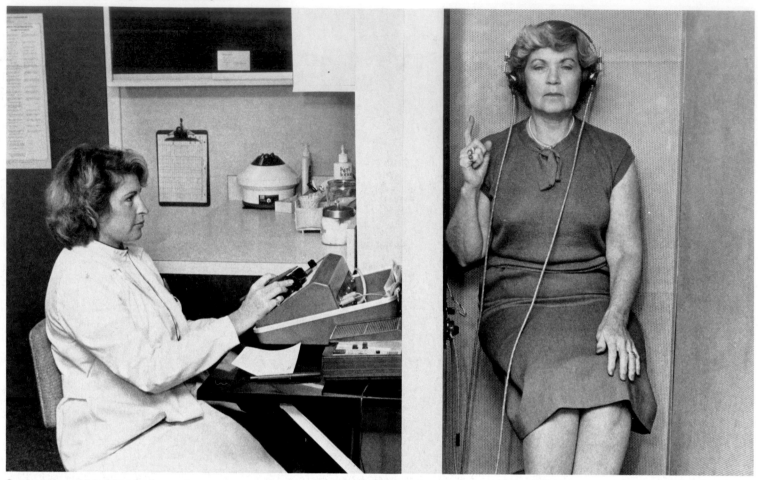

Occupational health nursing

As an occupational health nurse, you provide nursing care in the workplace. You use a wide range of nursing skills, particularly health teaching skills, to protect and promote worker health. If you're successful, you'll benefit employees *and* employers, by improving employee health and, consequently, morale and productivity.

Some of your major responsibilities are:
• in larger companies, working with a health team made up of a nurse, doctor, safety officer, management and labor representatives, and other health-care professionals, as necessary; in smaller companies, working independently and referring patients to other health-care professionals, as necessary.
• collaborating with the doctor to develop a written medical policy and working within its framework.
• providing emergency care for medical problems occurring at the workplace and referring the patient to other health-care professionals, as necessary.
• conducting health surveillance such as hearing tests (shown above), preemploy-

ment and annual physical examinations; identifying those at risk for disease by screening for such conditions as hypertension, cardiovascular disease, and diabetes; and monitoring patients with particular health problems.
• collaborating with the doctor to manage patient health problems.
• monitoring an employee's return to work after serious illness to determine whether he can meet job requirements.
• teaching first aid, cardiopulmonary resuscitation, and other health-related topics.
• developing such protective programs as noise and pollution abatement.
• conducting classes in the physiology of aging and the psychological impact of retirement, as part of employee retirement planning.
• interviewing and counseling an employee regarding his physical and psychosocial problems (such as alcoholism).
• maintaining a working knowledge of community resources for patient referral.
• fostering open communication with the community health nurse, who may see the patient in his home setting.

• maintaining accurate records to help detect health-problem patterns in the employee population. (These records must meet legal and confidentiality requirements.)
• acquiring a working knowledge of potentially toxic materials used in the workplace, including their effects; tests to detect harmful exposure; and nursing care after harmful exposure.
• conducting periodic surveys of the plant to detect physical and chemical hazards, such as loose rails, slippery floors, and chemical mists and dusts; communicating any hazards to a safety officer or appropriate authority; and participating in planning to eliminate hazards.
• maintaining knowledge of the Occupational Safety and Health Act (OSHA), the National Institute of Occupational Safety and Health (NIOSH) regulations, and the workmen's compensation laws in the state where the company's located.
• serving as consultant to labor and management in formulating policies that influence workers' health.
• working with management to provide adequate health-care facilities.

Problem-oriented assessment

"My throat's so sore and scratchy," John Hodges, a 60-year-old train conductor, tells you. "It's been this way for 3 days, and I think I have a fever."

Mr. Hodges is seeking help for the first time at the community health clinic where you work. You're responsible for identifying his presenting problem— and for deciding whether you can manage it or whether referral is necessary.

In the next few pages, we show you how to use the problem-oriented approach in assessing your patient and managing his care. This approach helps you *focus* on your patient's initial problem, so you can deal with it systematically. It also helps you sort out multiple problems, so you can give each the attention it requires.

To document your problem-oriented approach, use the SOAPIER format. This format helps ensure thorough documentation, for clearer communication between co-workers and better legal protection.

To learn the basic guidelines you need to assess and document *any* patient problem, read on.

Learning about the problem-oriented approach

What is the problem-oriented approach? Consider it a systematic method of identifying your patient's problems—one by one—and organizing them for nursing intervention.

To apply the problem-oriented approach, you'll need to use your basic skills of observation and assessment. As you assess your patient, you gather data to identify problems. Then, you develop a plan for each problem and put your plans into action. You must consider your patient's total family situation as an additional source of problems and solutions.

Be sure to familiarize yourself with your agency's policy and state's nurse practice act. This way, you can quickly and accurately distinguish problems that call for nursing intervention—either directly or through referral to interdisciplinary agencies.

Sound confusing? With practice it won't be. You'll find the problem-oriented approach puts you in closer touch with your patient. You'll be able to focus on the problem presented by the patient, perform a complete nursing assessment, and establish priorities.

Before explaining the problem-oriented approach further, let's define *problem:* A problem is a concern that affects the patient and/or his family. Keep in mind that your view of the patient's problem may differ from his assessment of his problem. Be as objective as possible when listening to, observing, and assessing your patient's problems.

To carry out the problem-oriented approach, follow these steps:
• *Assess your patient to identify the problem.* In so doing, you'll gather, examine, and interpret both subjective and objective information. What will you use for data? The patient's reason for the visit, present and past medical history, physical assessment findings, family profile and health history, environmental factors, emotional needs, financial situation, level of function, and nutritional needs.

Use your findings to identify and state the problem. This requires careful analysis, attention to detail, and the ability to differentiate relevant information from irrelevant information.
• *Develop a care plan.* The problem-oriented approach allows you to develop a care plan geared toward patient and family needs. Developing a plan involves considering alternatives and then deciding on and implementing a course of action. The care plan should include problem treatment or management, ongoing assessment, and patient and family education. In addition, be sure the plan is patient goal-oriented, to help you measure his progress.
• *Evaluate and revise the plan.* This includes monitoring results of nursing intervention through accurate documenting and reassessment as well as revising the care plan, as necessary. For guidelines on documenting a problem-oriented assessment, see the text on the following pages.

Reviewing problem categories

Wherever you work in the community, you must be prepared to deal with a wide range of problems, including some that aren't *strictly* medical. In addition to physical problems, your patient could have psychological, social, and financial problems that directly or indirectly affect his health. As you and your patient become more comfortable with each other, you'll be better able to gather and evaluate subjective and objective data. In turn, you'll probably uncover more problems.

Your patient's problems could fall into one or more of the following categories:
• nursing diagnoses based on presenting signs and symptoms; for example, ineffective airway clearance
• medical diagnoses of present and past conditions; for example, hypertension
• laboratory and radiology findings; for example, a positive chest X-ray
• demographic and environmental factors; for example, a language barrier
• socioeconomic problems; for example, lack of funds to provide adequate nutrition
• psychosocial problems; for example, recent divorce.

Problem-oriented assessment

Performing problem-oriented assessment

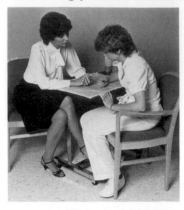

1 To learn how to perform a problem-oriented assessment, consider the following situation:

Martha Hobert, a 31-year-old accountant, enters the clinic where you work. Two days ago, she injured her right index finger in a car door. She tells you, "My finger's throbbing and the pain just keeps getting worse." Ms. Hobert's statement of the problem makes up the *subjective* portion of the assessment.

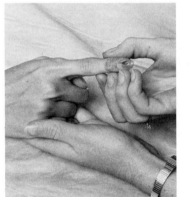

2 When you inspect her finger, you observe an accumulation of blood under the fingernail. Her fingertip is edematous and inflamed but not warm. These findings are the *objective* component.

What's your *assessment*? That she has a subungual hematoma (one under the fingernail) on her right index finger.

Now, you develop a *plan:* to relieve the hematoma and instruct the patient on wound care.

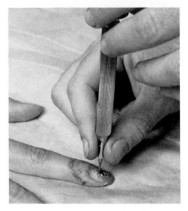

3 To accomplish this, you *intervene* by incising and draining the hematoma, cleansing the wound with povidone-iodine solution, and applying a dry, sterile dressing. You also administer a tetanus toxoid injection, if necessary.

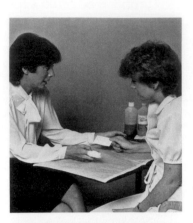

4 Now, tell Ms. Hobert to keep her wound dry and to return to the clinic in 2 days. Be sure to give her a card indicating the day and time of her appointment.

Advise her to go to a hospital emergency department or call her family doctor immediately, if she has any of these signs and symptoms: swelling, increased redness, severe pain, drainage or bleeding, or a temperature above 100° F. (37.7° C.).

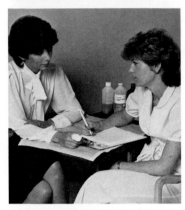

5 Before Ms. Hobert leaves the clinic, briefly *evaluate* your nursing intervention. In so doing, you note that she tolerated it well, understood all instructions given, and plans to return in 2 days.

Document your findings, using the SOAPIER format, explained in the following text, as the nurse is doing here.

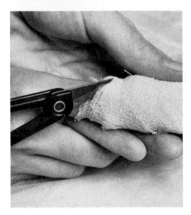

6 On your patient's return visit, reassess her status.

She tells you her pain has decreased. After removing the dressing, you note that the hematoma's drained. Your assessment: The hematoma's resolved. Your plan: Discharge her from care. Your intervention: Instruct her to return to the clinic or her doctor, if further problems develop. Your evaluation: She understands your instructions, so no revision's necessary.

Understanding problem-oriented documenting

How does documenting fit into the problem-oriented approach? Well, if you think about it, documenting is what makes the approach work. When your problem-oriented assessment is documented properly, it provides:
• the data needed to plan the patient's care and ensure continuity of this care.
• written evidence of why the patient received the nursing intervention he did, what response he had to this intervention, and what revisions were made in his care plan, if the intervention proved ineffective.
• a way for health-care professionals to communicate with one another.
• a way to review, study, and evaluate the patient's care in preparation for an audit.
• a legal record that can be used to protect the patient, the agency, and the health-care professional delivering the care.
• data for research and education.

To document a problem-oriented assessment, organize the data as follows:
• S - *subjective:* the patient's or family's statement of the problem; patient's symptoms
• O - *objective:* what you observe, either personally or through test results; patient's signs
• A - *assessment:* combination of subjective and objective data to identify a problem
• P - *plan:* evaluation of the problem and development of immediate and future nursing intervention to manage it

- I - *intervention:* implementation of nursing measures necessary to manage the problem, directly to, for, on, or with the patient (including patient and family teaching)
- E - *evaluation:* assessment of the effects of your immediate and ongoing nursing intervention.
- R - *revision:* based on your evaluation, revision of the care plan, as necessary.

How does problem-oriented documenting differ from narrative documenting? In narrative documenting, you note your observations of the patient's condition. For example, you might record that Mr. Brown complained of nausea and received 10 mg of Compazine I.M., with good results. But as we've explained, in problem-oriented documenting you attempt to identify possible problems and determine their causes and appropriate nursing intervention. Covering this information in an organized fashion—and keeping it updated—helps you better manage your patient's problems.

Progress notes

Progress notes contain a continuous evaluation of your patient's problem. The notes describe how your patient and his family respond to the care plan you've developed for each identified problem. Each time you make an entry in your progress notes, follow the SOAPIER format, organizing and recording the data as subjective, objective, assessment, plan, intervention, evaluation, and revision.

Be sure to cover changes in your patient's condition (improvement or decline), nursing intervention, laboratory findings, treatment and medication effects, unexpected side effects, unusual occurrences during therapy, changes in patient and family behavior resulting from health teaching, and relevant changes in your patient's personal life and family structure.

Flowsheets

You may use flowsheets to keep the documenting up to date. Flowsheets are specially designed progress notes built around the established care parameters you've identified. By recording only essential day-to-day data, you can document quickly and efficiently. In addition, you and other health-care professionals can evaluate patient progress—or lack of it—at a glance.

To learn how to document a problem-oriented assessment, see the care plan and progress notes at right. Here we show documenting for the patient's initial visit. First, assign each problem a number. On the *care plan,* write down the goal you've established for the problem. Then, jot down the letters SOAP.

Record actual intervention and evaluation carried out at the same visit on the *progress notes.* Notice that no information is entered under the letter R, because no revision is necessary at this time. When your patient returns for a follow-up visit, you'll document an entry under each SOAPIER letter (including R, if revision's necessary), using progress notes.

CARE PLAN

Client: Martha Hobert   Date: 9-17-82

Problem: # 1

Goal: Patient will have resolution of subungual hematoma through proper nursing intervention. Patient will have healing of subungual hematoma through compliance with established care plan.

S: "I slammed a car door on my right index finger about 2 days ago. My finger is throbbing and the pain keeps getting worse. I thought it would be better by now."

O: Right index fingertip inflamed and edematous
Accumulation of blood approximately ¼" in size under finger nail of right index finger
Temperature 98.6°F.
Pulse rate in affected hand, 16; rhythm, normal

A: Subungual hematoma right index finger

P: Relieve subungual hematoma of right index finger and instruct patient on proper wound care. *O.J. Strauch RN*

Client Consent: I have read the above Care Plan. I understand and agree with the Care Plan.
Martha Hobert
Signature of Client

PROGRESS NOTES

Date	Prob. No.	
9-17-82	1	I: Incise and drain subungual hematoma of right index finger. Clean wound with povidone-iodine solution. Apply dry, sterile dressing to wound. Administer tetanus toxoid injection. Instruct patient to keep dressing dry and to immediately report the following signs and symptoms of infection: swelling, increase of redness, severe pain, drainage or bleeding, fever above 100°F. Instruct patient to return to clinic on 9/19/82 at 10:00 a.m. Give patient written appointment card. E: Patient tolerated procedure well, understands all above instructions, and has signed consent to the established care plan. R: *O.J. Strauch RN*

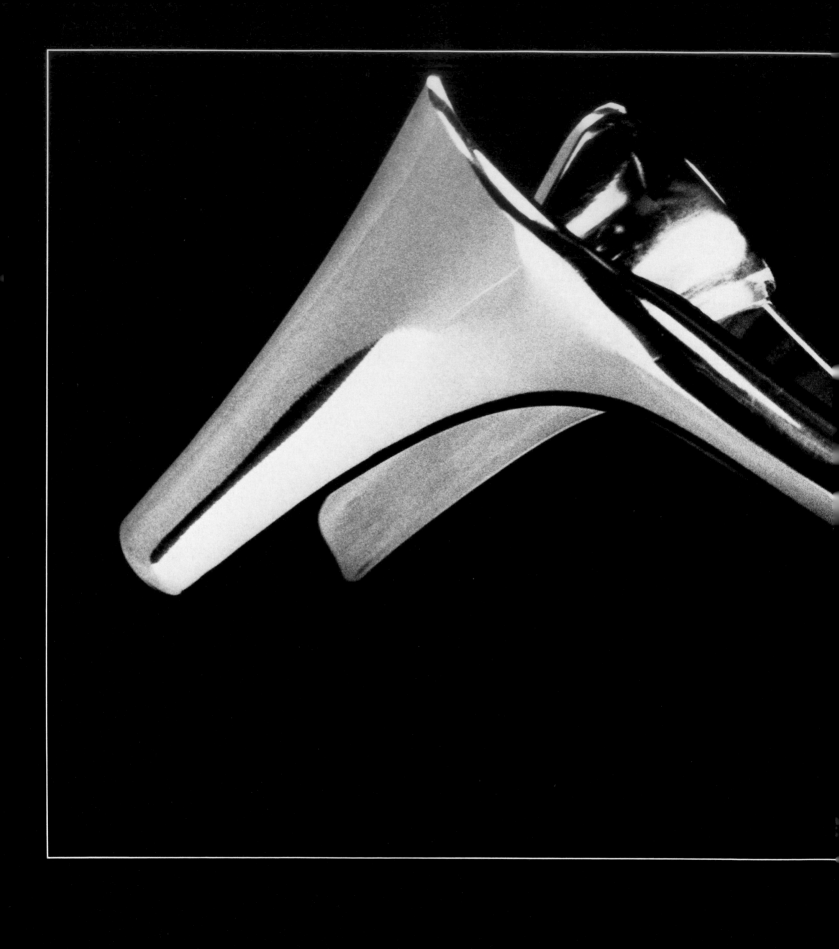

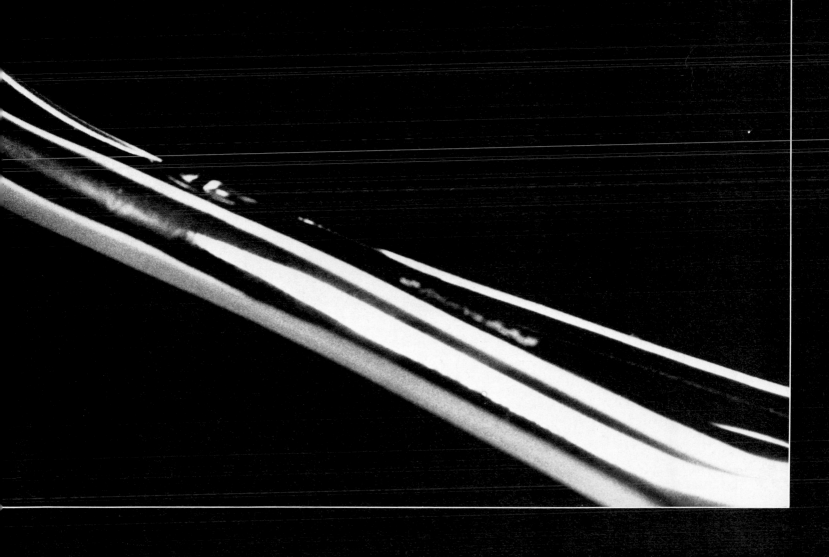

Managing Head and Neck Problems

Eye

Ear

Nose, mouth, and throat

Head

Eye

As a nurse treating ambulatory patients, you probably care for many types of eye injury. Whether your patient's injury is caused by a fistfight or by flying glass, your nursing skills may save his sight.

To care for your patient quickly and efficiently, you need to identify and manage his injury. In the next few pages, you'll learn how. For example, we tell you how to identify a contusion and treat it effectively.

Do you know how to perform emergency eye-care procedures? On the following pages, we show you the most important ones. You'll learn how to:
• remove a foreign particle by everting the eyelid
• check for corneal abrasion by performing corneal staining
• patch an eye without causing additional injury
• irrigate a chemical burn injury.

In addition, we provide you with valuable eye safety tips to review with your patient.

Do you feel you have a lot to learn about caring for eye injuries? Then, read the next few pages carefully.

Treating an eye injury

Are you ready to care for a patient with an eye injury? To help you prepare, review the chart on the following page, which outlines appropriate care for several types of eye injury. Some less critical problems, such as corneal abrasion, cause severe pain and stinging, whereas more urgent injuries, such as a chemical burn, may produce severe pain only briefly. But the decrease in pain doesn't minimize the need for immediate attention.

Begin treatment by reassuring your patient, who's probably concerned about losing sight in his affected eye. Then, take a quick but complete eye history and thoroughly inspect the patient's eye.

Important: If your patient has a serious emergency condition, such as a chemical burn, treat the problem *immediately*. Take the history only *after* giving the necessary care. Then, inspect the eye thoroughly to determine the extent of damage.

In giving eye care, keep in mind these general guidelines:
• Explain the procedure to your patient before beginning inspection or treatment.
• Wash your hands before touching your patient's eye.
• If your patient can't open his eyes independently, separate his eyelids with your thumb and forefinger.
• If your patient's wearing hard contact lenses, remove them before performing any procedures.
• Be gentle when performing all eye-care procedures. Keep pressure off the orbital bone and eyeball.
• Assess the eye completely, including the inside of the lower and upper eyelids. If necessary, evert the upper lid, as instructed on page 22.
• If your patient has an object embedded in his eye, don't attempt to remove it. Patch his eye and have him transported to an emergency department for immediate care.
• If you see any blood or blood clots in your patient's eye, apply a patch and refer the patient to an emergency department or a doctor. Don't attempt to remove the blood or blood clot.
• Use a clean, moistened handkerchief or the end of a moistened cotton-tipped applicator to remove a non-embedded object from the conjunctival surface. Never use a match, toothpick, or any other sharp object that could perforate your patient's eye.
• When irrigating a patient's eye, position his head so you're irrigating from the inner canthus to the outer canthus of the affected eye. This way, solution from the affected eye won't flow into the unaffected eye.
• After caring for your patient's eye injury, limit the use and movement of his affected eye by covering it with a patch or dressing, unless your patient has a chemical burn. If necessary, apply a patch to the unaffected eye.
• Remind your patient to keep his fingers away from his affected eye. Rubbing his eye may drive an object deeper and make it harder to remove.
• Avoid giving your patient anything to eat or drink if you suspect he'll need immediate eye surgery.

Taking an eye history

As you prepare to assess your patient's eye injury, you'll need to take a careful history. The information you gather helps you determine the extent of the injury and deliver the best possible care. Ask your patient these questions:
• Do you feel like something's in your eye?
• Did an object strike your eye?
• Do you work around chemicals or toxic fumes? Explain what contact you have with them. Did a chemical splash into your eye? Do you know what the chemical was or can you show me the container? Did you attempt to rinse out the chemical? What rinsing fluid did you use?
• Are one or both eyes affected?
• Do you have any eye pain? When did you first notice it? Describe the pain. Is it a sharp pain or a burning sensation?
• Have you experienced any vision changes since the injury? What kind? Any rapid vision loss or vision reduction? Are you having or have you had any blurred vision or double vision? When did this occur?
• Do you wear corrective lenses, such as glasses or contacts? At what age did you start wearing them? When was your last routine eye exam? Did the doctor detect any problems? What were they?
• What medication (if any) do you take? How often do you take it? How long have you been taking it? Are you allergic to any medications? Which medications and how do they affect you?
• Are you allergic to any foods? Which foods and how do they affect you? Have you recently eaten any foods you don't usually eat?
• Have you recently been exposed to pollen, dust, or mold?

Nurses' guide to eye injuries

Consider the eye a small globe of tissue, blood, and nerves arranged in layers around a firm, fluid-filled center. Normally, the sclera and cornea provide protection for the eye's inner layers. However, the sclera and cornea *can* be penetrated by foreign objects, such as wood splinters. Five of the most common eye injuries and the immediate care for each are on the following pages.

Recognizing eye danger signals

Your patient knows he must get medical attention immediately when he injures an eye. But can he recognize the onset of an eye disorder or infection? Tell him that any of the signs and symptoms listed below may indicate an eye problem and requires medical attention. Of course, if you note any of these during routine assessment, refer him to a doctor.

Eye danger signals include:
• persistent redness.
• continuous discharge, crusting, or tearing.
• pupil irregularities; for instance, if the pupils are not equal in size or the shape of either is distorted.
• visual disturbances, such as blurring, double vision, peripheral vision loss, and floating spots.
• continuing discomfort or pain in or around the eye, especially after an injury.
• opaque spots in normally transparent parts of the eye.
• eye crossing (strabismus), especially in children.

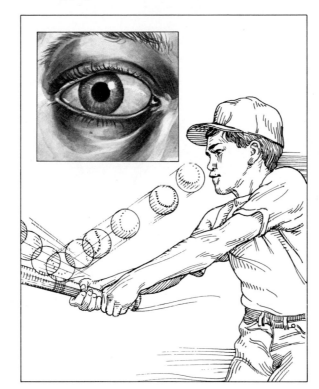

Blunt injury or contusion

Signs and symptoms
• Moderate to severe pain
• Orbital edema
• Ecchymosis
• Blurred vision, spots, or light flashes; all signs of possible retinal detachment
• Intraocular hemorrhage

Possible cause
• Severe direct blow to the eye or face, as from a fist or hard-thrown ball

Nursing intervention
• Keep a cool, wet compress on the patient's eye until edema decreases. Replace the compress with a fresh one every 15 minutes. For ecchymosis, keep a cool compress on the area continuously for up to 24 hours.
• No matter how minimal the damage appears, refer the patient to a doctor. Contusion can cause retinal tear or separation.

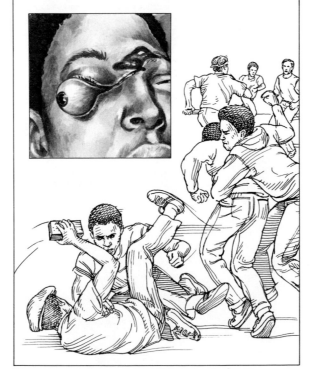

Avulsed eye

Signs and symptoms
• Eye protruding from its socket
• Hemorrhage
• Severe pain
• Possibly shock

Possible cause
• Traumatic blow to the eye

Nursing intervention
• Place moistened sterile 4"x4" gauze pads around the avulsion.
• Cover the avulsed eye with a crushed paper cup to protect it from any pressure. Secure the cup to your patient's face with tape or gauze roller bandage.
• Apply a patch over the unaffected eye to prevent eyeball movement.
• Have the patient transported to a doctor or a hospital immediately. Be sure he remains supine during transport.

Eye

Nurses' guide to eye injuries continued
Eyelid laceration

Signs and symptoms
- Profuse bleeding
- Eyelid edema

Possible cause
- Blow to the supraorbital area, as from a sports injury

Nursing intervention
- Cleanse and assess the wound and the orbital area.
- Observe for the presence of a foreign object, for laceration of the eyelid, and for penetration of the eyeball.
- Apply gentle direct pressure or a pressure patch over the affected area to stop the bleeding.
- If you're certain the eyeball's undamaged and no foreign object's present, place a clean dressing over the affected eye.
- Immediately apply cold compresses to treat soft-tissue bruises above and below the eye. Continue until the edema decreases.
- Place any detached fragments of eyelid skin in a container with normal saline solution, and transport the container to the doctor or hospital, along with the patient.
- Cover the unaffected eye with a patch.
- Transport patient to hospital.

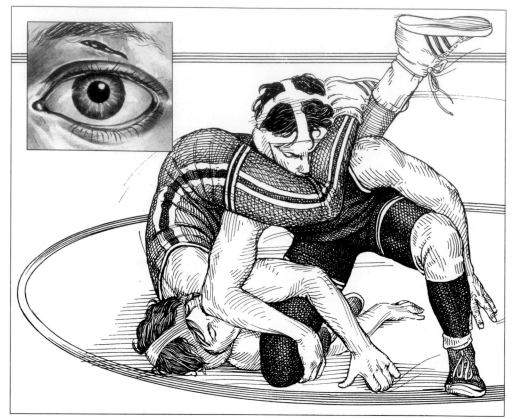

Eyeball laceration

Signs and symptoms
- Severe pain
- Reduced vision
- External leakage of ocular fluid
- Intraocular bleeding
- Retinal tear or detachment

Possible cause
- Penetration of a foreign object, such as a stick, glass, rock, or piece of metal, into the sclera or cornea

Nursing intervention
- Don't attempt to remove the object or irrigate the eye.
- Don't attempt to remove any blood or blood clots on the eyeball. Doing so may cause further damage.
- Stabilize the object, such as a stick, with a paper cup. Cut a hole in the cup and slip the cup around the object. Then, secure the cup to your patient's face with tape or gauze roller bandage.
- If the object's small, cover the affected eye with a patch. Then, apply an eye shield over the patch to prevent any pressure on the eyeball.
- Patch the unaffected eye.
- Have the patient transported to a doctor or a hospital immediately.

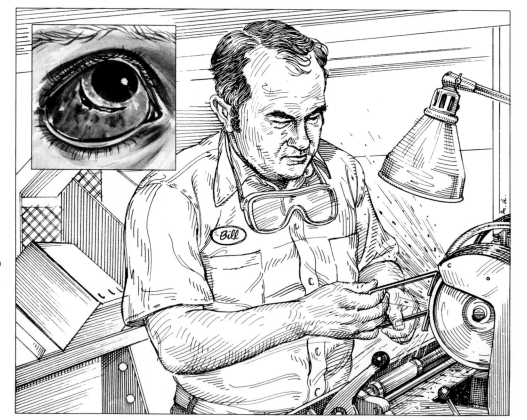

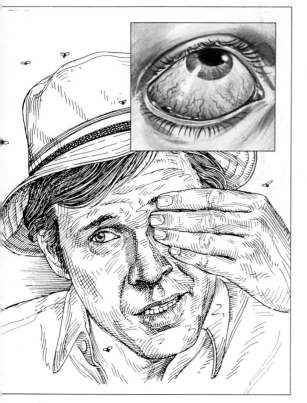

Superficial eye irritation

Signs and symptoms
• Sensation of foreign body
in eye
• Reddened conjunctiva
• Excessive tearing
• Moderate pain or stinging
• Blurred vision

Possible causes
• Particle (such as eyelash, cinder, or insect) on
conjunctiva
• Particle on inner surface of eyelid or in lower
conjunctival sac
• Particle on cornea
• Corneal abrasion
• Acute corneal infection

Nursing intervention
• If the object's on the cornea, gently patch the eye
and have your patient transported to a doctor or a
hospital.
• If the object's on the sclera and not embedded,
gently remove the object, using a moistened cotton-
tipped applicator, the end of a moistened clean
handkerchief, or a facial tissue.
• If the object's on the inner surface of the upper
eyelid, evert the lid and remove the object.
• After the object's removed, perform corneal
staining to assess damage. If corneal abrasion exists,
apply a pressure patch and refer the patient to a
doctor.
• If the object can't be removed or irritation persists,
gently patch the eye and have your patient transported to a doctor or a hospital.

Nurses' guide to eye burns

Caustic injury

Signs and symptoms
• Severe pain, which may *decrease*
after trauma because of destroyed
nerve endings
• Blurred vision or complete vision
loss

Possible causes
• Alkaline agents, such as those found
in household drain cleaners, paint
thinner, lime, plaster, mortar, cement,
and whitewash
• Acid agents, such as those found in
bleaches, antiseptics with phenol,
silver polish, and battery acids

Nursing considerations
• Be aware that a caustic injury can
cause extremely serious damage to the
cornea, conjunctiva, sclera, and lens,
which may lead to vision loss. The
injury's severity depends on chemical
type, length of exposure to the chemical,
and time elapsed before emergency
care is given. Acids cause immediate
damage; then a tissue protein forms,
which becomes a barrier against
further acid penetration.
• Immediately irrigate the affected eye
with sterile normal saline solution or
water.
• Manually separate the eyelids to
irrigate if patient can't open them
independently.
• After you've begun irrigation, try to
have someone identify the chemical
from the container label.
• Irrigate acid burns for at least
20 minutes, depending on the severity
of exposure.
• Irrigate alkaline burns for at least
30 minutes, and continue longer
if needed.
• Inspect for residual chemical particles
by everting the eyelid.
• Be aware that in a chemical burn,
pain's a poor indicator of the extent of
tissue damage. The most serious
injuries produce little pain.
• Perform corneal staining to assess
the degree of damage. Never cover the
affected eye.
• Have the patient transported to a
doctor or a hospital.

Surfactant injury

Signs and symptoms
• Intense stinging
• Superficial damage to the corneal
epithelium
• Corneal abrasion or infection

Possible causes
• Solvents, such as alcohol and ether

• Detergents, such as those found
in home and industrial cleaners,
antiseptics, cosmetics, and shampoos

Nursing considerations
• Be aware that solvents rarely cause
permanent eye damage.
• Follow the same procedure as for
treating a caustic injury.
• Irrigate the eye for at least 10 minutes.

Thermal burn

Signs and symptoms
• Edema of eyelid tissue
• Necrosis of eyelid area
• Scarring of cornea, on direct contact

Possible causes
• Exposure to flame
• Contact burns from flying ash or
molten metal

Nursing considerations
• Perform corneal staining to assess
the degree of damage.
• Apply cool, wet compresses to the
affected eye to reduce pain and edema.
• Instill antibiotic eye drops or ointment, if ordered, to prevent secondary
infection.
• Refer the patient to a doctor.
• You may apply a metal or plastic eye
shield over the eye patch at night, to
prevent further irritation.

Ultraviolet burn

Signs and symptoms
• Severe eye pain beginning 4 to
6 hours after exposure and lasting up
to 24 hours

Possible cause
• History of overexposure to bright
sunlight, sunlight reflected off snow,
sunlamp, electric flashes, welding
arc, or germicidal lamp

Nursing considerations
• Perform corneal staining to assess
the degree of damage.
• Apply cool, wet compresses to
reduce edema.
• Administer analgesic medication, as
ordered.
• Instill topical antibiotic ointment or
eye drops, as ordered.
• Encourage the patient to rest in a
quiet, darkened area.
• Tell the patient to keep a patch over
the affected eye for at least 24 hours,
as ordered.
• Reassure the patient that the pain
will probably diminish greatly within 24
hours.
• Refer the patient to a doctor.

Eye

Assessing the eye and removing a foreign particle

Let's assume you're an occupational health nurse at a pharmaceutical company. Forty-eight-year-old Paul Detweiler, a carpenter working at the company, enters your office complaining of intense pain in his left eye. He tells you he was sawing wood when he first felt the pain. You see the eye is red and tearing.

Because you'll be assessing his eye, you must wash your hands thoroughly. As you do, begin taking an eye history, following the guidelines on page 18. First, find out if he's wearing contact lenses. If he is, help him remove them. Then, explain to him that you'll be inspecting his eye for sawdust, splinters, and any other foreign particles.

Important: *Use the procedure shown here only to remove foreign particles on the conjunctival surface. Never attempt to remove a foreign particle on the cornea. Instead, follow the instructions in the eye injury chart on page 19.*

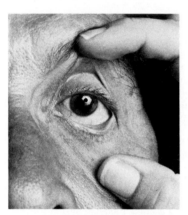

1 Now, with your thumb and forefinger, separate the eyelids of Mr. Detweiler's affected eye.

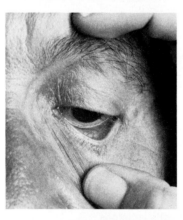

2 Assess the eyeball for foreign particles. Then, have him look up. Observe the inner surface of his lower eyelid, as the nurse is doing here.

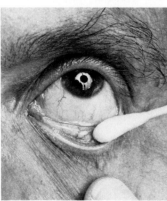

3 You locate a particle of sawdust on the lower conjunctival surface of Mr. Detweiler's eye. To remove it, use the moistened end of a cotton-tipped applicator, as shown.

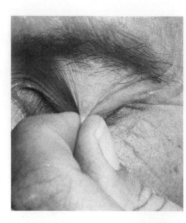

4 Although you've removed one particle, you want to check further to make sure no other foreign particles are in his eye.

First, grasp the upper lid of his affected eye and gently pull it *down* over the lower lid and *away* from the eyeball. This may dislodge particles on the eyeball or on the upper eyelid's inner surface, by allowing tears to wash over the eye's surface.

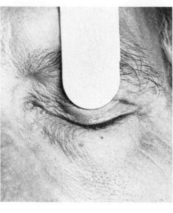

5 To check the inner surface of the upper eyelid, evert the eyelid. Here's how:

Place a tongue depressor about ⅜" (1 cm) above the edge of the lid, as shown. Be sure it rests against the edge of the eyelid's upper tarsal plate. Pushing down on this plate makes eversion easier.

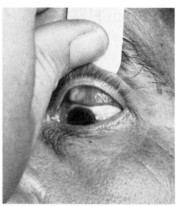

6 Before everting, assure Mr. Detweiler that you'll be gentle. Then, tell him to look toward the floor. This relaxes the levator muscle, making eyelid eversion easier. Encourage him to relax and remind him to avoid squeezing his eyelid shut.

To evert the eyelid, gently pull it over the tongue depressor, as the nurse is doing here. Then, inspect his upper eyelid for foreign particles.

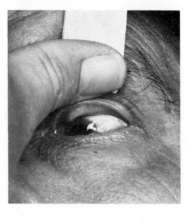

7 Return the everted lid to its normal position by having your patient look up as you gently pull his lid forward. Don't allow the lid to fall back over the eye suddenly.

Suppose you haven't found the source of irritation. Then, cover your patient's affected eye with an eye patch and refer him to a doctor or a hospital.

Finally, document all your findings, treatment, and instructions on the appropriate form.

Learning about corneal staining

How familiar are you with corneal staining? As you may know, you'll perform this procedure to detect such eye injuries as corneal abrasion. Staining also helps identify such corneal disorders as herpes simplex and keratitis.

To stain your patient's cornea, use fluorescein dye. Fluorescein is a green-yellow-orange indicator dye that changes color with pH changes. It stains the eye's surface orange or yellow. Although it doesn't adhere to intact corneal epithelium, it does adhere to abrasions, staining the abraded area bright green.

Note: The staining is temporary and washes off within a few minutes.

To instill the dye, use a strip of fluorescein paper. Then, view the eye through a slit lamp equipped with a cobalt blue filter. To identify corneal damage, look for areas that are stained green.

Keep in mind that fluorescein dye won't harm the eye, but it does temporarily hamper the corneal epithelium's protective function. Also, if the eye *is* injured, it will be more susceptible to infection. To prevent cross-contamination, which could lead to eye infection, use a new strip of fluorescein paper for each patient.

Performing corneal staining

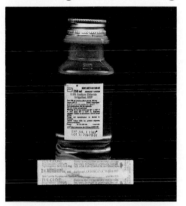

1 Now that you've removed the particle of sawdust from Mr. Detweiler's eye, you'll want to check for abrasions. To do this, perform corneal staining. Here's how to proceed:

First, obtain sterile normal saline solution and a strip of fluorescein paper.

Explain to your patient what you're going to do. Then, wash your hands thoroughly to reduce the risk of contaminating his eye.

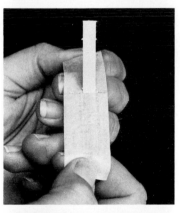

2 Next, remove the fluorescein paper strip from its packet by peeling away both sides of the packet.

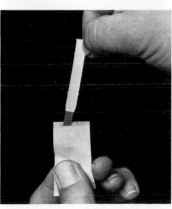

3 Pull the strip out of the packet halves without touching the orange area on the bottom of the strip, to avoid contaminating the dye.

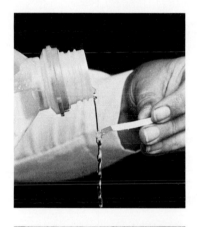

4 Then, wet the fluorescein paper strip with sterile normal saline solution.

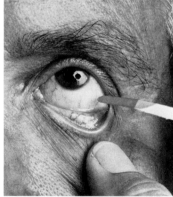

5 Now ask Mr. Detweiler to look at the ceiling. Gently touch the fluorescein paper to his sclera. As you do, a thin film of fluorescein dye will spread over his cornea.

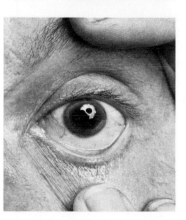

6 When the dye's covered the cornea, use a slit lamp to look for areas stained green. If you see any, patch Mr. Detweiler's eye and refer him to a doctor or a hospital.

When you complete the procedure, document your findings on the appropriate form.

Eye

Applying a pressure eye patch

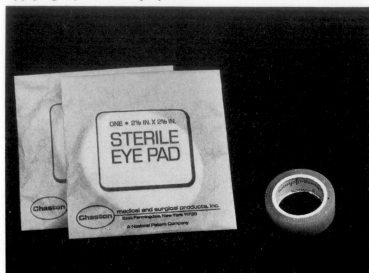

The corneal staining you performed on Paul Detweiler reveals a corneal abrasion in his left eye. The doctor wants a pressure patch applied to prevent Mr. Detweiler's eyeball from moving. This allows the eye to heal properly. Do you know how to apply a pressure patch?

First, obtain two sterile oval eye pads and a roll of ½" nonallergenic adhesive tape.

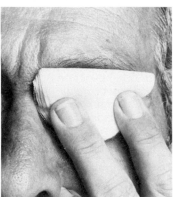

1 Now, explain to Mr. Detweiler what you're going to do. Tell him that the patch will protect his eye from further injury while the abrasion heals.

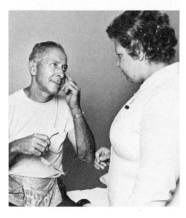

2 Have him close his affected eye. Next, take one of the eye pads, fold it in half, and position it horizontally over the affected eye. Gently hold it in place with one hand, as shown.

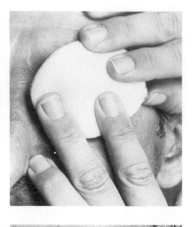

3 Then, with your other hand, take the second pad and place it at an angle over the folded eye pad, as shown.

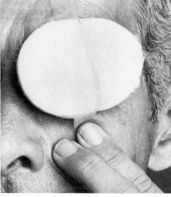

4 To secure the top eye pad, apply a strip of tape diagonally over the center of the pad. Secure one end to the patient's forehead and the other end to his cheek.

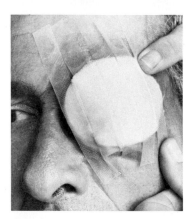

5 Apply the other four tape strips parallel to the first strip, placing two on each side of it.

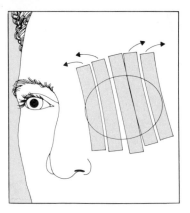

6 Pull the tape ends on the inner side of the pad firmly toward the nose (see illustration). Pull the tape ends on the outer side of the pad firmly toward the ear.

Ask your patient if he can open his patched eye. If he can, the patch isn't positioned properly. Reapply it and secure the tape strips more tightly. Tell Mr. Detweiler not to remove the patch and to return to the doctor for follow-up. Finally, document the procedure.

Applying an eye patch

Depending on the type of eye injury your patient has, you may need to apply a patch to the eye. A patch allows the eye to rest and protects it from outside sources of infection. Also, you can use a patch when you want to help prevent putting pressure on the eye; for instance, if the cornea's ulcerated or if blood is present on the eyeball (hyphema).

Important: A patch is contraindicated if your patient has a chemical burn, because it allows heat to build up in the affected eye, possibly reactivating the chemical residue that hasn't been removed with irrigation. A patch is also contraindicated if your patient has an eye infection, because the heat buildup can serve as an incubator for bacteria.

To prepare for the procedure, obtain two strips of ½" nonallergenic tape and a sterile eye pad.

Remember to wash your hands.

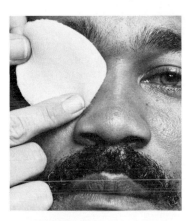

1 First, explain the procedure and the purpose of the patch to your patient. Then, ask him to close his affected eye.
  Next, position the eye pad over his affected eye.

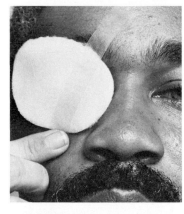

2 Place a strip of nonallergenic tape diagonally over the center of the pad, as the nurse is doing here. Secure one end to his forehead, close to the bridge of his nose, and the other end to his cheek.

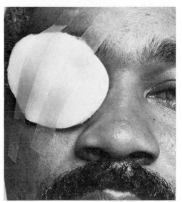

3 Then, place the other strip from the outer portion of his eyebrow to his cheek, as the nurse is doing here.
  Now, check the pad to make sure you haven't taped it too tightly. Loosen the tape strips, if necessary.
  Caution: Avoid applying pressure to the eyeball when taping.
  Finally, document the procedure on the appropriate form.

Teaching your patient how to apply an eye shield

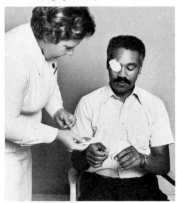

1 *Let's say your patient has a corneal ulceration of his right eye. To prevent any pressure on the eye and provide greater protection, you'll want to teach him how to apply an eye shield over his eye patch. Follow these steps:*
  First, have your patient wash his hands. Then, give him a metal or plastic shield wide enough to cover his eye, and four strips of ½" nonallergenic adhesive tape. He'll also need a mirror.

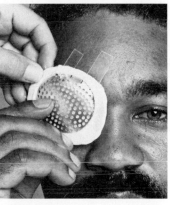

2 Now, have your patient stand in front of a mirror and position the shield over his eye patch, as shown. Tell him to be sure the edge of the shield rests on the bone surrounding the eye. If the shield you're using has a narrow edge, make sure it's placed toward the bridge of his nose.

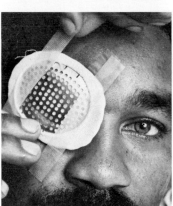

3 To secure the shield, tell your patient to apply two tape strips diagonally over each end of the shield. Have him secure the top ends to his forehead and the bottom ends to his cheek.

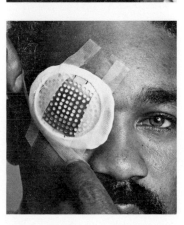

4 Now, tell him to cross the two remaining strips at 90° angles to the first two. He'll secure the top ends to his forehead and the bottom ends to his cheek and the side of his nose.
  Now, remind him to check the shield to make sure it's taped securely but not too tightly.
  Finally, document your patient teaching and observations on the appropriate form.

Eye

Protecting an avulsed eye

Ten-year-old Jade Harper, an elementary school student, is in the playground when a baton her girlfriend is twirling hits her in her right eye. The force of the twirling stick causes her eye to avulse. Do you know how to provide proper emergency care? Caution: Never attempt to push an avulsed eye back in its socket; instead, cover it with a paper cup. Doing so protects the eye from pressure and movement.

First, position your patient supine. Try to calm her, and explain what you're going to do.

At the same time, ask a teacher to go to your office and call an ambulance and get the following equipment: sterile 4"×4" gauze pads, paper cup, scissors or sterile suture set, container of sterile normal saline solution, and roller gauze bandage. Note: If you don't have a paper cup on hand, use a paper plate, a handkerchief, or a saucer.

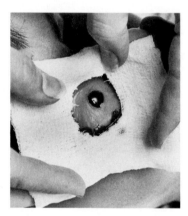

1 When the equipment arrives, begin by cutting a hole in one gauze pad. Make the hole large enough so the pad can fit over the avulsed eye. Next, moisten the pad with the sterile saline solution. (If none's available, you may use water.)

Place the cut pad over her avulsed eye, as shown.

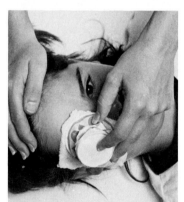

2 Now, crush the paper cup with your hand. Doing so prevents further eye damage caused by accidentally crushing the cup during transfer. Position the cup over the affected eye.

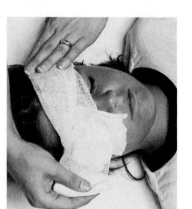

3 Finally, secure the cup with gauze bandage, as shown. Also, place a patch over your patient's unaffected eye. Then, have your patient transported to a hospital immediately. Document the procedure on the appropriate form.

Treating a mild chemical burn

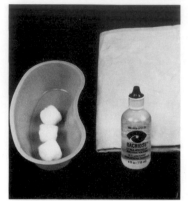

1 Stephanie Dailey, a 35-year-old assembly-line worker, accidentally sprays ether in her left eye while cleaning her equipment. After assessing her eye, you decide to irrigate it with an eye irrigation solution.

First, obtain eye irrigation solution at room temperature, emesis basin, bed-saver pad, and sterile cotton balls. Wash your hands thoroughly. Reassure Ms. Dailey and explain to her what you're going to do.

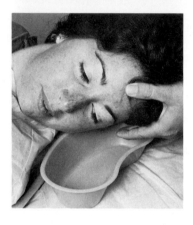

2 Place her in supine position, with her head turned toward her affected side. Now, position the bed-saver pad and emesis basin under her head, as shown.

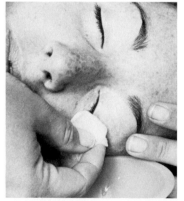

3 Next, moisten a cotton ball with the irrigation solution and gently cleanse the outer surface of her eyelids.

Then, ask your patient to open her affected eye. If necessary, assist her by using your thumb and forefinger.

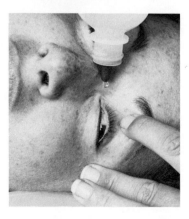

4 Now, using your other hand, direct a stream of solution toward her eye's inner canthus and allow it to flow over her eyeball, to the outer canthus. As you irrigate, avoid touching Ms. Dailey's eyeball or eyelids with the tip of the solution container.

After completing the procedure, dry her face with a sterile cotton ball and reassess her eye. Refer her to a doctor, as necessary. Finally, document the procedure and referral.

Treating a severe chemical burn

Parnell Stevens, a 42-year-old maintenance worker, is disinfecting equipment when he accidentally splashes cleaning fluid in his left eye. You've been called to the scene to give emergency care. You know that chemical burns, if not treated immediately, can lead to serious eye damage, including blindness. You need to act quickly to irrigate his eye. Follow the procedure below.

After irrigating his eye, ask your patient about the cleaning fluid. If he doesn't remember any details and the container's not at the scene, ask someone to retrieve it. Identifying the chemical involved will help you determine the likely extent of the injury.

Then, complete your assessment. Refer your patient to a doctor or a hospital. Document your care—including how the patient tolerated the procedure—assessment, and referral on the appropriate form.

Never cover a chemical eye burn with a dressing or patch.

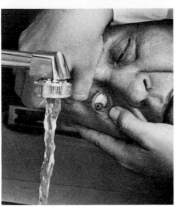

1 First, reassure Mr. Stevens, and explain what you're going to do. Then, turn on the faucet. Make sure the water's lukewarm and that it's flowing at a slow to moderate rate.

Next, position his head under the faucet, affected eye down, so the stream of water flows over the conjunctiva, from the inner canthus. This prevents the caustic solution from entering the unaffected eye.

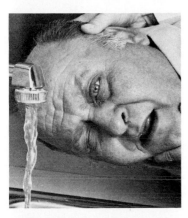

2 Now, ask your patient to open his affected eye. If he can't, assist him, using your thumb and forefinger, or both thumbs, as shown here.

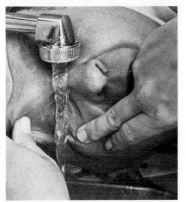

3 Begin irrigating his eye, and continue for at least 20 minutes. Make sure the water contacts all parts of his eye, including the inner and outer canthi and the inner surface of the eyelids, as shown here.

Note: If both eyes are affected, irrigate them alternately, repositioning the patient's head.

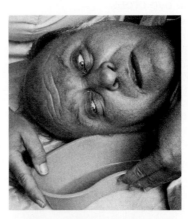

4 You may also irrigate a chemical burn with sterile normal saline solution. To do so, obtain a 1,000-ml I.V. bag of sterile solution. Make sure it's at room temperature. Attach I.V. tubing to the solution bag. Now, have your patient lie down and turn his head toward his affected side. Place an emesis basin just below the affected eye's outer canthus, as the nurse is doing here.

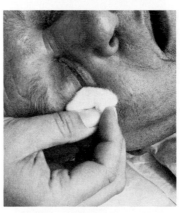

5 Next, ask him to open his eye; assist him, if necessary. Then, open the flow clamp on the tubing and irrigate his eye from the inner canthus to the outer canthus, as shown. Adjust the flow clamp to keep the solution flowing evenly but not forcefully.

Empty the emesis basin, as necessary.

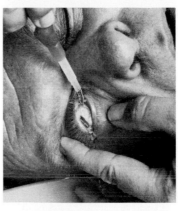

6 After you've finished irrigating Mr. Stevens' eye, gently dry his eyelids and face with a gauze pad or cotton ball.

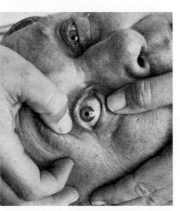

7 Then, inspect his affected eye for any residual chemical particles. Irrigate further, if necessary. Remove any nonembedded objects from his conjunctiva with a moistened cotton-tipped applicator.

Eye

Instructing your patient to instill eye drops

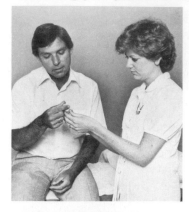

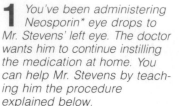

1 *You've been administering Neosporin* eye drops to Mr. Stevens' left eye. The doctor wants him to continue instilling the medication at home. You can help Mr. Stevens by teaching him the procedure explained below.*

First, remind your patient to wash and dry his hands thoroughly before starting. Tell him the procedure will be most effective if he lies flat on his back.

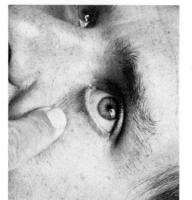

2 Now, have him remove the cap from the eye drop container and place it on its side, to avoid contaminating the inside.

Because he's instilling eye drops in his left eye, he should use the fingers of his left hand to pull down gently on the skin under his lower left eyelid, as shown here.

3 Next, tell him to hold the solution container in his right hand and invert it directly over his left eye.

◚ *Nursing tip:* He can stabilize the container by resting his right hand on the bridge of his nose.

Remind him not to touch his eyelid or eyeball with the container tip during the procedure. Doing so could contaminate the tip or injure his eye.

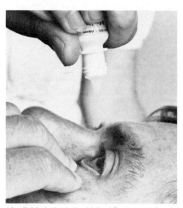

4 Now, tell Mr. Stevens to look directly at the eye drop container and gently squeeze a drop into his lower conjunctival sac, as shown. Instruct him to blink several times to distribute the solution over his eye.

Note: If the drop misses his eye, instruct your patient to repeat the procedure.

When he's finished, tell him to replace the cap on the eye drop container. Finally, document the teaching you've done.

*Available in both the United States and Canada

Teaching eye safety

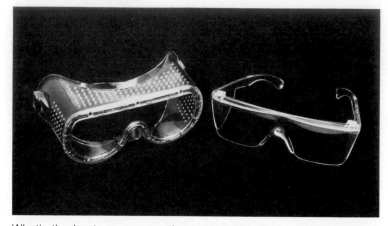

What's the best way your patient can practice eye safety? By wearing protective eyewear, such as goggles, whenever his eyes are vulnerable to injury. Encourage your patient to wear protective eyewear when he's performing these activities:
• Working around chemicals, ash, superheated material, and open flames
• Riding a motorcycle or a similar fast-moving vehicle that lacks a windshield
• Participating in sports that involve racquets and rapidly propelled objects; for example, racquetball, tennis, and squash
• Using outdoor power equipment, such as a chain saw
• Using indoor power equipment, such as an electric saw
• Working in a school shop class or in a vocational-technical setting.

As you probably know, eyewear that meets quality and strength standards is required at many job sites. But some employers may be lax in implementing safety measures for employees. If you're an occupational health nurse, recommend protective eyewear for anyone who works near machinery or chemicals or in any other dangerous setting.

Remind your patient that prescription eyeglasses alone don't provide adequate protection. But tell him he can continue to wear his glasses under specially designed safety goggles. Assure him that protective eyewear is inexpensive, and that the newer models are relatively comfortable and attractive.

Eye safety extends beyond protective eyewear. Instruct your patient always to make sure machinery parts are tightened properly before starting equipment. If he works with dry chemicals, he should make sure the area's well ventilated. He should also check that all chemicals are properly stored in appropriate containers.

Remind your patient to follow safety rules when participating in such active sports as racquetball and tennis.

Instruct your patient to seek aid immediately if an eye injury occurs. If a chemical splashes in his eye at home, tell him to rinse his eye with running water for at least 20 minutes. He should get to a doctor or an emergency department as quickly as possible.

Document any patient teaching on the appropriate form.

Ear

"I keep hearing ringing in my right ear," 46-year-old Steve Toth, a bank manager, tells you. "I don't notice it as much at work as I do at home. In fact, I can hardly sleep at night. It scares me. Am I going deaf?"

Some patients will come to you with ear problems similar to this one. They'll need reassurance and proper care. Can you provide for their needs?

Perhaps the ringing in your patient's ear is an early symptom of hearing loss. If so, you'll need to assess his hearing. On the following pages, we show you how to assess your patient's hearing using two tuning fork tests. And we show you how to use an audiometer to administer a pure tone audiometry test.

In reading the following pages, you'll also learn:
• how noise damages your patient's hearing
• how protective ear equipment, such as earplugs, can prevent noise-induced hearing loss
• how to irrigate your patient's ear with a water–jet-spray appliance
• how to teach your patient to instill ear drops.
• how to identify and manage common ear problems.

Study the information carefully.

Understanding hearing

You know that the ear's primary function is to channel sound to the brain for interpretation. But do you remember how the hearing process occurs? Could you explain the process to your patient?

Hearing begins with airborne sound waves entering the external ear canal. These waves move through the tubelike canal to the tympanic membrane (eardrum), causing it to vibrate. On the other side of the tympanic membrane is the middle ear, a tiny chamber containing three bones: the malleus, the incus, and the stapes. Sound waves pass through each of these bones in succession and become amplified.

From the middle ear, sound moves through the footplate of the stapes and then across the oval window to the internal ear. Here the waves enter the cochlea. Within this hearing organ are thousands of delicate hair cells arranged along a membrane. These cells convert sound waves to electrochemical impulses, which then proceed along the auditory nerve to the brain. Whenever these hair cells stop functioning, either from disease or trauma, a person's hearing will be disrupted.

Learning about hearing loss

As you probably know, sound waves must complete their pathway through the ear for your patient to hear. Any disruption of this pathway results in hearing loss. This loss may be *conductive* or *perceptive* (sensorineural).

Conductive hearing loss

Conductive hearing loss occurs when sound waves are blocked in the external ear or the middle ear. If the blockage is caused by an accumulation of cerumen (earwax), you should be able to remove it. The problem may be more serious, however, necessitating more extensive treatment—possibly surgery. For instance, your patient might have:
• a perforated tympanic membrane (eardrum)
• accumulated pus or fluid in the middle ear (otitis media)
• a formation of spongy bone in the middle ear (otosclerosis).

Perceptive hearing loss

Perceptive hearing loss affects the inner ear. In geriatric patients, the most common problem is presbycusis, a natural deterioration of cochlear hair cells. Other causes of perceptive loss include a lesion of the inner ear (cochlear lesion), of the eighth cranial nerve, or of the higher neural pathways (retrocochlear lesion).

In many cases, aural rehabilitation (for example, a hearing aid or speech therapy) can resolve or diminish these problems. For detailed information on hearing aids, see the NURSING PHOTOBOOK HELPING GERIATRIC PATIENTS.

Taking an ear history

You're on duty in the clinic when 17-year-old Theodore Krill enters the office. He tells you his ear feels as though it's blocked. To find out what's causing his hearing problem, you'll need to examine his ear with an otoscope. (For more information on using an otoscope, read the NURSING PHOTOBOOK ASSESSING YOUR PATIENTS.)

While examining Theodore's ear, take a brief history. Ask him these questions:
• Are you experiencing any pain? Describe the pain.
• How would you describe your hearing? Excellent? Adequate? Fair? Poor?
• Do you have a loss of hearing now? Describe what you can hear and how it sounds.
• Have you ever had dizzy spells or any trouble maintaining your balance? When does it occur and how frequently?
• Have you had previous problems with either ear, such as ringing, pain, or discharge? How often? Did you receive any treatment for the problem?
• Have you ever had an ear infection? When? How was it treated? Does it recur?
• Has either ear ever been injured?
• Have you ever been examined by an ear specialist?
• Have you ever had ear surgery? What type of surgery? Have you had tonsil, adenoid, or other nose or throat surgery?
• Do you clean your ears regularly? What do you use to clean them?
• Do any family members have a history of hearing problems or deafness?
• Do you spend much time around loud noise; for example, amplified rock music? Is your workplace or home very noisy?
• Have you been swimming recently?
• When did you last fly in an airplane?
• Are you allergic to any drugs? Which ones?
• Are you currently taking any medication?
• Have you ever received antibiotic injections, such as gentamicin sulfate or streptomycin sulfate?
• Have you ever taken large doses of aspirin, Anacin, Bufferin, or quinine?

Ear

Nurses' guide to common ear problems

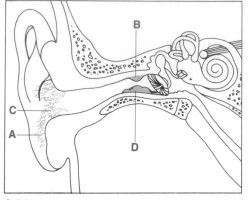

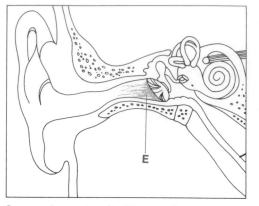

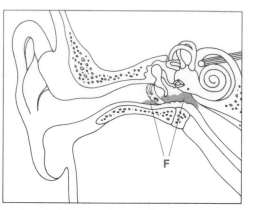

Otitis externa
(external otitis or swimmer's ear)
Inflammation of the external ear canal and auricle; usually caused by bacteria; most common in the summer; may be acute or chronic

Possible causes
Chronic moisture in canal; chronic drainage from a perforated tympanic membrane; excessive ear manipulation while cleaning, which can irritate the ear canal and introduce an infecting micro-organism; foreign bodies (such as insects) in the ear canal; overuse of earphones, earplugs, or earmuffs, which trap moisture in the ear canal, creating a culture medium for bacteria

Signs and symptoms
• Moderate to severe pain that worsens when the patient clenches his teeth, opens his mouth, and chews, and during auricle and tragus manipulation
• Possibly fever
• Foul-smelling aural discharge
• Localized cellulitis (A)
• Partial hearing loss
• Redness (B), swelling, and flaking of external ear canal (C), and a clear to cheesy discharge (D) from the ear canal
• In chronic form, intense pruritus, leading to scaling and skin thickening

Nursing interventions
• In severe conditions (acute and chronic), cleanse the ear and remove all debris, using a soft washcloth and warm water. Apply wet soaks intermittently on draining lesions or infected skin.
• For all forms, instill antibiotic ear drops or apply antibiotic cream or ointment, as ordered.
• Have the patient wear specially fitted earplugs while showering, shampooing, and swimming.
• Advise the patient not to clean his ears with cotton-tipped applicators, bobby pins, or other foreign objects.

Serous (secretory) otitis media
Middle ear inflammation resulting from eustachian tube obstruction; most common in children; occurs most frequently during the winter; may be acute or chronic

Possible causes
Recent or current viral upper respiratory tract disease, incomplete resolution or inadequate treatment of acute purulent (suppurative) otitis media, nasopharyngitis, purulent rhinosinusitis, allergy, chronic sinus infection

Signs and symptoms
• Severe hearing loss
• Irritability
• Sensation of ear fullness or tinnitus
• Child pulls on his ears
• Popping, cracking, or clicking sound with swallowing and jaw movement
• Clear, straw-colored drainage (E)
• Echo heard when speaking
• Sensation of top-heaviness
• Mild earache (otalgia)
• Pain
• In a child, may present as suspected hearing loss, language development delay, abnormal pure tone audiometry results, or abnormal findings on routine otoscopy

Nursing interventions
• Take measures to correct causes.
• Administer antibiotics, as ordered, to eliminate any existing infection.
• Have the patient perform Valsalva's maneuver several times daily to inflate the eustachian tube.
• Give nasopharyngeal decongestants to open a blocked eustachian tube, as ordered. Continue at least 2 weeks, but extend therapy if reassessment indicates. If therapy fails, aspiration of middle ear or myringotomy may be necessary.
• If surgery's anticipated, prepare patient and family accordingly.
• Instruct the patient in the correct use of nasopharyngeal decongestants. Encourage compliance with prescribed treatment.
• Advise the patient with the acute form of this disorder to report any pain or fever immediately.
• Encourage early treatment of upper respiratory tract infection.
• To prevent infected secretions from being pushed into the middle ear, advise the patient to blow his nose gently.

Perforated tympanic membrane
Damage to the tympanic membrane; defined as marginal or central, depending on location; marginal perforation considered more serious because it may allow movement of keratinizing squamous epithelium into middle ear

Possible causes
Untreated otitis media and, in children, acute otitis media; tympanic membrane retraction pockets caused by blocked eustachian tube, previous myringotomy, or trauma from deliberate or accidental insertion of sharp objects (for example, cotton-tipped applicators and bobby pins) or from sudden excessive changes in pressure (for example, from a blow to the head, flying, or diving)

Signs and symptoms
• Pain
• Bleeding from the ear
• Hearing loss
• Tinnitus
• Vertigo
• History of purulent aural discharge (mucopurulent otorrhea [F])

Nursing interventions
• If your patient's bleeding from the ear, use a sterile, cotton-tipped applicator to absorb the blood. Assess for purulent drainage or evidence of cerebrospinal fluid leakage. Obtain a culture specimen, as ordered. Apply a loose sterile dressing over the outer ear, and refer the patient to an ear specialist immediately.
• Administer a mild analgesic to relieve pain or a sedative to decrease the patient's anxiety, as ordered.
• Give antibiotics, as ordered, if the patient has a middle ear infection.
• Remind the patient to keep the affected ear dry and clean during the healing period. Tell him not to blow his nose until the perforation heals.
• Refer the patient with persistent signs and symptoms or suspected perforation to the doctor, for further evaluation and care.

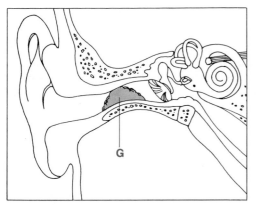

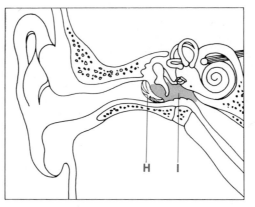

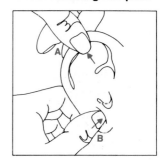

Differentiating ear pain

Ear canal obstruction
Ear canal blockage that interferes with proper auditory function; may lead to infection and inflammation

Possible causes
Ceruminal impaction (G), caused by excess cerumen secretion or narrowness of ear canal; foreign object, such as an insect, bead, or eraser

Signs and symptoms
• Pain, especially if the obstruction's located deep in the ear canal
• Hearing loss, with severity depending on the size of obstruction
• Annoying buzzing sound or sensation of movement, if the obstruction's an insect

Nursing interventions
• If cerumen's causing the obstruction, you may need to remove it by gently scraping the ear canal with a cerumen spoon or by irrigating the canal.
• Irrigate the internal ear canal with an ear syringe or water–jet-spray appliance, as ordered. Before irrigating, instill ear drops (for example, warm glycerin or a ceruminolytic) to soften firmly impacted cerumen.
Caution: Irrigation is contraindicated in a patient with suspected tympanic membrane perforation. Stop irrigation immediately if the patient experiences pain, nausea, or dizziness.
• If an insect's causing the obstruction, instill 70% alcohol solution or a few drops of mineral oil in the ear canal to kill the insect; then, remove the insect with a forceps or a cerumen spoon.
• Remind the patient to avoid cleaning his ears with cotton-tipped applicators or similar objects.
• Refer the patient with a large or firmly embedded object in the ear canal to an otolaryngologist for extraction of the object under general anesthetic.
• Instruct the patient (especially if he's a child) to avoid inserting any foreign objects in his ears.

Suppurative otitis media
Middle ear infection, resulting from disruption of eustachian tube patency; most common in children; may be acute or chronic

Possible causes
Respiratory tract infection, allergic reaction, and positional changes (such as holding an infant supine during feeding). Predisposing factors include the normally shorter, wider, and more horizontal eustachian tube and increased lymphoid tissue found in a child and anatomic anomalies (such as cleft palate). Chronic cases result from inadequate treatment of acute otitis media episodes or from infection by resistant bacterial strains, such as pneumococcus, *Hemophilus influenzae,* beta-hemolytic streptococci, staphylococci, and gram-negative bacteria.

Signs and symptoms
• Malaise and sensation of ear fullness
• In the acute condition, severe, deep, throbbing pain; signs and symptoms of upper respiratory tract infection, such as runny nose and sore throat; mild to extremely high fever; mild hearing loss; dizziness; nausea; vomiting. However, many patients may be asymptomatic.
• Child pulls on his ears
• Bulging of the tympanic membrane (H), with accompanying redness
• Purulent drainage behind the tympanic membrane (I) or in the ear canal, if tympanic membrane is ruptured
• Irritability

Nursing interventions
• Give antibiotics, as ordered.
• Administer acetaminophen or aspirin to control pain and fever.
• Give oral or local nasal decongestants to improve eustachian tube patency.
• Suggest to the patient that the application of heat to his external ear may relieve pain.
• Advise the patient with acute condition to immediately report pain and fever—both signs of secondary infection.
• Instruct parents not to position their infant supine when feeding him or to put him to bed with a bottle.
• To prevent recurrence, encourage early treatment of upper respiratory tract infection and discourage forceful nose blowing.

Suppose your patient's signs and symptoms indicate that he has either otitis externa or otitis media. To distinguish between these two, apply auricular traction (also known as the helix maneuver) to the ear canal.

To proceed, pull on the helix (A) of the ear's auricle or press on the tragus cartilage (B), as shown. If tension on the inflamed ear canal skin produces pain, suspect otitis externa.

But if your patient doesn't experience pain (but has other ear-related signs and symptoms), suspect a middle ear disorder; for example, otitis media. Document your findings.

Ear

Understanding sound's frequency and intensity

When you evaluate your patient's hearing, you're actually assessing how well he distinguishes the frequency and intensity of sound. Has it been awhile since you reviewed these terms? If so, read on.

Frequency is the number of sound waves per second produced by a sounding body. You use the unit of measure hertz (Hz) to determine frequency. If your patient has normal hearing, he can detect sound frequencies between 20 and 20,000 Hz. To recognize most words spoken in a quiet environment, however, he needs only to hear frequencies in the 500- to 2,000-Hz range.

Intensity is the loudness of sound. You measure intensity in decibels (db).

To help you relate decibel amounts to everyday situations, consider the following:
- A faint whisper is 10 to 15 db.
- Normal conversation is 50 to 60 db.
- A shout registers 70 to 80 db.

How to perform Weber's test

Your patient, 36-year-old Brenda Ballance, tells you she's experiencing ringing in her ears and, occasionally, has a sensation of ear fullness. She reports that she's had these symptoms for several weeks and has never had an ear problem in the past. Ms. Ballance also tells you that her father has a hearing loss.

To help you determine whether Ms. Ballance has a hearing loss, perform Weber's test. This test assesses your patient's hearing acuity by bone conduction. Although a positive test result usually indicates a hearing loss, you'll want to confirm the results by performing pure tone audiometry.

First, select a quiet room or area for the test. Then, explain to Ms. Ballance why you're performing this test. Familiarize her with the testing routine, and seat her on a chair or an exam table. Assure her that it's painless and takes only a few minutes to complete.

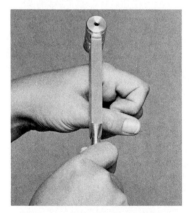

1 To obtain the most accurate results, use a low-frequency tuning fork; in this case, a 256-hertz fork.

Set the tuning fork vibrating by striking it against your fist, as shown here.

Note: You can also produce a tone by pinching the fork's prongs together or by stroking the prongs upward.

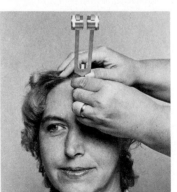

2 Now, hold the vibrating tuning fork between your thumb and forefinger and touch its base to the midline of your patient's forehead, as shown here.

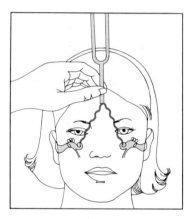

3 Then, ask her whether she hears the tone louder in her left ear, louder in her right ear, or equally loud in both ears. Document the results as Weber left, Weber right, or Weber negative, respectively.

To understand what occurs in Weber's test, study this illustration. If your patient has normal hearing, she can hear the tone equally in both ears.

If the tone's louder in either ear, she may have a hearing problem.

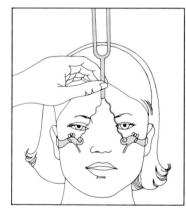

4 Let's say your patient hears the tone louder in her left ear. Then she may have *conductive* hearing loss in this ear. Why? Because in conductive hearing loss, extraneous sounds in the environment are blocked in the affected external ear canal or the middle ear. This allows the cochlea to transmit only the sound of the test tone to the brain, making it louder.

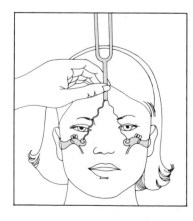

5 If your patient hears the tone louder in her right ear, she may have *perceptive* hearing loss in her left ear. That's because perceptive hearing loss affects the inner ear (cochlea), allowing her to hear better with her unaffected ear.

How to perform the Rinne test

To assess Ms. Ballance's hearing acuity by bone conduction and air conduction, perform the Rinne test. This test works by comparing air conduction with bone conduction. To review, air conduction is the transmission of sound to the auditory nerve through the ear canal, tympanic membrane, and ossicular chain, whereas bone conduction is the transmission of sound to the auditory nerve through the bones of the skull.

A patient with normal hearing will hear the sound twice as long by air conduction (with the tuning fork held opposite the external meatus) as he will by bone conduction (with the tuning fork held on the mastoid bone).

Begin by explaining the test to Ms. Ballance and answering any questions she may have. Assure her that it's painless and takes only a few minutes to perform. Note: *Confirm abnormal results with pure tone audiometry testing.*

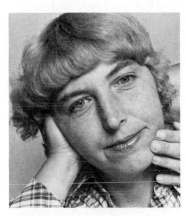

1 First you'll test bone conduction. Ask your patient to cover her right ear with her hand, as shown here.

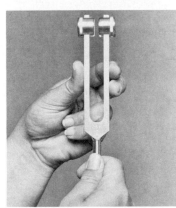

2 The nurse in this photo is vibrating the fork by stroking the prongs upward.

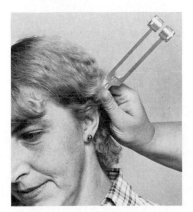

3 To test your patient's hearing acuity by bone conduction, place a vibrating tuning fork against her left mastoid process, as shown. Then, ask her to tell you when she stops hearing the tone. Note the length of time she heard it.

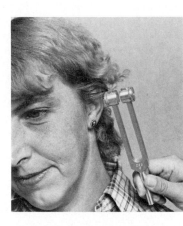

4 Immediately, without revibrating the tuning fork, place the prongs about 1″ (2.5 cm) from Ms. Ballance's left ear canal, to test her hearing acuity by air conduction.

Again, ask your patient to tell you when she no longer hears the tone. Document the results.

Repeat the procedure on her right ear. Make sure she covers her left ear with her hand.

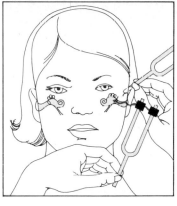

5 If all's well, Ms. Ballance will hear the air-conducted sound twice as long as the bone-conducted sound. Record the result as *Rinne positive.*

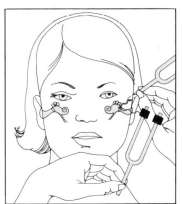

6 If Ms. Ballance hears the bone-conducted sound longer, suspect *conductive* hearing loss in her left ear. Record abnormal results as *Rinne negative.*

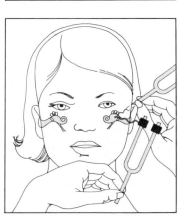

7 If she hears the air-conducted sound as long or only slightly longer than the bone-conducted sound, she probably has *perceptive* hearing loss in her left ear.

Ear

Learning about pure tone audiometry

Pure tone audiometric testing is a valuable tool for assessing your patient's hearing acuity. By performing this test, you can accurately determine hearing loss severity and type (conductive, perceptive, or mixed).

The most important feature of this test is that it detects hearing loss in its early stages. This way, you can refer your patient to an audiologist for specific evaluation, for treatment to prevent further deterioration, and for aural rehabilitation, if necessary.

Your testing schedule should coincide with your patient's needs. For example, test him annually as part of his routine physical examination. But if you suspect hearing loss or your patient works in a noisy setting that could affect his hearing, you may need to test him more frequently, to monitor his condition.

To perform pure tone audiometric testing, you'll use a machine called an audiometer, which can produce a set of test tones (called pure tones) at various frequencies. The machine increases the decibel level for each frequency until your patient hears the tone. By recording the lowest intensity at which your patient can hear these tones, the audiometer determines his hearing threshold. A graph of hearing thresholds is called an *audiogram*. See the chart below for a comparison of audiograms for persons with different levels of hearing ability.

The audiometer establishes air conduction and bone conduction thresholds. To perform air conduction testing, place the audiometer earphones on your patient's head and direct the tones through his auditory pathway. For bone conduction testing, remove the earphones and place the audiometer vibrator on the mastoid process of his unaffected ear. A comparison of air conduction and bone conduction thresholds confirms hearing loss and indicates type and severity. Further testing by an audiologist may determine the cause.

When possible, perform the test in a soundproof room to ensure accurate test results. Also, have your patient sit where he can't see your hand movements on the audiometer and react to *them*.

To prepare your patient for testing, first explain what you're going to do. Tell him the procedure takes about 20 minutes and that you'll test each ear separately, beginning with the unaffected ear. Inform him that he'll hear tones at various intensities.

Instruct him to indicate when he hears each tone by giving you a prearranged signal. Tell him also to signal when he no longer hears the tone. For example, he can raise his hand when he first hears a tone and lower it when the tone stops. Or, he can use the response cord (see page 35), if the machine has one. Emphasize that he should respond even if the tone is faint.

Before starting the test, ask your patient to remove anything from his head that may prevent him from putting on the earphones correctly; for instance, eyeglasses or a hearing aid.

Caution: Don't perform this test if, within the past 16 hours, your patient's been exposed to noises loud enough to cause tinnitus. By waiting, you obtain more accurate results.

Gaining familiarity with the audiometer

Suppose your patient requires pure tone audiometric testing. Do you know how to operate an audiometer correctly? The audiometer shown at right is an Autotech GRS-1A, a microprocessor-controlled model.

As you look from left to right across the top front panel, you'll see two digital display boxes: the TEST FREQUENCY display and the TONE LEVEL/FAULT display. During the test, the audiometer indicates the frequency of the tone your patient's hearing in the left box and the intensity of the tone in the right box.

Located to the right of the display boxes are four lights, aligned vertically. The two lights corresponding to the right and the left ears indicate when the respective ear's being tested. The other two lights, marked VALID, are lit when the testing of the ear is complete and a valid test result has been obtained.

The audiometer measures your patient's air conduction threshold at seven frequencies: 1,000; 2,000; 3,000; 4,000; 6,000; 8,000; and 500 hertz (Hz). *Note:* After 8,000 Hz, the audiometer performs an automatic retest at 1,000 Hz. After your patient's threshold at each frequency is determined, the matching light located below the display boxes is lit.

Learning about the controls

To perform a pure tone audiometry test, you'll operate the controls on the lower front panel. First, let's review the four buttons arranged horizontally in the top row of the panel. The START/STOP button's located at the far left. The MANUAL button allows you to switch modes from automatic to manual. The PULSE button is used to control the number of pulses your patient hears in a tone. When the PRINT button is depressed, the printer (if your model's equipped with one) begins transcribing the results on paper after the test's completed. *Note:* You can also obtain the results manually, as we explain in the photostory that follows.

In the bottom row, at left, you'll find the PRESENT TONE button, which is used to select the form in which the patient hears the tone. (The audiometer may sound either one or two tones at a time.) The READ button, which is located in the middle of the row, allows you to direct the tone to the ear you want to test first. The READ button also functions in recording, as explained in the photostory. At right is the MANUAL ADVANCE button, which you'll use only if you switch to the manual mode. Use it to advance the tone manually to each succeeding frequency.

Depress the RESET button, located on the far right of the panel, to clear all data from the audiometer's memory bank and prepare

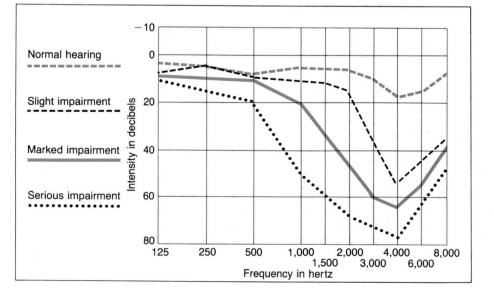

Normal hearing

Slight impairment

Marked impairment

Serious impairment

it for the next test or for a retest.

The OPERATOR ALERT light, located above the RESET button, is lit when one of the system's validity checks detects an error requiring intervention. The TONE RESPONSE light (below the RESET button) is lit whenever your patient responds to a tone.

The STOP light is lit when the machine stops—either because the test's finished or a problem has arisen. The PRESENT TONE light is lit when you produce a tone in manual mode. The MANUAL light above the manual button indicates a switch to manual mode. The PULSE light indicates a switch to a continuous pulse tone.

At the rear of the unit, on the left side, you'll see the POWER switch. In the middle, you'll see a plug for the audiometer's accessories, which include:

• *headphone*, which your patient wears to hear the tones
• *a response cord*, which your patient uses to indicate that he hears a tone

• *a microphone*, which you can use to talk to your patient during the test
• *a printer*, which prints the test results. (The machine you use may not be equipped with this accessory.)

When operating in automatic mode, the audiometer begins testing at each frequency, with a 30-decibel (db) tone. In turn, the intensity level increases 30 db until your patient signals that he's heard the tone

by pushing the button on his response cord. The intensity level then decreases in 10-db steps until your patient fails to respond. Then, the level increases in 5-db steps until he responds again. These increases and decreases continue until the audiometer validates the correct threshold. When this occurs, the results are stored in the memory bank, and the machine moves to the next frequency.

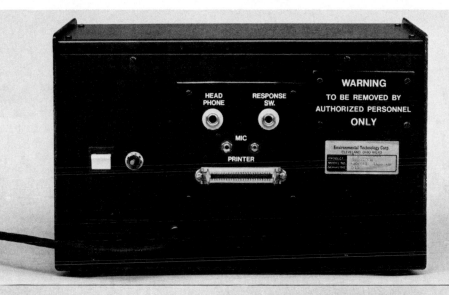

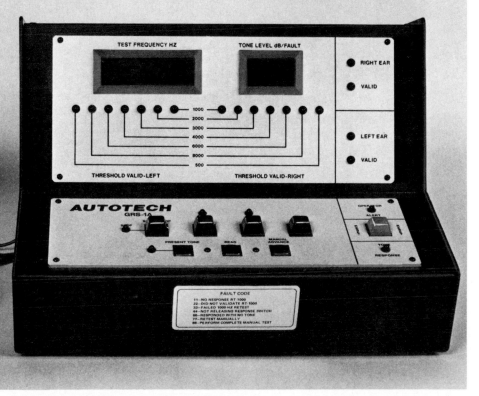

Ear

Performing a pure tone audiometry test

After assessing Brenda Ballance's hearing acuity with a tuning fork, you suspect conductive hearing loss. To more accurately evaluate her hearing, perform a pure tone audiometry test. Note: In this photostory, we use the Autotech GRS-1A microprocessor audiometer.

First, choose a quiet area, away from distractions, in which to perform the test. Use a soundproof room, if possible. Position Ms. Ballance so she can't see you set the digital display boxes on the unit, which could influence her response. Now, turn on the power and plug the response cord, the headphones, and the microphone jacks into the back of the unit.

Explain to Ms. Ballance that her right ear will be tested first and then her left ear. Tell her the test is painless and takes only about 6 minutes. Then, hand her the response cord and instruct her to push the button on top of it as soon as she hears a tone.

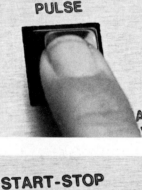

1 Now, place the headphones over her ears.
Important: Make sure you match the headphones with the correct ears. Remember, the audiometer automatically tests the right ear first, unless you direct otherwise.

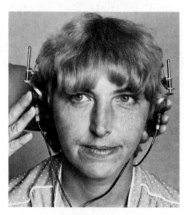

2 The audiometer allows you to test your patient's hearing by producing either a single pulse tone or a series of three short tones. The nurse in this photostory has selected the single tone. To make this selection, push the PULSE button, as shown here.

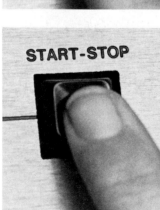

3 Because you're testing your patient in the automatic mode, press the START/STOP button to begin the test.
Note: For instructions on operating the audiometer manually, see the manufacturer's guidelines.
Position yourself at the audiometer so you can both observe Ms. Ballance and follow the test's progress by watching the front panel of the unit.

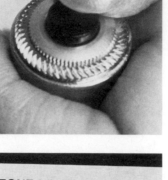

4 To begin, the machine produces a 1,000-hertz (Hz) tone at 30 decibels (db). If Ms. Ballance hears the tone, she'll push the response button. The next tone she'll hear is 1,000 Hz at 20 db.
If she didn't respond to the 30-db tone, the next tone she'd hear would be at 60 db. The audiometer proceeds through the following sequence of frequencies: 1,000; 2,000; 3,000; 4,000; 6,000; 8,000; a retest at 1,000; and 500 Hz.

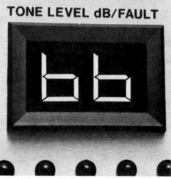

5 Suppose the STOP and OPERATOR ALERT lights light up, and you hear a loud beeping. This means the audiometer has detected a problem. Check the TONE LEVEL/FAULT display box. Note the fault code indicated in this box, and refer to the manufacturer's guide to correct the problem. Then, press the START button and proceed. When the test's completed, the lights will flash again and you'll hear a 10-second tone.

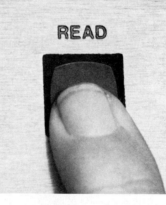

6 To record the test results, push the READ button, and observe the digital display boxes. The audiometer shows the frequency in the left box and the accompanying threshold in the right box. Record the threshold. Then, push the READ button to advance to the next frequency and threshold. Remember, the audiometer displays the right ear results first.

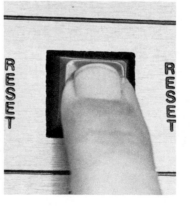

7 After you record the valid results, clear the audiometer's memory bank by pushing the RESET button.
Finally, document the results of the test on the appropriate form. If the findings indicate hearing loss, refer your patient to an audiologist.

Noise-induced hearing loss: An insidious process

Are you familiar with the effects of noise on your patient's auditory system? Can you recognize environments that may cause noise-induced hearing loss? By understanding how noise can damage the inner ear, you can better teach your patient how to prevent hearing loss.

Until recently, the severest cases of hearing loss resulting from noise exposure occurred in industry. Today, the problem is more wide-spread (see chart below).

The noise level in the city and around the home is rising annually. Some persons—especially teenagers—prefer to listen to contemporary music played at a high volume and compound the noise level by listening through earphones.

The result is noise-induced hearing loss—an especially dangerous condition, because it causes no pain and changes are so subtle that it may go undetected for months or years. During this time, your patient may exhibit such signs and symptoms as irritability and fatigue. But he probably won't realize that exposure to loud noise may be causing irreversible hearing loss.

What determines your patient's rate of hearing loss? Many factors, including:
• length and frequency of noise exposure
• noise intensity
• susceptibility to exposure; for example, work-related noise.

Noise-induced hearing loss can be temporary. For instance, short-term exposures to an intensity of 160 decibels (db) can rupture the eardrum and drive the stapes through the oval window. This condition is called auditory fatigue, and full hearing commonly returns the next day. Because exposure to high-intensity noise lowers your patient's tolerance level, continued exposure can cause permanent damage.

Prolonged exposure to loud noise causes degeneration of the cochlear hair cells. Initially, this damage impairs your patient's ability to hear sounds in the 4,000-hertz (Hz) range. Eventually, hearing loss also occurs in the normal speech range of 2,000 Hz and below.

The Occupational Safety and Health Act has set standards to combat work-related hearing loss. For example, employees must wear protective equipment, such as earplugs or ear-muffs, if the noise level exceeds 90 db. To prevent high-intensity hearing loss, employees must protect their ears if they're exposed to at least 115 db for longer than several minutes.

To better understand your role in protecting your patient against noise-induced hearing loss, read the information at right.

Preventing noise-induced hearing loss

Because ear damage resulting from loud noise doesn't cause pain and hearing loss usually occurs gradually, your patient may not realize his hearing's being affected. This is why you need to increase his awareness of the effects of noise and of how he can prevent hearing loss.

To do so, follow these steps:
• Explain how noise-induced hearing loss occurs.
• Perform audiometric testing annually. But if he's working in a noise-polluted area, assess him more frequently.
• Identify noise sources inside and outside the workplace.
• Encourage the consistent use of protective equipment for the ears.

To demonstrate how the noise level at his workplace is affecting his hearing, suggest that when he arrives at work, he set the volume of his car radio at a barely audible level. He should not turn off the radio. When he starts his car after work, tell him to listen for the radio. He should be able to hear it without adjusting the volume. If he can't hear it, his ears are probably fatigued from noise exposure.

Audiometric testing can help you determine if your patient's hearing is regressing. Ideally, you should test his hearing when he's first hired, and then retest him 90 days later. These results provide a baseline for future testing.

Note: If your patient's experiencing tinnitus from exposure to high-intensity noise, wait at least 16 hours before performing audiometric testing. This allows you to assess the extent of the damage.

As you probably know, your patient's hearing can be impaired by prolonged exposure to loud noise as well as by high-intensity noise bursts. Take noise level readings around machinery and in other work areas to determine where protection is needed. After you locate these areas, stress to your patient the importance of wearing protective equipment. Make sure he knows how to apply the earwear correctly.

Assure him that because the earwear filters out only high-intensity noise, he'll still hear other sounds.

	Sound level in db	Sound source
Danger range	140	Jet aircraft
	130	Pneumatic hammer
	THRESHOLD OF PAIN	
	120	Turbine generator
Risk range	110	Steam shovel
	100	Circular saw
	90	18-wheel truck
	80	Electric typewriter
	70	Automobile
	60	Normal conversation
Safe range	50	
	40	Soft music
	30	Whisper
	20	Quiet suburban home
	10	
	THRESHOLD OF HEARING	

Ear

Learning about common protective equipment for the ears

You'll want to teach your patient how to prevent noise-induced hearing loss. One way he can do this is with protective equipment.

When you recommend hearing protection for your patient, be sure to tell him it'll take time for him to adjust to the equipment. Stress the importance of selecting equipment that's comfortable, because he'll need to use it consistently for effective protection.

Also, keep in mind that whether or not protective equipment is necessary depends on the surroundings. An employee may feel that being able to hear safety warnings is more important than preventing noise-induced hearing loss.

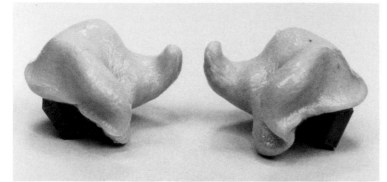

Permanent earplugs
Description
Usually made of plastic or silicone rubber; available in all sizes and shapes
Advantage
Reusable
Disadvantages
• Necessitate initial fitting by trained person
• Must be cleaned thoroughly with mild soap and water before each use
• Feeling of pressure in the ear possible with tight fit
• Lead to formation and trapping of moisture in the ear canal

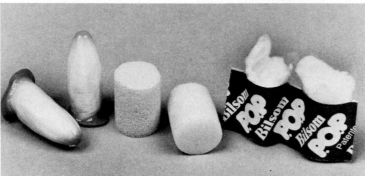

Disposable earplugs
Description
Made of mineral down or foamed plastic. Mineral down is available in bulk or as preformed earplugs.
Advantages
• Most hygienic, because they're worn once and then discarded
• Can change shape in the ear canal during jaw movement because of high resiliency
• Permeable; allow air and moisture to pass through the ear canal, preventing them from becoming trapped
Disadvantage
• Possibly more expensive, because they must be replaced daily

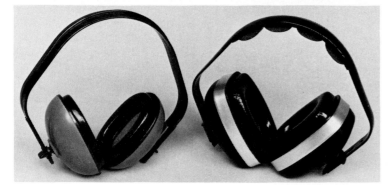

Earmuffs
Description
Hard cups lined with a liquid or plastic foam cushion that forms a tight seal over the ears; connected by a headband
Advantages
• Provide most effective noise barrier
• Cushions are soft and easily replaceable.
• Headband designed to maintain a firm but comfortable fit.
• Can be worn over earplugs to increase noise resistance
• Some models attach to a safety helmet and can combine with an earphone headset to provide music or messages, as well as protect hearing.
Disadvantages
• May be uncomfortable if fitted too tightly.
• Ear cushions may become soiled or brittle with extended use, necessitating replacement.

PATIENT TEACHING

Helping your patient adjust to earplugs

Just because your patient has earplugs doesn't guarantee he'll use them. Why? Because they may feel uncomfortable or strange until he gets used to wearing them. Suggest that he start by wearing his earplugs 30 minutes in the morning and 30 minutes in the afternoon. Instruct him to increase the wearing time the 2nd day to 1 hour in the morning and in the afternoon and the 3rd day to 2 hours before and after lunch. Then, tell him to try wearing them all day.

Advise him that the plugs will probably feel uncomfortable the first few days. In addition to the sensation of something in his ears, his own voice may sound distant. Explain that as he gets used to the plugs, the discomfort will subside.

Each time he inserts the earplugs, have him check to make sure they fit snugly. Tell him to return for reassessment if the plugs fit loosely or if he has any discomfort throughout the 1st week.

Teaching your patient how to insert earplugs

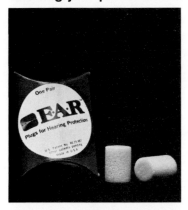

1 John Sears is a machinist at the company where you're employed. Because he works around loud machinery, you'll teach him how to insert earplugs.

Note: In this story, Mr. Sears is inserting E-A-R™ plugs. Some models of E-A-R plugs have a connecting cord that prevents the plugs from dropping into the patient's work area. If your patient *does* drop his earplugs on the floor, tell him to obtain new ones.

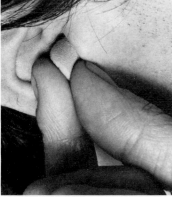

2 First, explain to Mr. Sears that the earplugs will help protect his hearing.

Then, have him wash and dry his hands thoroughly before preparing and inserting his earplugs.

Now, give him a plug and instruct him to prepare it for insertion by rolling and squeezing it with his fingers, as shown.

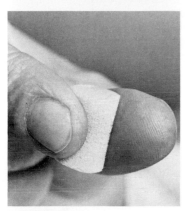

3 Next, tell him to straighten his right ear canal by pulling the top of his ear upward and backward. Tell Mr. Sears to insert the prepared plug into his ear canal, quickly but gently, as shown. Then, have him hold it in place lightly until the plug begins to expand.

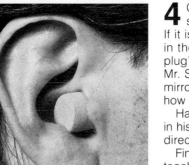

4 Check the plug to make sure it's inserted correctly. If it is, the plug will fit snugly in the ear canal. When the plug's inserted correctly, ask Mr. Sears to look at himself in a mirror to become familiar with how the plug should look.

Have him put the other plug in his left ear, following the same directions.

Finally, document your patient teaching on the appropriate form.

Teaching your patient to instill ear drops

Larry Frankenfeld, a 51-year-old electrician, is at your clinic for his annual physical examination. While examining his right ear with an otoscope, you detect a large ceruminal impaction. Because a ceruminal impaction may affect his hearing, it will have to be removed. To do so, you'll irrigate the ear canal.

But before extremely hard or firmly impacted cerumen can be removed by irrigation, it may require preliminary softening with a ceruminolytic; for example, carbamide peroxide (Debrox*). To soften the cerumen, the doctor orders Debrox ear drops to be instilled in Mr. Frankenfeld's right ear three times a day for 2 days. The doctor instructs him to return to the clinic on the 3rd day, so you can perform ear irrigation.

To teach Mr. Frankenfeld how to put the drops in his ear, follow the procedure shown in the photostory below. Caution: Some ceruminolytics may cause an inflammatory reaction.

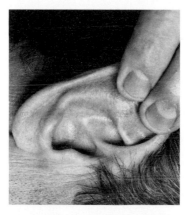

1 First, instruct your patient to wash his hands thoroughly. Tell him to shake the container of ear drops, as the package directs, and open it. To prevent contamination, tell him to place the cap on its side.

Next, have him lie on his unaffected side, with his affected ear facing toward the ceiling. Ask him to gently pull the top of his affected ear upward and backward, as shown here, to straighten the ear canal.

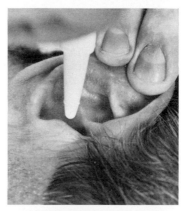

2 Now, have him position the container tip just above the ear canal. Remind him to avoid touching any part of his ear with the container tip, which could contaminate the tip and lead to ear infection.

Next, have him squeeze the container gently until he feels a drop in his ear. Tell him to repeat the procedure until he's administered the prescribed number of drops.

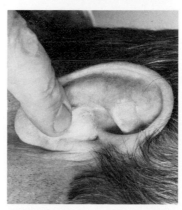

3 To keep the drops in his ear, tell him to insert a piece of cotton. Or, he may remain lying on his unaffected side for 10 minutes.

If the doctor directs, have him repeat the procedure for his other ear.

Instruct him to recap the container and store it in a dark, cool location. Remind him to keep a record of the time he instills the drops and the amount instilled.

Document your teaching.

*Available in both the United States and Canada

Ear

Using a WaterPik® for ear canal irrigation

Larry Frankenfeld's returned to your clinic for right ear canal irrigation. To remove the softened, impacted cerumen from his ear, use a water–jet-spray appliance, such as a WaterPik®. Do you know how? Read the following photostory.

First, gather the necessary equipment: WaterPik, bed-saver pads or plastic drape, emesis basin, and cotton balls. Set up the appliance in a secure location, near an electrical outlet. Then, explain to your patient what you're going to do. Tell him the procedure takes approximately 20 minutes.

Caution: Never attempt to irrigate the ear of a patient with a perforated tympanic membrane. Also, instruct your patient to tell you immediately if he experiences pain, nausea, or dizziness. If these effects occur, stop the procedure and notify the doctor. Note: If the impaction remains after irrigation, refer your patient to an ear specialist.

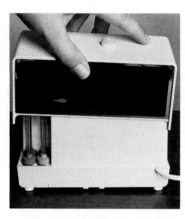

1 Wash your hands thoroughly. Then, remove the cover (tray) from the appliance and take it to the sink. Invert the tray and fill it halfway with water warmed to 95° F. to 105° F. (35° C. to 40.5° C.).

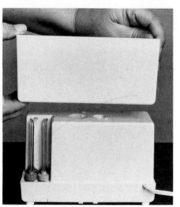

2 Now, fit the tray to the appliance so the protruding and indented areas match. Then, push the tray on the appliance, so it's securely attached, as the nurse is doing here.

Check to be sure the pressure control's set at *low*. A higher pressure could cause pain or ear damage. Then, drape bed-saver pads or a plastic drape around Mr. Frankenfeld's shoulders.

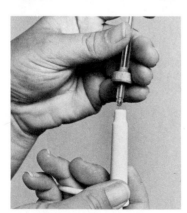

3 Next, take the tubing out of the appliance's storage compartment. Lift out an irrigating jet tip (nozzle) and push it into the fitting on the end of the tubing. When you hear a click, you'll know the nozzle is secure.

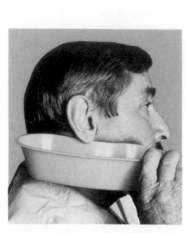

4 Next, have him sit close to the WaterPik and tilt his head slightly toward his left side. This position allows the irrigating solution to circulate behind the impaction in his affected ear.

Give him an emesis basin, and ask him to hold it below his right ear, as shown.

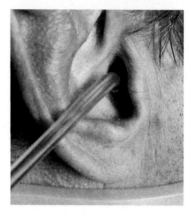

5 Then, gently pull upward and backward on the top of the ear, to straighten the ear canal. This creates a direct passageway for the irrigating solution.

Important: If your patient's a child, gently pull his ear downward and backward.

Grasp the WaterPik's handle and position the nozzle just inside the patient's ear canal.

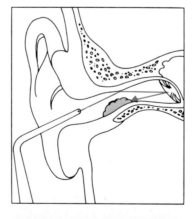

6 Now, turn on the appliance. Aim the stream of irrigating solution toward the top of your patient's ear canal, as illustrated. As you perform irrigation, observe Mr. Frankenfeld for any signs of pain, nausea, or dizziness.

Stop the procedure periodically and reexamine his ear for cerumen with an otoscope. Discontinue irrigation when you're satisfied you've removed the impaction or if you can't dislodge it.

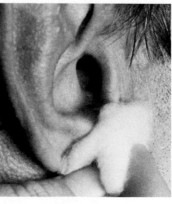

7 After the procedure, remove the bed-saver pads or plastic drape from his shoulders and dry his ear and face with cotton balls. Dispose of the basin's contents and the remaining water.

Finally, document the procedure on the appropriate form, including the amount of solution used, color and consistency of the irrigating solution return, your patient's tolerance of the procedure, and the results of the irrigation.

Nose, mouth, and throat

Providing good nose, mouth, and throat care for your patients is a tall order. You may be called on to remove a foreign body from a young child's nose or to collect a throat culture specimen for laboratory analysis. Or, you may have to perform emergency procedures; for example, clearing an obstructed airway.

On the following pages, we give you the information you need to manage your patient's nose, mouth, and throat problems. Read the information carefully.

MINI-ASSESSMENT

Assessing the nose

Suppose your patient comes to you with a nose problem. Before examining his nose, ask him these questions, which may help you identify the disorder.
• Do you have pain or discomfort in your nose? Can you describe how it feels? When does it occur? Does anything relieve it?
• Do you ever feel as though your nose is blocked? On one side or both? How do you clear it?
• Do you breathe through your nose or through your mouth?
• Do you snore?
• How would you describe your sense of smell? Can you tell one odor from another?
• Do you ever have nosebleeds? How often? Do they occur more frequently at a certain season or time of day? Do they follow a pattern? Can you stop the bleeding? How?
• Do you ever have a runny nose? Does the fluid usually come out of one or out of both nostrils? Or does it drip down the back of your throat? Is this condition more prevalent at a certain time of day or night? Does it occur more frequently during a particular season? What color and consistency is the nose discharge? Does it have an odor?
• Do you have colds and sore throats frequently? How often? What do you take to relieve the discomfort?
• Has your nose ever been injured? Describe what happened.
• Have you ever had sinus trouble? Do you have hay fever or other allergies? Do you take medication to relieve the symptoms? What kind?
• Have you ever had surgery on your nose or sinuses? If so, for what reason? When was it? Do you know what procedure was used?
• Do you take any medication by mouth for your nose problems?
• Do you use nose drops or nasal sprays? What kind and how often?
Note: For complete details on assessing the nose, see the NURSING PHOTOBOOK ASSESSING YOUR PATIENTS.

Foreign objects in the nose: Reviewing the basics

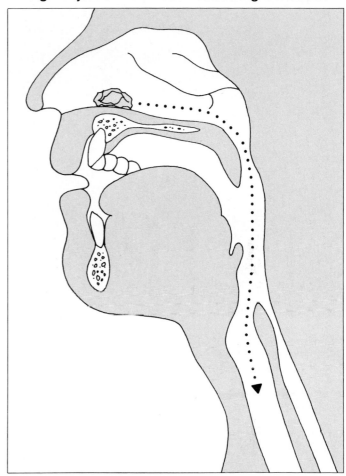

As happens with many 4-year-olds, Cynthia Stokes' curiosity sometimes gets the better of her. Although her mother tells her not to put things in her mouth or nose, Cynthia decides to test the smell of paper by inserting a wad of it in her left nasal cavity. While trying to remove the wad herself, she pushes it farther into her nasal cavity (see illustration above).

Each year, many children between the ages of 18 months and 6 years find themselves in the same predicament as Cynthia: placing an object in the nose and not being able to remove it. When the child can't remove the object, he avoids telling his parents about the incident, because he's afraid he'll be punished.

What is a child likely to put in his nose? Usually small, smooth objects; for example, beads, buttons, round toy parts, corn kernels, peas, beans, and wads of paper or other compressible materials.

Unless the child tells someone about the object or the object's visible, it'll remain undetected until the child develops such complications as unilateral purulent nasal mucous discharge (rhinorrhea), inflammation, and infection, which can cause severe halitosis.

Before inspecting your patient's nose to determine whether an object's inside, take a complete history from him (or from his parents if he's a child). Then, use a nasal speculum to examine his nasal cavities for the foreign object. (For more information on using a nasal speculum and recovering a foreign object, see pages 42 and 43.)

Nose, mouth, and throat

Using a nasal speculum

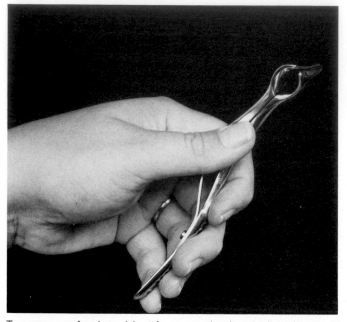

To remove a foreign object from a patient's nasal cavity, you'll use a nasal speculum, which allows you to see the inside of the nose. In the following photostory, we show you how to remove a foreign object from a patient's nose. But first, you must learn how to use the nasal speculum properly.

Hold the speculum between your thumb and index finger, as shown above. To open the blades, squeeze the handles between your palm and fingers, as shown below.

Insert the speculum—blades closed—about ½" (1.3 cm) into the nasal cavity. As you do, place your right index finger on the lower side of your patient's nose to stabilize the blades.

As you open the blades, the speculum elevates the tip of the nose. When you're finished, close the blades gradually and withdraw the speculum from your patient's nasal cavity.

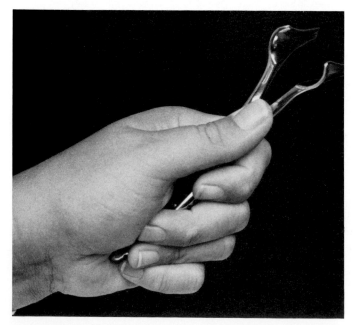

How to remove a foreign object

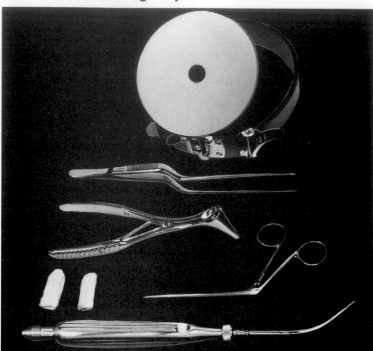

Remember Cynthia Stokes? Her mother brings her to the clinic where you work and asks you to check Cynthia's red, swollen, and draining nose. After observing her nose, you suspect she may have a foreign object in one of her nasal cavities. Do you know how to proceed? If you're unsure, follow the steps in this photostory.

Begin your assessment by taking Cynthia's history (see page 41). Then, tell Cynthia and her mother you'll inspect the inside of Cynthia's nose for foreign objects. Assure them the procedure's painless and that it won't injure her nose further. But advise them that Cynthia's nose may bleed slightly after the exam.

Next, gather the equipment you'll need: a nasal speculum, bayonet forceps, nasal forceps or curved hemostat, head mirror, nasal suction tip, and cotton pledgets. You'll also need a topical anesthetic and vasoconstrictor (for example, a mixture of 2% tetracaine and 0.5% phenylephrine) and a small anterior nasal pack.

Put on your head mirror. Then, wash your hands. Make sure Cynthia is seated comfortably.

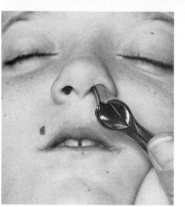

1 Tilt Cynthia's head back with your right hand and insert the speculum with your left hand, as the nurse is doing here. Make sure the blades are closed.

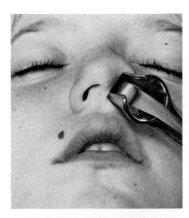

2 After you've inserted the speculum, slowly squeeze the handles together to open the blades. Inspect Cynthia's left nasal cavity.

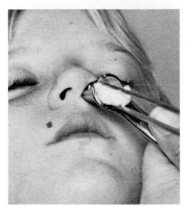

3 Moisten the pledgets in the tetracaine and phenylephrine mixture. Use the bayonet forceps to pick up a pledget. Insert the pledget in Cynthia's left nostril *gently*, to avoid pushing any object *farther* into her nasal cavity. Repeat the procedure for her right nasal cavity.

Leave the pledgets in place for 10 minutes. Then, remove them with the forceps.

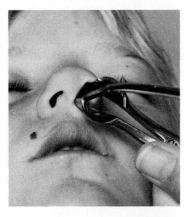

4 Carefully examine Cynthia's nasal cavity. If any purulent secretions are present, gently remove them with nasal suction, as the nurse is doing here.

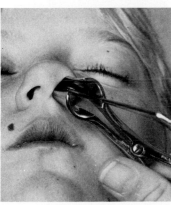

5 Suppose you see the wad of paper. Get ready to remove it. Gently insert the nasal forceps—with blades closed—into Cynthia's nostril.

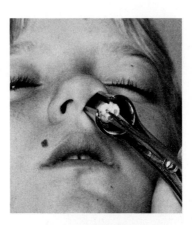

6 Then, open the forceps blades, position them around the wad, and gently pull it out. Take care not to push the wad into her trachea. It could become lodged there, requiring removal by bronchoscopy under general anesthetic.

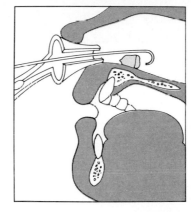

7 But suppose Cynthia had inserted a corn kernel in her nose. Because this type of object's soft and decomposable, use suction to remove it. If you can't remove the object by suction, use a right-angle blunt hook. Place the hook's tip just behind the kernel, as shown in the illustration.

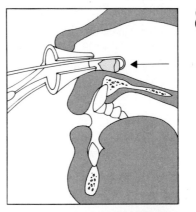

8 Then, slowly and gently pull out the kernel.

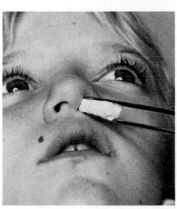

9 After you remove the foreign object, check to see if Cynthia's nasal cavity is bleeding. If it is, insert a small anterior nasal pack. Remove the speculum.

Tell Mrs. Stokes and Cynthia that any swelling should subside in a few days. Instruct them to return to the clinic if intermittent bleeding continues for more than 24 hours or if bleeding's excessive. Finally, document the procedure and any patient teaching.

Nose, mouth, and throat

_____ SPECIAL CONSIDERATIONS _____

Learning about epistaxis

Epistaxis (nosebleed) is usually resolved quickly with proper medical attention. But keep in mind that severe epistaxis can be life-threatening. In all cases, you need to assess the cause and type of epistaxis quickly and then provide the necessary care.

What causes epistaxis? Here are some possibilities:
• Habitual nose picking or rubbing (usually in children)
• Upper respiratory tract or sinus infections, which lead to forceful nose blowing
• Low indoor humidity (usually during the winter), which dries out the nasal membranes
• Cardiovascular disease (including hypertension), especially in the elderly
• Head trauma, such as a nose fracture
• Medications that thin the blood, such as aspirin and anticoagulants
• History of bleeding tendencies associated with leukemia and aplastic anemia
• Allergies, which dilate blood vessels and cause congestion, making the patient more susceptible to epistaxis
• High altitude.

In most cases, epistaxis begins in the *anterior* nasal septum. Blood may flow from one or both nasal cavities. You can usually control bleeding from the anterior nasal septum by squeezing your patient's nostrils or having him squeeze them.

When epistaxis originates in the *posterior* nasal septum, the condition's more serious. In this type of epistaxis, blood may flow from both nasal cavities into the mouth and throat, possibly obstructing the airway. Epistaxis in the posterior nasal septum occurs more frequently in the elderly than in younger persons.

Of course, if your patient has severe epistaxis resulting from trauma, control the bleeding before taking his history. But if the epistaxis is mild, you may want to ask him these questions before treatment:
• When did the bleeding begin? Is the blood flowing from one or both nostrils?
• Have you had nosebleeds in the past? How frequently do they occur? When was the last time your nose bled?
• Do you usually have trouble stopping the bleeding?
• Were you hit in the face recently, particularly in the area around your nose and sinuses?
• Have you had a cold or sinus problems recently, causing you to blow your nose forcefully? Have you noticed any sores or tenderness inside your nose?
• Do you have any allergies?
• Have you been treated for hypertension, heart disease, or a blood disorder?
• Have you noticed any other bleeding; for example, from your gums?
• Have you had oral or nasal surgery recently?
• Are you taking any medications regularly? What? How often?

How to control epistaxis

Suppose you work as an industrial nurse at a large metropolitan newspaper. Sixty-two-year-old Charlie Grabowski, a pressman, enters your office with epistaxis. Nervously, Mr. Grabowski tells you he frequently has nosebleeds, and usually, he can stop the bleeding. But this time he can't. What can you do to help?

First, ask Mr. Grabowski to sit down. Reassure him and help him relax. Then, have him tilt his head slightly forward to prevent blood from running down his throat. By doing so, you'll reduce the risk of his swallowing blood, choking, or aspirating blood into his lungs.

Next, obtain several 4"x4" gauze pads, an emesis basin, cold compresses, and a drape to protect Mr. Grabowski's clothing. Take his history (see page 41) and explain what you're going to do. Record his vital signs, and closely monitor them for changes.

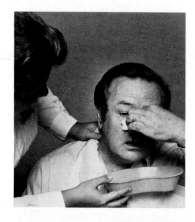

1 Now, give Mr. Grabowski a 4"x4" gauze pad. Instruct him to use his thumb and forefinger to squeeze the pad over the soft part of his nose. Tell him to apply steady pressure to both nostrils for 10 minutes. Urge him to breathe through his mouth while he's holding his nose and to spit out any blood that accumulates in his mouth.

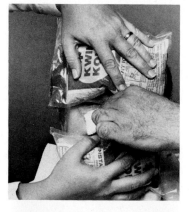

2 As Mr. Grabowski holds the gauze pad over his nose, apply cold compresses above and below his nose, as the nurse is doing here. The compresses cause vasoconstriction, which decreases bleeding.

After 10 minutes, have Mr. Grabowski remove the pad from his nose. Determine whether the bleeding has stopped. If it hasn't, have him repeat the procedure.

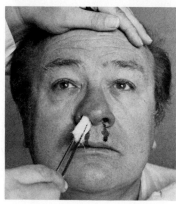

3 If bleeding still hasn't stopped, roll up two clean gauze pads and insert one in each nostril. Make sure part of each pad remains outside his nostrils to make removal easier. Take Mr. Grabowski's vital signs again. Refer him to a doctor or have him transported to a hospital *immediately* if his vital signs are unstable or if you can't stop the bleeding after a second attempt.

Home care

Recovering from a nosebleed

Dear Patient:
Now that your nosebleed has been controlled, you'll want to take special care of your nose to prevent it from bleeding again.

Important: If your nose begins to bleed again, contact your doctor immediately or go to your local hospital's emergency department.

To help your nose heal properly, follow these instructions during the next 7 days:

• Keep your hands away from your nose. Avoid picking or rubbing your nose, even if it itches. Also, don't try to put anything inside your nose, such as cotton-tipped swabs or tissues.

• If you have to sneeze, do so with your mouth open. *Don't* blow your nose.

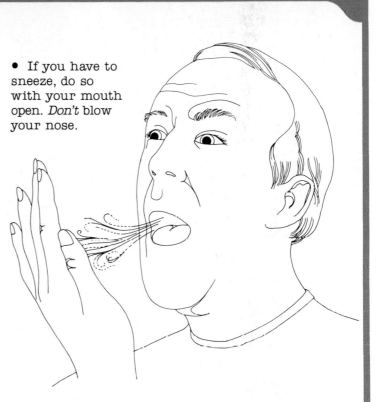

• If you have to pick up something from the floor, bend your knees and keep your head upright. When you lie down, prop your head on two or three pillows. Remember, don't exert yourself.

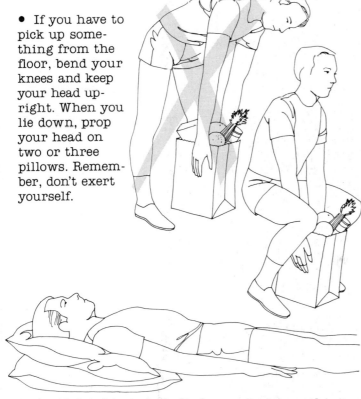

• Avoid drinking alcoholic beverages or anything hot.
• Don't smoke, or take aspirin or medications containing aspirin.
• If you're constipated, take a laxative. Avoid straining when you move your bowels.

• Every day apply a small amount of petrolatum just inside your nostrils. This keeps them moist and softens any crusts that form after the nosebleed. If your home is heated with hot air, set up a cold-mist humidifier at night to moisten the air and prevent your nostrils from drying out while you sleep.

Nose, mouth, and throat

Inspecting your patient's mouth and throat

As you probably know, the mouth and throat function as the entrance to the digestive tract and as one of the entrances to the respiratory tract. Considering that air, food, liquids, and, in some cases, cigarette smoke constantly pass through the mouth and throat, you can see why these areas may harbor bacteria that cause diseases.

Assessment of your patient's mouth and throat can help detect various abnormalities; for example, tonsillitis, herpes simplex I virus, and candidiasis.

Begin your assessment by asking your patient the questions listed below. (For complete details on assessing the mouth and throat, see the NURSING PHOTOBOOK ASSESSING YOUR PATIENTS.)

• Have you noticed severe or persistent pain in your mouth? Do you have difficulty chewing or swallowing?
• Are all your teeth natural? Do you wear upper or lower dentures or a partial plate? Are any of your teeth loose or missing? Which ones, and how long have they been so?
• When was your last dental examination? What did the dentist find at that time?
• Do you have toothaches frequently? Do you brush and floss your teeth daily?
• Do your gums bleed? Do you ever have sores inside your mouth or on your tongue? How long do they last?
• Has your jaw ever been broken or have your mouth and teeth been injured? Describe what happened. Have you ever had oral surgery? Why?
• Has your saliva ever been bloody? How long did this condition last? Was it constant or intermittent?
• Do you ever have bad breath?
• Does your tongue ever feel sore? Do you have difficulty distinguishing one taste from another? Describe the problem.
• Do you have frequent sore throats? When did you last have a sore throat? About how many times a year do you have a sore throat? Do you take any medication to relieve it? Do you or members of your family have a history of streptococcal infections?
• Does your voice ever sound hoarse or your throat feel scratchy? How long does the feeling last?
• Do you ever have any problem speaking? Describe what happens.
• Have your tonsils or adenoids been removed? When and for what reason?
• Are you allergic to any medications or foods? What are they? Are you currently taking any medications? What kind?
• Do you smoke or did you ever smoke? If you smoke, how many cigarettes or cigars do you smoke a day? Do you smoke a pipe? If you no longer smoke, when did you stop?
• Do you usually breathe through your mouth?

Nurses' guide to dental problems

Nursing-bottle caries

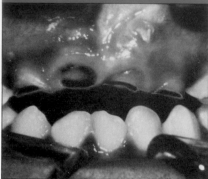

Causes
• Improper dental hygiene
• Liquids containing sugar (milk, soft drinks, and fruit juices) in the child's mouth, such as from giving a bottle just before bedtime and from bottle- or breast-feeding beyond age 12 months

Signs and symptoms
• Teeth hypersensitive to heat and cold; usually affects upper front teeth
• Sore and bleeding gums

Fractured tooth

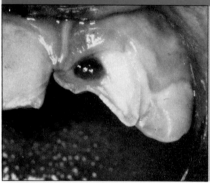

Cause
• Trauma; for example, injury from a contact sport or a fall

Signs and symptoms
• Slightly displaced tooth
• Bleeding from gums or pulp
• Pulp visible around injured area

Loose or displaced tooth

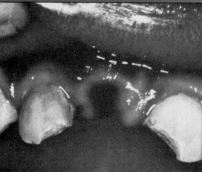

Causes
• Blow to the mouth or tooth
• Bone and gum disease, such as periodontitis
• Vitamin deficiency, such as scurvy

Signs and symptoms
• Tooth easily shifted within socket
• Tooth shorter than adjacent teeth or not visible (intrusion)
• Tooth longer than adjacent teeth or out of position (extrusion)
• Tooth missing from socket (total displacement)
• Possibly bleeding from gums (especially with disease)

Avulsed tooth

Cause
• Blow to the tooth or mouth from a contact sport, a fall, or an automobile accident

Signs and symptoms
• Tooth torn from socket
• Bloody gums around affected area

Nursing considerations
• Tell parents to begin weaning child from bottle-feeding about his first birthday.
• Instruct parents to avoid giving child a bottle before his bedtime. If they must, however, tell them to fill it with water, rather than milk or juice.
• Tell parents not to give child a pacifier sweetened with soda or syrup
• When child's first tooth erupts, advise parents to wipe it with a clean, damp cloth after each feeding. Have them repeat the procedure with successive teeth.
• Recommend that parents take child to a dentist as soon as possible.
• When child's age 18 months, tell parents to begin cleaning his teeth with toothpaste and a soft-bristled toothbrush. Encourage parents to have child participate in this procedure as much as possible.
• Suggest to the parents that they try to provide snacks that contain little or no processed sugar (for example, fruits, carrots, and celery).

Nursing considerations
• Check patient's mouth and airway for tooth fragments and other objects that may obstruct his airway.
• Tell patient to seek treatment from a dentist immediately.
• Advise patient to bring the piece of tooth to the dentist, if possible.

Nursing considerations
• With intrusion, don't try to pull the tooth into position, especially if the patient's a child. The tooth may return to its normal position in about 1 month.
• With extrusion, try to push the tooth into its socket, using gentle but firm pressure. Have patient hold the tooth in position until he's examined by a dentist.
• If the tooth is totally displaced, try to locate it. Then, rinse it with sterile normal saline solution and reimplant it.

Nursing considerations
• Check patient's mouth and airway for tooth and other objects that may obstruct his airway.
• Tell patient to seek treatment from a dentist immediately.
• Teach patient ways to avoid this type of injury; for example, not putting his mouth too close to water fountains, wearing a protective mouthpiece when playing contact sports, and wearing seat belts while riding in an automobile.

Relieving dental pain
Dental pain may be a symptom of dental caries, pulpal or gingival disease, pressure from prostheses, mandibular fracture, sinusitis, fractured or avulsed teeth, or teeth that have not erupted. Accompanying signs and symptoms depend on the cause. If your patient has caries, his teeth may be hypersensitive to heat and cold; if he has a periodontal disease, his gums may bleed; if he has sinusitis, his maxillary sinuses may be congested.

To help relieve dental pain, take the following measures:
• Apply cold compresses on the cheek or lip over the patient's affected tooth.
• Administer aspirin or acetaminophen in recommended dosages.
• Instruct your patient to avoid hot or extremely cold food and drinks.
• If the pain's being caused by sinusitis, administer antihistamines.
• Refer the patient to a dentist for evaluation and treatment.

Teething pain
Whenever a tooth erupts through the gums, pain and often irritability accompany the eruption. Your patient may complain that his face or jaw aches, and that he lacks interest in food. You may note that he moves his mouth excessively when chewing and has a low-grade fever.

In addition, if your patient's a child, he may also drool, be irritable and lethargic, and have diarrhea.

What can you do to help relieve teething pain? Take these steps:
• Administer aspirin or acetaminophen in recommended dosages.
• Apply a teething liquid or ointment to anesthetize your patient's gums.
• Advise your patient or his parents that soft foods are less painful for him to ingest than foods that require chewing, such as red meats. If your patient's a young child, warn his parents that his food should be cut in large pieces so he doesn't aspirate them.
• Eating cold foods, such as ice cream, and sucking on ice chips may help relieve gum pain. For an infant, use a teething ring that's been chilled in the refrigerator.

Nose, mouth, and throat

Saving an avulsed tooth

Imagine this situation: A group of teenagers suddenly bursts into the medical clinic where you work. One member of the group, 15-year-old Bobby Morgan, has been hit in the mouth by a baseball while playing at a nearby baseball diamond. Bobby's right central incisor has been knocked out and his left central and right lateral incisors are chipped.

How would you manage this situation? Obviously, your first priority is to get Bobby to a dentist as soon as possible. But you can provide prompt emergency care in the interim. This care involves locating the avulsed tooth, cleansing it (if it's dirty), and either reimplanting the tooth or placing it in a transport medium to preserve it. By doing so, you'll increase the chances of successful tooth reimplantation.

To learn more about caring for an avulsed tooth, read the following photostory.

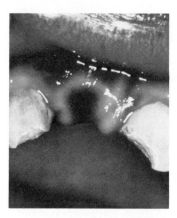

1 First, reassure Bobby that he'll be OK. Then, determine the extent of his injury. Check his gums for bleeding and his mouth and pharynx for pieces of teeth and for other objects that could obstruct his airway.

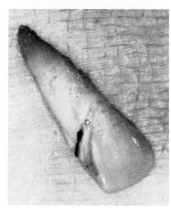

2 Next, try to find the avulsed tooth. If possible, gently rinse the tooth with water or sterile normal saline solution. *Important:* Don't scrub or wipe the tooth after you rinse it, because you may remove tissue. Place the tooth on a clean, dry surface.

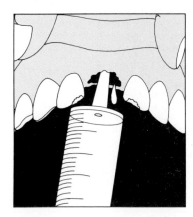

3 Now, you'll want to irrigate the gum socket. To do this, fill a 5-cc syringe with normal saline solution. Place the syringe tip at the gum socket, as shown in this illustration. Depress the plunger to direct the stream of solution toward the socket. If you don't have a syringe on hand, have your patient rinse his mouth with water.

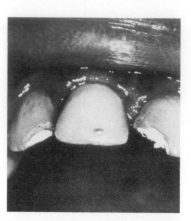

4 After rinsing the avulsed tooth, reinsert it in its socket. This way, the dentist may be able to permanently reimplant the tooth in the alveolus socket. Make sure the tooth is held in place while Bobby's transported to the dentist.

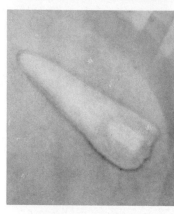

5 If you can't reimplant the tooth, put it in a paper cup or on a towel. If possible, pour normal saline solution in the cup or on the towel, to help preserve the tooth.
⬛ *Nursing tip:* Because of its natural components, cold milk also helps preserve an avulsed tooth. Milk's more effective than saliva, water, or air.

Document the care you've given.

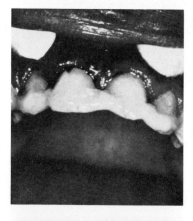

6 As you can see in this photo, the dentist's applied an acrylic splint over the avulsed and chipped teeth. The splint holds the teeth in position to ensure proper healing.

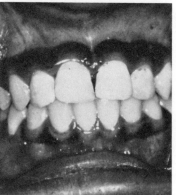

7 After the dentist removes the splint, reassess Bobby's mouth periodically to make sure it's healing properly. Check for malalignment and for any signs and symptoms of infection. If you notice any problems, refer Bobby to his dentist. Document your findings.

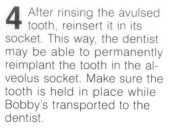

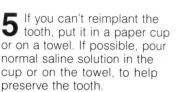

How to obtain a specimen for throat culture

Suppose your patient, Bill McNamara, has a sore throat. To help determine appropriate treatment, you need to obtain a specimen for throat culture, as ordered. The specimen helps identify the causative organism; for example, group A beta-hemolytic streptococci. And by early treatment of the disorder, you can help prevent such complications as rheumatic heart disease and glomerulonephritis.

Important: Ask Mr. McNamara if he's taking any medications, particularly antibiotics. If he is, find out what he's taking and how often he takes it. Remember, antibiotics may affect test result validity by masking the infection's cause.

Before you begin the procedure, gather the equipment you'll need: sterile culture swab with culture medium (Strep Culturette®), tongue depressor, and penlight.

Note: The Strep Culturette® is a cotton-tipped swab encased in a soft plastic tube. At the tube's base is transport medium, which preserves the specimen for culture.

Now, explain the procedure to Mr. McNamara. Tell him he may feel the urge to gag during the procedure. Reassure him that the sensation's temporary. Instruct him to concentrate on breathing through his nose.

Then, wash your hands.

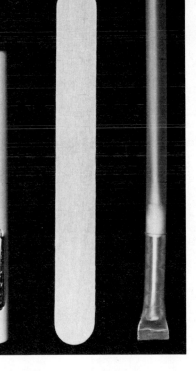

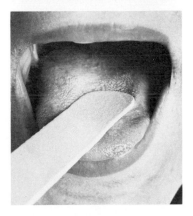

1 Now, ask Mr. McNamara to sit on a chair, facing you. Have him tilt his head back, open his mouth wide, and stick out his tongue. Use the tongue depressor to hold down his tongue, as shown. If he starts to gag, remove the tongue depressor. Tell him to breathe deeply through his nose and relax. Then, try using the tongue depressor again, but avoid positioning it as far back as before.

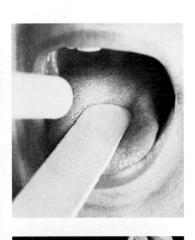

2 Shine the penlight into his throat and check for inflamed, purulent, and ulcerated areas.

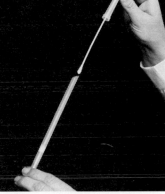

3 Next, grip the culture swab by its handle and carefully remove it from its tube. To prevent Mr. McNamara's tongue from touching the swab, hold it down with the tongue depressor. Doing so also keeps the specimen free of oral secretions, which may invalidate the specimen and make the causative organism difficult to identify.

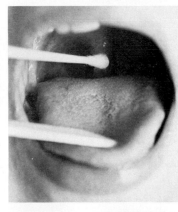

4 Now, insert the swab in the patient's mouth. Using a rolling motion, quickly swab the infected area. Take care not to touch the patient's cheeks, teeth, or tongue with the swab. Doing so may invalidate test results. Then, carefully withdraw the swab.

Place the swab in its plastic tube, making sure you don't touch the outside of the tube with the swab.

Slide the hard plastic cover over the tube's base.

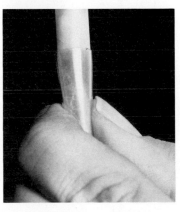

5 Holding the tube's base between your thumb and index finger, crush the ampul—which contains the culture medium—inside the tube.

Push the swab into the culture medium, making sure it's immersed. Wash your hands. Label the specimen tube with your patient's name, the date and time of collection, and the specimen's origin. Then, send the specimen to the lab immediately. Document the procedure.

Nose, mouth, and throat

Learning about airway obstruction

Are you aware that each year, in the United States, 2,500 people die of airway obstruction caused by foreign objects? Other causes of airway obstruction include edema, trauma, strangulation, bilateral vocal cord paralysis, near-drowning, tumor, drug overdose, and laryngospasms. If the patient's unconscious, his tongue may be obstructing his airway.

A number of these conditions—for example, edema, strangulation, and drug overdose—necessitate intensive nursing measures carried out in a hospital. In these cases, try to maintain a patent airway until help arrives. *Remember:* Some signs of airway obstruction are similar to those of a myocardial infarction. Always assess your patient carefully.

But when you suspect a foreign object's the cause of your patient's airway obstruction, carefully assess your patient's signs and symptoms. By doing so, you can pinpoint the level of obstruction (see illustration). For example, if your patient has:

• hoarseness, coughing, aphonia, hemoptysis, wheezing, dyspnea, cyanosis, apnea, drooling, dys-phagia, or stridor, the foreign body's lodged in his *laryngeal area.*
• audible slaps, palpatory thuds, asthmatic wheezes, and possible hoarseness, the foreign body's lodged in his *trachea.*
• coughing, choking, wheezing, possibly cyanosis, and chest pressure or pain, the foreign body's lodged in his *bronchial tubes.*

Suppose you've established that your patient has an obstructed airway. To help identify the cause of your patient's airway obstruction, look for clues; for example, if your patient was eating, the cause may be a piece of food.

More common foreign objects that cause airway obstruction in adults include fish bones and large pieces of meat; in children, coins, peanuts, pins, small toys, and buttons are frequent causes.

When you've determined the cause, take effective measures to expel the object. These include a series of back blows and manual thrusts (either abdominal or chest). You'll intervene with the methods shown in the following pages.

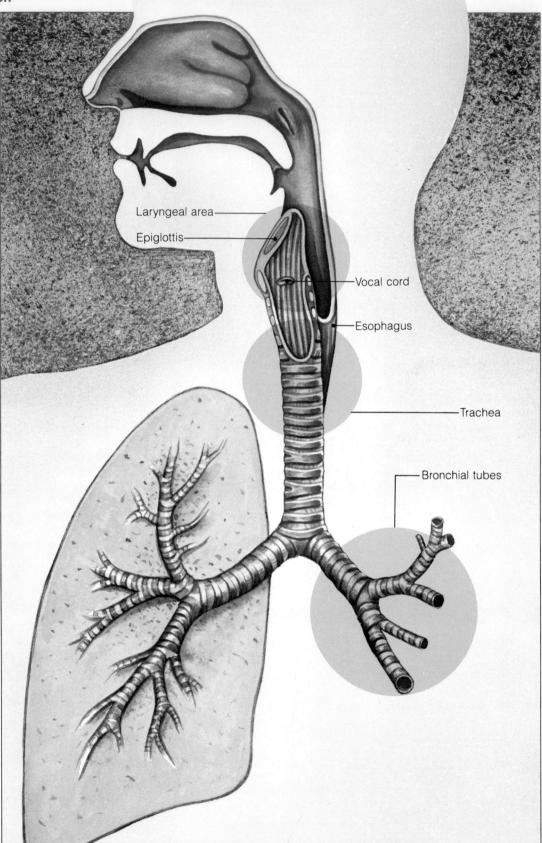

Laryngeal area
Epiglottis
Vocal cord
Esophagus
Trachea
Bronchial tubes

Clearing the airway of a conscious patient

You're walking through the cafeteria at the college where you work when you see Mike Heath, a student, eating lunch. Suddenly, he jumps up from his chair, begins coughing, and clutches his throat. Noting his actions, you assess that food is obstructing Mike's airway. You know you must act quickly, because every second counts.

In this photostory, you'll learn how to perform back blows and manual thrusts to loosen the foreign body and expel it from the airway.

First, ask your patient if he can speak. If he can speak or cough, he has some air exchange and only partial obstruction. Encourage him to continue coughing, because he may expel the foreign object on his own.

But if your patient can't speak or cough, is making crowing sounds, or is cyanotic, he may have complete obstruction.

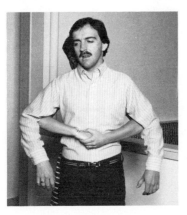

1 Call for assistance right away. Then, quickly position yourself at Mike's side, slightly behind him. Place one hand on his sternum and lean him forward. (Ideally, position his head lower than his chest, to take advantage of gravity.) If your patient collapses, you can lower him slowly to the floor.

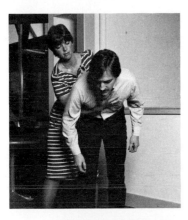

2 With the heel of your other hand, deliver four sharp blows over Mike's spine, between his shoulder blades. Use the same amount of force for each blow. Doing so increases pressure in his airway, which may partially or completely dislodge the foreign body.

Remember: You can perform back blows with your patient standing, sitting, or lying.

Again assess your patient's air exchange. If it's still poor, deliver abdominal thrusts.

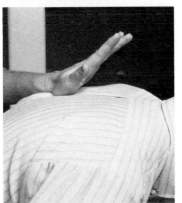

3 To do this, stand behind Mike and wrap your arms around his waist. This stance affords both leverage and maximum arm reach. With your right hand, form a fist, tucking the thumb inside so it doesn't injure your patient. Clasp the fist with your left hand.

Place your clasped fist against Mike's abdomen, midway between his waist and rib cage.

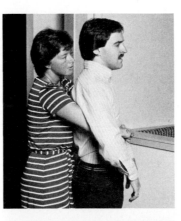

4 Then, quickly thrust your fist inward and upward against his abdomen. To make sure you're pressing upward at the correct angle, imagine you're trying to hit yourself in the chin. Keep your fist above the patient's navel but below his xiphoid process.

Perform four successive abdominal thrusts, using the same amount of force for each. By doing so, you force air out of the lungs, helping to expel the foreign object.

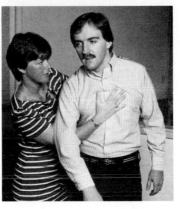

5 Reassess Mike's air exchange. If he doesn't have good air exchange, continue delivering the series of back blows and abdominal thrusts until he does.

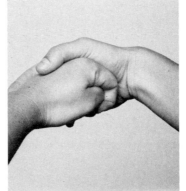

6 If your patient's a young child, pregnant, or obese, use chest thrusts instead of abdominal thrusts. Why? Because abdominal thrusts may injure a child's internal organs or a pregnant patient's fetus and will be ineffective in an obese patient.

To perform chest thrusts, stand behind him and wrap your arms around his chest, beneath his axillae. With one hand make a fist and grasp it with the other hand, as shown.

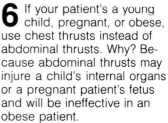

7 Position your clasped fist approximately 2 finger-breadths or 1½" to 2" (3.8 to 5 cm) up from his xiphoid process. (To avoid injuring your patient, never deliver chest thrusts directly over his xiphoid process or the margin of his rib cage.) Support your patient against your body and deliver four thrusts of equal force. Avoid tightening your arms around his rib cage.

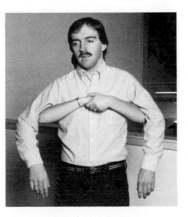

Nose, mouth, and throat

Clearing the airway of an unconscious patient

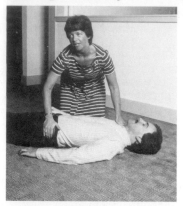

1 Suppose, despite your best efforts, Mike Heath—your patient in the previous photo-story—loses consciousness. When that happens, his throat muscles relax and the foreign object may become partially dislodged. Now, full and forceful mouth-to-mouth ventilation can push air past the obstruction, keeping him alive. To do so, first position Mike on his back on a firm, flat surface.

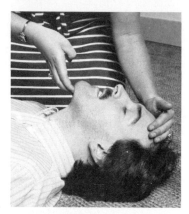

2 Then, using the head-tilt/chin-lift method, open his airway. To perform this maneuver, place one hand on his forehead and tilt his head back. Place the fingertips of your other hand under his lower jaw, on the bony part near his chin. Gently lift up his chin, taking care not to close his mouth.

3 Now, look, listen, and feel for any signs of air exchange. Observe his chest to see if it's rising and falling, and listen and feel for air coming from his nose.
 If you don't detect signs of breathing, prepare to ventilate him.

4 To ventilate your patient, pinch his nostrils closed with the index finger and thumb of the hand on his forehead. Remember to maintain slight pressure on his forehead to keep his airway open. Then, open your mouth wide and place it over his mouth, pressing down firmly so no air can escape. Try to blow air into his lungs. If you're unsuccessful, reposition his head and neck to move his tongue out of his airway and try again.

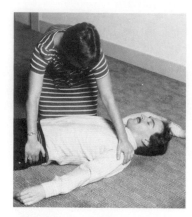

5 If you still can't ventilate Mike, you know something other than his tongue's obstructing his airway. To dislodge the obstruction, perform a series of maneuvers, including back blows, manual (abdominal or chest) thrusts, and a finger sweep.
 First, place one hand on Mike's shoulder farthest from you and your other hand on his hip farthest from you, as shown here.

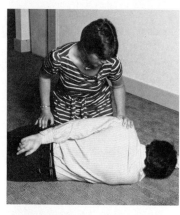

6 Now, roll him toward you and support him against your thighs.

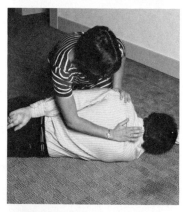

7 Using the heel of your hand that's on his hip, deliver four sharp back blows over his spine, between his shoulder blades.
 Quickly but gently return him to his back and assess his air exchange. If it's still poor or if he's not breathing, prepare to deliver manual thrusts (either abdominal or chest).

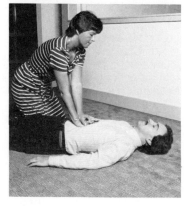

8 To deliver abdominal thrusts, kneel close to Mike's side, with your knees even with his hips. Or, straddle his hips or one of his thighs. Place the heel of one hand on his abdomen, halfway between his waist and rib cage. Cover this hand with your other hand and interlock your fingers. Align your fingers directly over his abdomen and deliver four sharp thrusts inward and upward, as the nurse is doing here.

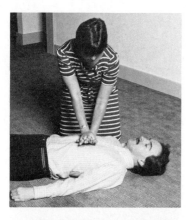

9 To deliver chest thrusts, kneel beside your patient, between his waist and shoulders. Clasp your hands together and position them as you would for cardiac compression; that is, with the heel of one hand on the lower half of his sternum. Then, administer four downward thrusts.

After delivering manual thrusts (either abdominal or chest), quickly move to your patient's head to reassess his air exchange.

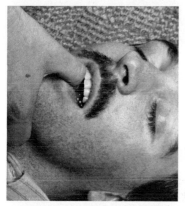

10 If your patient's air exchange is still poor, perform a finger sweep. To do this, open his mouth by grasping his tongue and lower jaw with the thumb and fingers of your hand closest to his feet and lifting. This maneuver will pull his tongue away from the back of his throat, which may partially relieve the obstruction.

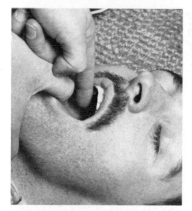

11 Next, insert the index finger of your other hand in his mouth and move it along the inside of his cheek and deep into his throat, to the base of his tongue. Use a hooking action to dislodge the foreign object and move it into his mouth so you can remove it. But take care not to force the foreign object deeper into his throat.

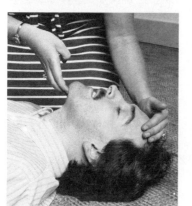

12 Now, reposition Mike's head and try again to ventilate him.

If you *can't* ventilate him, repeat the series of back blows, manual thrusts, and finger sweep until you can ventilate him or until advanced care's available.

If you can ventilate Mike, continue with the steps of cardiopulmonary resuscitation.

Preventing airway obstructions

You can help your patients avoid airway obstruction by teaching them preventive measures and reviewing these precautions:
• Cut your food in small pieces.
• Chew your food slowly and thoroughly.
• Don't talk or laugh while chewing or swallowing.
• Don't drink an excessive amount of alcohol before and during meals. The depressant effect of alcohol on your throat muscles makes you more susceptible to choking.
• Don't let children run, walk, talk, or play with objects or food in their mouths.
• Try to keep small objects away from toddlers (ages 1 to 3).
• If you wear dentures, make sure they fit correctly.
• Secure or remove (if appropriate) loose teeth.

Positioning a child to clear his airway

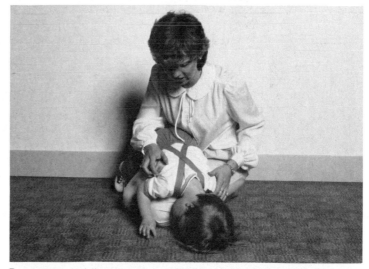

Because a toddler or young child frequently puts small objects in his mouth, you may encounter a child with an airway obstruction. To relieve the obstruction, you'll perform a series of back blows and chest thrusts similar to those shown in the preceding two photostories. However, you'll position a child differently than an adult to deliver back blows.

To position a child properly for the procedure, kneel, and drape the child across your thighs, as shown here. Keep his head lower than his trunk, and support his head and chest with one hand. Doing so uses gravity advantageously and helps you hold on to the child.

Caution: Never let a child's head hang over the edge of a table or bed when you deliver the back blows. You may seriously injure him.

For more information on relieving a child's airway obstruction, see the NURSING PHOTOBOOK NURSING PEDIATRIC PATIENTS.

Head

No matter what type of head injury or disorder your patient has, most of your nursing care is directed toward providing patient comfort and reassurance, preventing complications, and performing follow-up measures. That's why on the next few pages we tell you how to:
• identify common head injuries
• perform an emergency assessment of a head-injured patient
• take an on-the-scene history
• differentiate a vascular headache from glossopharyngeal neuralgia.
   To find out more, read these pages carefully.
   (For more information on head injuries and disorders, see the NURSING PHOTOBOOK COPING WITH NEUROLOGIC DISORDERS.)

Nurses' guide to head injuries

As you know, a head injury can have grave, even life-threatening consequences; for example, irreversible brain or spinal cord damage. To prevent complications, proper emergency care is essential. Read the guidelines that follow to review your role in caring for a patient with a head injury.
• Check patient's airway, respirations, pulse rate, and level of consciousness.
• Carefully examine patient for other injuries, such as fractures, lacerations, and abrasions. Pay particular attention to his scalp.
• Immobilize patient's head and neck with a cervical collar, backboard, or sandbags. *Remember:* Don't move him until he's properly immobilized.
• Dress any open wounds.
• Call for medical assistance and stay with patient until help arrives.
   Now, study the chart that follows to familiarize yourself with the causes, and signs and symptoms of common head injuries.

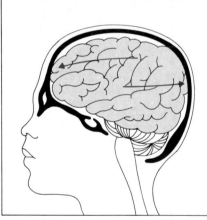

Cerebral contusion
(bruising of the brain)
Two types: Coup-contrecoup and acceleration-deceleration
Causes
Blow to the head that bruises the brain directly; for example, from being hit with a blunt instrument. Such a blow drives the brain into the opposite side of the skull, causing more bruising (coup-contrecoup injury). Or, a person's head may be jolted forward, such as in a car accident, causing the brain to slap against the back of the skull. Then, the head stops abruptly, causing the brain to slap against the front of the skull (acceleration-deceleration injury).
Signs and symptoms
• Variable respirations; may range from normal to ataxic, periodic, or rapid
• Rapid pulse
• Drowsiness
• Disorientation and confusion

• Possibly agitation or violent behavior
• Deteriorating level or loss of consciousness
• Usually small, equal, and reactive pupils
• Loss of normal eye movement
• Hemiplegia or, if injury's severe, quadriplegia
• Fever, accompanied by diaphoresis
• Possibly severe scalp wounds
• Decerebrate or decorticate posturing

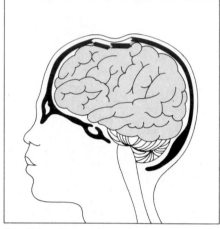

Skull fracture
Cause
Blow to the head, possibly resulting from a fight, fall, or motor vehicle accident
Signs and symptoms
• Scalp wounds, abrasions, contusions, lacerations, or avulsions. *Note:* Linear fractures may be insidious and require X-ray confirmation.
• Profuse bleeding, especially with an open fracture
• Persistent, localized headaches
• Changes in respiratory patterns; possibly respiratory distress
• Alterations in level of consciousness; possibly loss of consciousness
• Possibly agitation and irritability (with a depressed fracture)
• If bone fragments pierce the dura mater or cerebral cortex, possibly subdural, epidural, or intracerebral hemorrhage or hematoma
• With intracranial or intracerebral hemorrhage, hemiparesis, dizziness, convulsions, projectile vomiting, and decreased pulse rate
• With cranial vault fracture, soft-tissue edema in area of fracture
• With basilar fracture, hemorrhaging from the nose, pharynx, or ears; cerebrospinal fluid drainage from the nose or ears; periorbital ecchymosis without a history of eye trauma; supramastoid ecchymosis (Battle's sign); and sometimes bleeding behind the tympanic membrane (hemotatympanum)
• With sphenoidal fracture, optic nerve damage, possibly resulting in blindness
• With temporal fracture, possibly unilateral deafness or facial paralysis

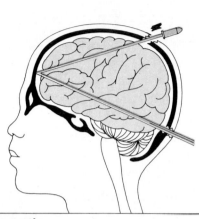

Concussion
(functional impairment of the brain)
Cause
Blow to the head or face; for example, from a fall, punch, or motor vehicle accident
Signs and symptoms
- Headache
- Dilated pupils
- Restlessness or combativeness
- Drowsiness
- Vertigo
- Nausea
- Weak pulse
- Unusually rapid or slow breathing
- Brief unconsciousness
- Possibly transient amnesia
- Disorientation
- Blurred or double vision (diplopia)

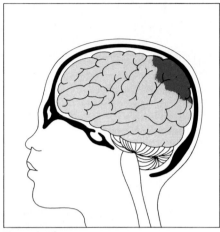

Penetrating skull injury
(foreign object in the brain)
Cause
An object, such as a bullet, passing through the skull and lodging in the brain
Signs and symptoms
- Headache
- Bleeding
- Open wound with protruding object
- Irritability
- Restlessness
- Loss of normal eye movement
- Loss of consciousness

Laceration
(penetration of skull and brain by an object)
Causes
Blow to the head, such as from a baseball bat, that may fracture the skull and cause bone fragment to tear brain tissue; in other cases, an object, such as a bullet, passing through the skull and brain but not lodging there
Signs and symptoms
- Visible open wound at entrance and exit sites
- Loss of consciousness
- Bleeding

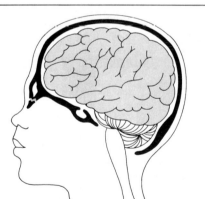

Facial fractures
Cause
Direct blow to one of the facial bones, such as the nasal, mandible, maxillae, or zygomatic, usually from trauma, such as from a fall, motor vehicle accident, or contact sport
Signs and symptoms
- Epistaxis, ranging from trickling to full nasal hemorrhage
- Ecchymoses at the affected site
- Soft-tissue edema
- Head and neck pain
- Facial asymmetry from fracture or soft-tissue edema
- Malfunctioning or loss of function of the affected area
- Possibly blood or cerebrospinal fluid drainage from the nose and ears

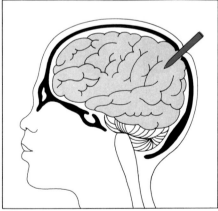

DOCUMENTING

Head injuries: Taking the patient's history

If your head-injured patient's conscious, take a brief history while performing the assessment. Be sure to tailor your questions to the patient's condition. For example, if he's having difficulty speaking, ask questions that require only a yes or no answer. If the patient appears alert and oriented, however, ask open-ended questions, such as, "How did the accident happen?"

As you take your patient's history, be alert for signs and symptoms of secondary injuries or complications. For example, suppose your patient has hemiplegia opposite to the injury, as well as dizziness and vomiting. He may have an intracerebral hematoma. Because this condition's associated with increasing intracranial pressure and may result in convulsions, take seizure precautions and continue with the history.

Note: For complete details on secondary brain injuries, see the NURSING PHOTOBOOK COPING WITH NEUROLOGIC DISORDERS.

Of course, if the patient's unconscious, you'll need to gather some of this information from witnesses.

What information do you need? Besides determining the type and extent of your patient's injury, find out how and when the accident happened. Then, you'll need answers to these questions:
- Does the patient have any allergies, diseases, or disorders? How has he been treated for these conditions?
- Does he take any medications?
- Who is his doctor?
- What is the patient's present consciousness level? If he's unconscious, try to find out how long he's been this way. If he regains consciousness, ask him if he remembers what happened.
- Is the patient experiencing blurred or double vision (diplopia), headache, dizziness, nausea and/or vomiting, weakness, or numbness?
- Is blood or cerebrospinal fluid draining from the patient's nose or ears?
- Had anyone provided emergency care before you arrived on the scene? Check to see if your patient's wearing a Medic Alert™ bracelet or necklace. If necessary, search his wallet for a medical identification card.

When help arrives, advise them of your observations and the information you collected. If possible, accompany the patient to the hospital.

Head

How to remove a helmet from a neck- or spinal-injured patient

You're on your way to the clinic where you work, when you spot a motorcycle overturned at the side of the road. As you get out of your car, a bystander tells you that the motorcyclist, Linda Harrison, lost her balance and can't get up. You immediately suspect a neck or spinal cord injury and ask someone to call an ambulance.

Because Linda is conscious, you decide to remove her helmet so you can continue your assessment. Do you know how to do this correctly, without causing further injury?

First, enlist the help of another person to keep Linda's spinal cord properly aligned. Her head and neck must remain rigid while the helmet is maneuvered over her nose and ears.

Important: If the patient complains of pain while you're attempting to remove the helmet, stop the procedure immediately and leave the helmet in place.

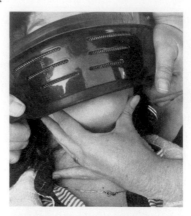

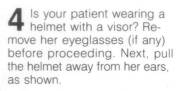

4 Is your patient wearing a helmet with a visor? Remove her eyeglasses (if any) before proceeding. Next, pull the helmet away from her ears, as shown.

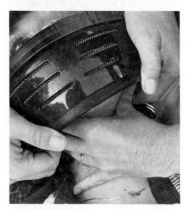

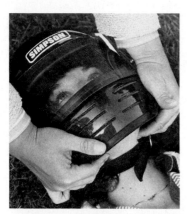

1 Position yourself behind your patient, as shown, with your hands on the sides of her helmet and your fingers on her jaw. Doing so will keep her head from slipping if the helmet is accidentally moved.

2 As you maintain traction on your patient's head, ask your helper to unfasten or cut the helmet's chin strap. Don't remove your fingers from her jaw or attempt to reposition them.

3 When the chin strap is out of the way, instruct your helper to place one of her hands on your patient's jaw, keeping her thumb on one side and her index and middle fingers on the other side (see photo). Tell her to place her other hand underneath your patient's neck, using gentle pressure to maintain traction.

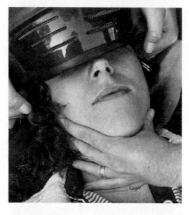

5 Now, still positioned behind her, carefully begin sliding the helmet toward you. Continue to pull outward slightly on the helmet's sides.

As you work, take care not to twist her head or neck or to jostle your helper's hands from their correct traction position. If for some reason you do, stop immediately and start over.

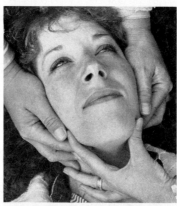

6 When you've removed the helmet, place it to one side, as your helper continues to keep your patient's head and neck properly aligned.

Then, place your hands on either side of your patient's head, with your palms over her ears and your fingers under her jaw.

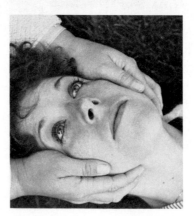

7 As you support your patient's head and neck, instruct your helper to apply a neck collar. Maintain proper head alignment and immobilization in this manner until someone comes with a long spineboard. Then, begin to assess your patient for other injuries.

Document the entire procedure, including your nursing assessment.

Assessing a patient with head injuries

Jim Tyler, a 22-year-old maintenance worker at the office supply company where you work, is struck in the head with a plank while replacing floorboards. When you arrive at the scene, you see Mr. Tyler lying on the floor. He appears to be unconscious. As you call for help, begin assessing the extent of his injury. Do you know how to proceed? If you're unsure, follow the steps in this photostory.

As you work, gather the information you need from his co-workers. Try to find out when the accident occurred, how long he's been unconscious, and if he has any medical problems, such as epilepsy or hypertension. Check to see if your patient's wearing a necklace. If so, remove it before applying a cervical collar. Note: For more detailed information on assessing and treating a patient with a head injury, see the NURSING PHOTOBOOK COPING WITH NEUROLOGIC DISORDERS.

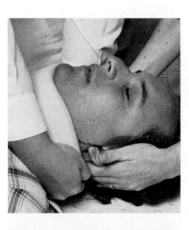

4 To avoid serious and perhaps irreversible complications, remember that a patient with a traumatic head injury may also have a cervical spine injury. Immobilize Mr. Tyler's head with the proper equipment. To do this, have a co-worker maintain traction as you apply a cervical collar.

Note: Never attempt to move the patient until he is immobilized.

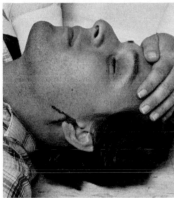
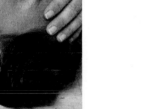

1 First, position Mr. Tyler's head as shown here, to check for airway patency and to maintain an open airway.

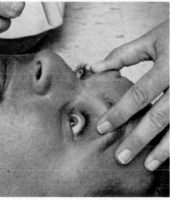

5 To check Mr. Tyler's pupils, lift both eyelids simultaneously and use a penlight to assess pupillary response. His pupils should be equal in size and constrict to light bilaterally. Also, check his eyes for evidence of trauma, excessive tearing, and pale or reddened conjunctivae. Tearing or reddened conjunctivae may indicate irritation from a foreign object or infection.

2 Assess his breathing. To do so, put your ear close to his mouth and nose. Try to detect air movement. Watch for the rhythmic rise and fall of his chest and abdomen. Also look for signs of respiratory distress, such as gasping, wheezing, cyanosis, and restlessness.

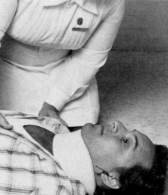

6 Now you're ready to check Mr. Tyler's level of consciousness. In a clear, strong voice, ask, "Can you hear me?" If he responds, ask, "What day is it?" and "What's the last thing you remember?" Also ask him his name and where he is. Note slurred speech or dysphasia. Also note any restlessness or irrational or combative behavior, which may indicate increasing intracranial pressure.

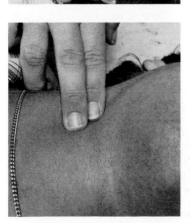

3 Now, locate your patient's carotid artery. Check his pulse rate and assess circulation, as the nurse is doing here. Look for signs of hemorrhaging and shock.

After your initial assessment, remember to reassess Mr. Tyler's vital signs every 5 minutes.

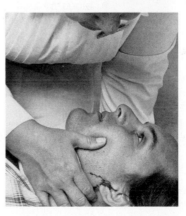

7 Examine Mr. Tyler's mouth, nose, and ears for blood or clear fluid drainage. Draining blood or cerebrospinal fluid may indicate a skull fracture.

Head

Assessing a patient with head injuries continued

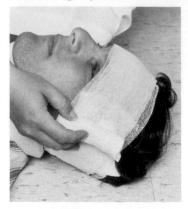

8 Suppose blood or cerebrospinal fluid is draining from your patient's left ear. Cover the ear with a loose dressing, and turn his head to the left side to allow for drainage.

What if your patient's also experiencing epistaxis? Position him on his side. Doing so allows for blood or mucus drainage.

Important: If you suspect a spinal injury, logroll your patient onto his side.

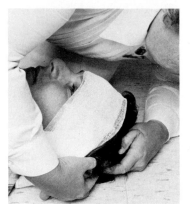

9 Check the patient's head and scalp, as the nurse is doing here. Look for bleeding, lacerations, avulsed tissue, deformities, or soft spots that could indicate a depressed skull fracture.

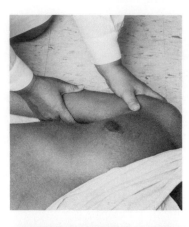

10 Examine your patient for other injuries. Remove his clothing and look for arm or leg fractures, open wounds, lacerations, and puncture wounds.

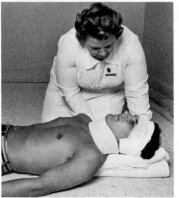

11 If your patient's conscious, elevate his head and upper body, as shown. Never position the patient's head lower than his feet. Doing so may cause cerebral edema.

Suppose your patient's unconscious. Position him on his side or stomach.

Now, carefully document your findings and the care you've given. Assist in transporting Mr. Tyler to the local hospital's emergency department.

Home care

Your head injury: What to watch for

Dear Patient:
As you know, you've suffered a head injury. Because the doctor has found no evidence of serious injury, you can go home at this time.

Of course, proper healing depends on your cooperation. For the next few days, watch your condition closely. Inform your family and friends of this precaution. Contact your doctor immediately or return to the emergency department at once if you note any of the following:
• increased drowsiness
• forceful or constant vomiting.

(If you vomit only once or twice, eat lightly until it stops.)
• continual or worsening headache
• neck stiffness
• blood or clear fluid draining from your ears or nose
• weakness in your arms or legs
• unsteadiness
• twitching
• slurred speech or inability to talk
• difficulty waking up. *Important:* During your first night at home, have a family member or friend awaken you every 2 hours.

• decreased pulse rate
• double vision or abnormal eye movements
• one pupil larger than the other
• convulsions (fits).

In addition, follow these instructions:
• Don't take anything stronger than aspirin or acetaminophen for a headache.
• Advise a family member or friend that if you have a convulsion (fit), he should place you on your side in an area where you can't fall or injure yourself. Tell him to stay with you until the convulsion subsides.

Nurses' guide to headaches

Headaches are one of the most common patient complaints you'll encounter. But are you familiar with the various types of headaches? If you feel you need to know more, study the following chart.

Vascular
Possible causes

Intracranial vasoconstriction, followed by extracranial vasodilation of cerebral arteries. May result from use of vasodilators (such as nitrates, alcohol, and histamines), systemic disease, hypoxia, hypertension, head trauma, tumor, or intracranial bleeding.

Characteristics

• Signs and symptoms may be aggravated by alcoholic beverages, oral contraceptives, menstruation, stress, and foods containing tyramine.
• *Classic migraine:* occurs unilaterally, primarily in the temporal or frontal area; usually periodic and recurrent; high hereditary incidence; personality factors may contribute.
• *Common migraine:* may be unilateral and spreading; gradual onset episodic; high hereditary incidence; signs and symptoms may be relieved by pregnancy; increases with each life crisis.
• *Cluster migraine* (histamine headaches): excruciatingly painful, unilateral headaches that occur at the same time each day for a few days. These attacks are followed by remission with no signs or symptoms and then occur weeks, months, or even years later. Cluster migraine headaches are more common in men than in women and are most likely to occur at night.

Signs and symptoms

• *Classic migraine:* transient visual field defects, such as flashing or zigzag lights, followed by severe unilateral pain in temporal or frontal area; transient paralysis; paralysis of an arm or leg; confusion; photophobia; nausea; vomiting; irritability; chills; sweating; constipation
• *Common migraine:* vague psychic disturbances for several hours or days before headache begins; nausea; vomiting; chills; nasal stuffiness; localized or generalized edema; diuresis
• *Cluster migraine:* intense, unilateral throbbing pain beginning high in the nostril and spreading to one side of the forehead, around and behind the eye on the affected side; possibly nasal and ocular lacrimation on this side, reddening of skin, and nasal congestion

Muscular contraction (tension)
Possible causes

• Sustained muscle contractions around the scalp, face, neck, and upper back; vasodilation of associated cranial arteries may contribute to muscle irritability and head pain on the affected side.

Characteristics

• May be unilateral or bilateral; pain frequently occurs in occipital and upper cervical areas and radiates over top of head.
• Headaches may be unrelieved for weeks, months, or years.
• Fleeting but recurrent headaches
• Gradual onset
• May be associated with depression or anxiety.

Signs and symptoms

• Dull, persistent ache
• Tender spots on head and neck
• Dizziness, tinnitus, lacrimation
• Feelings of tightness around the head (hatband sensation), pressure, or fullness; pain may be localized or vary in location as well as intensity.
• Nausea and vomiting

Traction and inflammatory
Possible causes

• *Traction:* direct nerve pressure from a disease or injury; for example, blood clot, brain tumor, or abscess
• *Inflammatory:* primary inflammation that affects specific structures in the head; for example, the meninges (meningitis), sinuses (sinusitis), cranial nerves (trigeminal or glossopharyngeal neuralgia)

Characteristics

• Headaches follow injury or disease (secondary sign)
• May lead to irreversible complications
• Exposure to cold may precipitate or aggravate headache.
• *Trigeminal neuralgia* (tic douloureux): unilateral headache involves the face and head and occurs in episodes lasting from 15 seconds to 4 minutes; most common in women over age 40
• *Glossopharyngeal neuralgia:* onset occurs at back of throat and tongue, spreading upward and outward to ears

Signs and symptoms

• Variable, depending on the underlying cause; in most cases, sudden onset, possibly fever (either accompanying the headache or following it)
• Possibly convulsions
• Visual disturbances
• Mental changes (apathy, euphoria, inattentiveness)
• Muscle weakness and paresthesia
• Pain ranges from mild and intermittent to sharp and stabbing.
• Nausea and vomiting
• *Tumor:* severe pain when patient awakens
• *Intracranial bleeding:* paresthesias and muscle weakness
• *Tic douloureux:* aching, burning, stabbing pain, usually unilateral
• *Trigeminal or glossopharyngeal neuralgia:* sharp, stabbing facial pain in one or more of the nerve's three branches; may be triggered by cold winds, touching, or talking.

Treating a headache: Some alternatives

What's the best way to manage your patient's headache? That depends on the type of headache, its severity, and the patient's age and condition. For many types of headache, medication offers effective pain relief. But if the headache is only a symptom of an underlying problem, your patient may find alternative pain relief measures beneficial. And when combined with medication, these measures can reduce the dosage your patient needs.

Remember: Many medications have side effects that may harm your patient. Tell your patient about these side effects.

Drugs

Analgesics, ranging from aspirin to codeine or meperidine, may provide symptomatic relief. A muscle relaxant, such as orphenadrine citrate (Norflex*), may help relieve a muscle tension headache. For migraine headaches, ergotamine tartrate alone or combined with caffeinic beverages may be the most effective treatment. Although migraine headaches can't be prevented, methysergide maleate (Sansert*) can help reduce their frequency and intensity. During acute headache attacks, your patient may find that a tranquilizer, such as diazepam (Valium*), or an antidepressant, such as amitriptyline hydrochloride (Elavil*), helps relieve his symptoms.

If your patient's taking medication to relieve a headache, encourage him to take it at the first sign of the attack. If nausea or vomiting makes it impossible for your patient to take the medication orally, advise him that most headache relief medications are available as rectal suppositories.

Alternative pain relief measures

Familiarize your patient with alternative pain relief measures to help prevent or treat his headache. *Remember:* Before administering any type of medication or treatment, try to identify the cause of your patient's headaches. As you take his history, look for clues of excessive stress, such as marital difficulties, job insecurity, or an illness in the family. If your patient's a child, find out whether he's undergoing stress in school or at home.

If you suspect that one of these problems may be the underlying cause of your patient's headaches, do your best to make him and his family aware of the situation. Explain the result of your assessment and refer him to the proper resource for help, as needed.

Also check for other causes of the headaches, such as recent or previous head trauma, high blood pressure, arthritis, allergies, and other chronic disorders. Refer your patient to a doctor for further evaluation and treatment.

Other pain-relieving measures include:
• simple relaxation techniques
• highly structured relaxation methods
• acupuncture or acupressure
• electrical stimulation.

*Available in both the United States and Canada

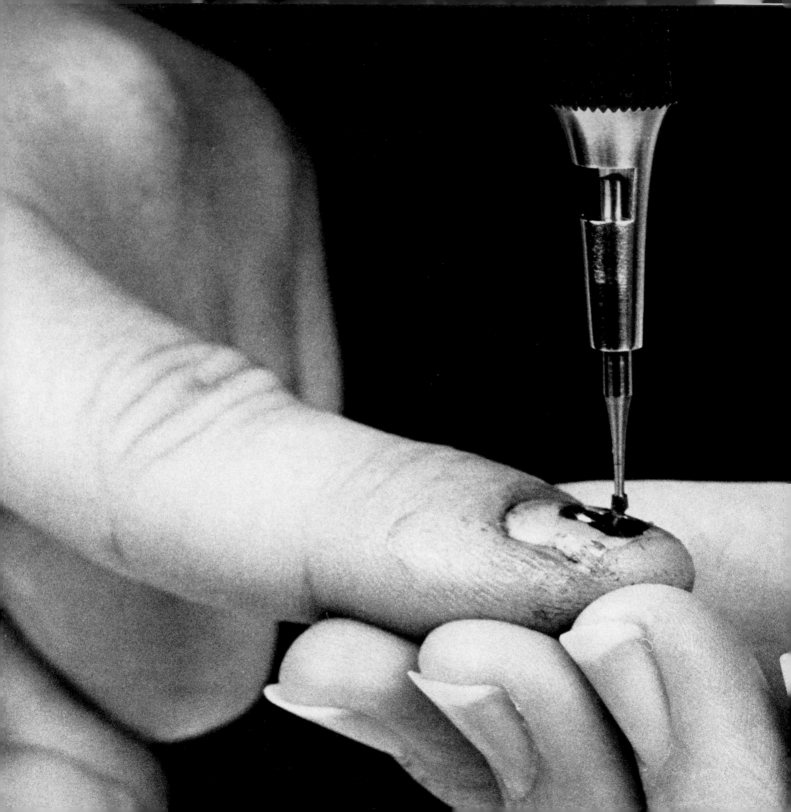

Managing Skin, Muscle, and Bone Problems

Skin

Muscle and bone

Skin

As the body's first line of defense, the skin is susceptible to a variety of disorders. To help refresh your memory of skin problems, read the following pages. In them, you'll find details covering:
• skin assessment
• common skin disorders and color changes
• management of parasites that may infest humans, such as lice or mites
• skin surface trauma
• local anesthetic
• wound-closure techniques, including a suturing procedure
• coping with minor trauma, such as an embedded barbed fishhook or a superficial splinter.

Taking a skin history

Suppose you're a clinic nurse working in a community health center. Raina Jacobs, a 40-year-old homemaker, comes to the clinic with a rash on her arms. As she rolls up her sleeves, you see small, red, oozing vesicles covering her arms from her elbows to her fingertips.

As you know, skin disorders are usually an ambulatory-care responsibility; they rarely require hospitalization. But because your patient may perceive the disorder as disfiguring, she may be hesitant to answer your questions (or tell you about the problem).

Be generous with your understanding and support. Remember, any uneasiness you feel toward your patient's condition will be projected to your patient. Reinforce your verbal messages by touching her. If you suspect she has a contagious skin disorder, touch an area without lesions. Keep in mind that the attention and care you give the patient and her family will help her cope with the disorder.

Taking the history

To determine whether your patient's problem is acute, chronic, or recurrent, as well as its specific signs and symptoms, take a history. Here are some questions you might ask:

• When did you first notice your skin problem?
• How did it begin? Were you using any new products when you noticed it? For example, did you change detergents, fabric softener, soap, or cleaning solution?
• If it recurs, how does a typical flare-up or attack begin? Does anything seem to trigger it?
• Does your skin itch?
• Do you have any pain?
• Do you ever have sores? If so, what do they look like? Do they ever drain? What color is the drainage? Does the problem or itching seem to increase with drainage?
• Are you allergic to any medicines or foods? If so, which ones? Have you begun taking any new medicines lately?
• Do you use any medication for your skin (oral, injected, or applied to your skin)? Do the medications relieve the problem or make it worse?
• Have you had any emotional upsets recently?
• Have you come in contact with poison ivy or poison oak recently?
• Do you have any direct contact with chemicals, dyes, dusts, or other irritants?
• Do any family members, friends, or other personal contacts have the same problem as you?

Assessing your patient's skin

After taking your patient's history, examine all her skin, including mucous membranes, hair, scalp, axillae, genitalia, palms, soles, and nails. You may use a magnifying glass, as necessary (see photo below). Note skin moisture, temperature, texture, thickness, turgor, and color irregularities. Check for edema and mobility of affected arms and legs.

Now, closely observe her skin lesions. Note color and location. Measure them, using a flexible pocket ruler or tape measure (see photo at right). Try to determine which lesion appeared first. Perhaps the patient can point it out. If the lesions are draining, note drainage color and consistency. Is the patient's skin excoriated from scratching?

Note the lesion distribution pattern. Is it localized, regional, general, or universal (involving her entire skin, hair, and nails)? Is it unilateral or bilateral? Symmetric or asymmetric? How are the lesions arranged? Singly? In clusters? In a linear configuration?

Be sure to document your findings thoroughly. To help distinguish your patient's particular skin problem from other common skin disorders, consult the chart on page 64.

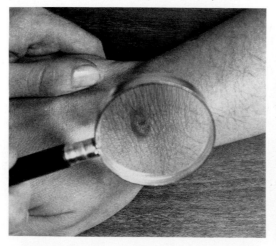

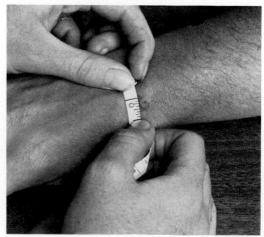

Assessing for skin color changes: Some guidelines

Even if your patient doesn't have a specific skin disorder, you'll want to assess his skin for signs and symptoms of systemic problems. Often these affect pigmentation, as well as vasodilation. Depending on his problem, your patient's skin might be flushed, blue, or yellow.

In the chart below, we describe skin-color changes you may observe and explain what they may indicate. We also tell you how to detect skin-color changes in dark-skinned patients, which may not be as obvious. But first, review these guidelines for skin-color assessment:

• Familiarize yourself with your patient's normal skin color, if possible. This way, you'll establish a baseline for detecting subtle changes.

• Perform your skin-color assessment in good light— daylight, if possible. Or, as an alternative, use a stand light with a 60-watt bulb, as shown in the photo below. Never use a flashlight or an overbed light, which may obscure subtle changes.

• Don't underestimate the importance of positioning. Position your patient so the light reflects off the skin area you're inspecting. Consider the effects of gravity, too. Depending on the position of an arm or leg in relation to the heart, either vasoconstriction or vasodilation

may occur, producing false color changes or enhancing the subtle color changes of early pathology. To know how raising or lowering an arm or leg affects skin color, first examine your patient's arm or leg at heart level. Then, unless contraindicated, elevate the extremity about 15° for at least 5 minutes and examine it, as shown in the top photo. Now, lower it 30° to 90° for at least 5 minutes and repeat your examination.

• Assess your patient's skin at room temperature. An air-conditioned room may induce a temporary cold cyanosis, in which lips and nail beds become blue; conversely, a warm room may cause superficial vasodilation.

• Assess your patient when he's calm. Anger or fright may make him pale; embarrassment may cause him to flush.

• If the patient's wearing lipstick, remove it by gently wiping the lips with a cream or lotion. Allow 20 to 30 minutes for the lips to regain their normal color before assessing.

• Clean the skin, if necessary, before inspection, because sweat and sebum may obscure signs and symptoms. As you do, take care not to scrub too vigorously or use harsh soaps.

• Note whether your patient's skin is edematous. Edema decreases skin-color intensity by increasing the distance be-

tween the surfaces and the pigmented and vascular layers. Dark skin may appear lighter, and anemia, jaundice, and erythema may be obscured or distorted.

• Keep in mind that body areas exposed to the sun and other climatic conditions may not be appropriate to use for skin-color determinations.

• Before documenting color changes in vascular flush areas (cheeks, bridge of nose, neck, upper chest, flexor surfaces of the extremities, and genital area), compare them with less vascular areas. As you know, a patient's vascular areas respond rapidly to changes in his emotions and in the temperature. However, your patient

may have a vascular disturbance in one of these areas; for example, arterial insufficiency.

• Determine when your patient who smokes last had a cigarette. The vasoconstrictive effects of smoking may induce subtle nail-color changes.

• Follow the guidelines given in the chart on the next page for assessing a dark-skinned patient. Although assessing skin-color changes in a dark-skinned patient is difficult, you'll find this usually becomes easier with practice. To ensure the greatest success, learn where to look for color changes, for example, the patient's conjunctiva, shown in the bottom photo, as well as how to identify the associated signs and symptoms.

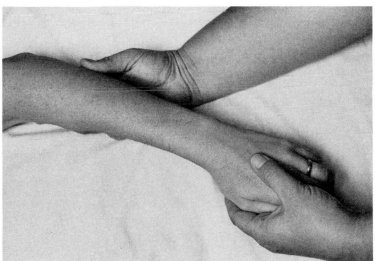

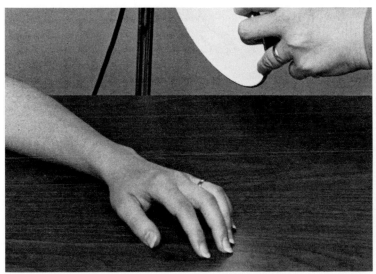

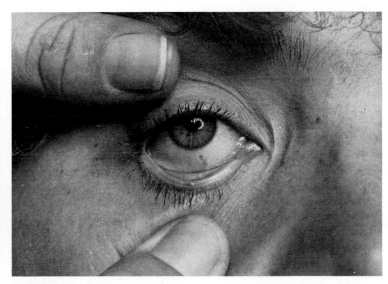

Skin

Interpreting skin color changes

If you're not sure what common skin color changes mean, study the following chart. It'll help you understand how these changes occur and tell you how to detect them.

Erythema (red or red-blue)
May be localized or generalized

Possible causes
• Dilation of or increased number of superficial blood vessels, as in blushing and with fever, increased alcohol intake, localized inflammation, and burns (including sunburn)
• Increase in the number of circulating erythrocytes and the concentration of hemoglobin in the blood, from exposure to cold

Nursing considerations
• If your patient has light skin, observe his face, upper chest, affected localized areas, and other exposed body parts (such as the ears, face, and hands) for red or red-blue color.
• Check the patient's lips for increased redness, which may accompany carbon monoxide poisoning or polycythemia.
• If your patient has dark skin, suspect erythema if you see purple skin tones. If the color change isn't obvious, palpate the skin for increased warmth, which can confirm inflammation. But remember that erythema isn't always associated with increased skin temperature.

Gray-tan or bronze
Usually generalized

Possible causes
• Deposition of melanin and hemosiderin resulting from liver disease, such as hemochromatosis
• Deposition of metallic salts (silver, gold, and bismuth) in blood from prolonged ingestion

Nursing considerations
• If your patient has light skin, check his exposed areas, genitalia, and any scars for color change.
• If your patient has dark skin, check his genitalia, palms, soles, and any scars.

Cyanosis (pale violet, blue, purple, or near-black)
May be peripheral or arterial

Possible causes
• Increased amounts of reduced hemoglobin secondary to hypoxia; may result from anoxia, anxiety or exposure to cold (mainly affects peripheral areas), lung abnormalities, and heart or lung disorders
• Abnormal hemoglobin, as in sulfhemoglobinemia and congenital or acquired methemoglobinemia

Nursing considerations
• If your patient has light skin, check the nail beds, lips, and mucous membranes for color changes. Cyanosis may be visible in the area around his mouth (circumoral cyanosis), his earlobes, and over his cheekbones.
• If your patient has dark skin, closely inspect his lips, nail beds, palms, and soles. Also check the circumoral area, buccal membranes, nostrils, eyelids, and vaginal walls.
• To help confirm suspected cyanosis, apply light pressure to the affected area to blanch it. Then, check how long the color takes to return from the periphery of the area to the center. If the patient is cyanotic, color return takes longer than 1 second.
• If the patient has dark skin and the color change isn't obvious, rely on other signs and symptoms. For example, restlessness, changes in levels of consciousness, and flaring of nostrils indicate possible heart and lung problems.

Pallor
May range from ash gray to pale yellow to brown, depending on individual's pigmentation

Possible cause
• Reduced visibility of oxyhemoglobin, possibly from decrease in flow to the superficial blood vessels (as in shock or syncope), in number of red blood corpuscles, and of oxyhemoglobin in blood or from nonfilling capillaries (as in lead poisoning)

Nursing considerations
• To help confirm pallor regardless of skin color, check the outer canthus as well as the inner canthus when examining the conjunctivae. The patient's pigmentation's often lighter near the inner canthus.
• If your patient's nails aren't pigmented, apply slight pressure on the far edge of the second or third fingernail to blanch the nail bed. If color returns to the nail bed slowly, vasomotor function may be poor. *Note:* If the patient's skin isn't too dark, you may assess lips and earlobes the same way.
• If your patient has light skin, check his face, conjunctivae, buccal membranes, lips, and nail beds for white tint.
• If your patient has dark skin, look for a yellow-brown tint in the conjunctivae, mucous membranes of the mouth, and nail beds. If you suspect he's in shock, check his tongue and the mucous membranes inside his cheeks. They will appear pale, gray, and waxy.
• Be aware that a lemon-yellow skin tint, slightly yellow sclerae, sensory neurologic deficits, and red, painful tongue accompany pernicious anemia. Other signs and symptoms accompanying severe anemia include dyspnea on exertion, fatigue, increased pulse rate, dizziness, and altered or impaired mental function.

Increased pigmentation

Possible cause
• Deposition of melanin; may result from genetic predisposition, sunlight, pregnancy, Addison's disease, certain pituitary tumors, or use of anovulatory medication

Nursing consideration
• To help confirm increased pigmentation regardless of skin color, check exposed body parts, points of pressure or friction, nipples, genitalia, palmar creases, and recent scars, which may indicate Addison's disease, pituitary tumors, or that patient's taking anovulatory medication; face, nipples and areolae, linea nigra, and vulva, which may indicate pregnancy; and unexposed body parts, if possible, which may indicate sunburn.

Decreased pigmentation

Possible causes
• Decreased melanin from congenital inability to produce melanin (as in albinism) or acquired loss of melanin (as in vitiligo or fungus infection)
• Edema (as in nephrotic syndrome), which masks the colors of melanin and hemoglobin and prevents the detection of jaundice

Nursing considerations
• To confirm decreased pigmentation regardless of skin color, check hair, eyes, and skin, which may indicate albinism, and chest, neck, and upper back, which may indicate a fungal infection.
• If your patient has dark skin, check exposed parts for depigmented patches with hyperpigmented edges; if present, suspect vitiligo.
• If depigmentation's present, also check for swelling.

Jaundice (yellow)

Possible cause
• Accumulation of bilirubin in the blood that can't be conjugated by the liver; excess collects in the skin; may result from disorders involving the hepatic cells and the biliary tract (hepatitis, cirrhosis, and pancreatitis) or from rapid rate of erythrocyte hemolysis

Nursing considerations
• To confirm jaundice regardless of skin color, check sclerae for early signs. Later, condition spreads to the mucous membranes and eventually becomes generalized.
• Light- or clay-colored stools and dark gold urine commonly accompany jaundice.
• If your patient has dark skin, inspect the portion of the corneas revealed naturally by open eyelids. If the sclerae appear yellow up to the edges of the corneas, confirm your findings by checking the posterior portion of the hard palate in natural lighting.

Carotenemia (orange-yellow)

Possible cause
• Excessive carotene pigment in blood, resulting from myxedema, hypopituitarism, diabetes, pregnancy, or increased intake of vegetables and fruits containing carotene (such as carrots)

Nursing considerations
• To help confirm carotenemia regardless of skin color, check the face, palms, and soles.
• To differentiate from jaundice, be aware that carotenemia doesn't involve the sclerae or the mucous membranes.

Nurses' guide to skin disorders

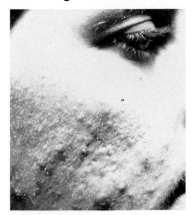

Acne vulgaris
Chronic inflammatory disease of the sebaceous follicles

Causes
- Unknown, although hormonal dysfunction and sebum oversecretion may be possible causes
- Predisposing factors include use of oral contraceptives, corticosteroids, adrenocorticotropic hormone, androgens, iodides, bromides, trimethadione, phenytoin, isoniazid, lithium, and halothane; exposure to heavy oils, greases, or tars; trauma or rubbing from tight clothing; cosmetics; emotional stress; an unfavorable climate; cobalt irradiation; total parenteral nutrition therapy

Signs and symptoms
- Whiteheads
- Blackheads
- Pustules and papules
- Cysts and abscesses (in severe cases)
- Scarring

Treatment
- Benzoyl peroxide, a topical antibacterial, may be used alone or with tretinoin, a keratolytic (skin peeling) agent
- Topical antibiotics, such as tetracycline, erythromycin, and clindamycin phosphate.
- Systemic antibiotics, such as tetracycline. (Erythromycin is used if patient is sensitive to tetracycline.)
- Exposure to ultraviolet light (but *never* when patient's receiving a photosensitizing agent, such as tretinoin)
- In severe cases, intralesional corticosteroid injections, cryotherapy, or surgery

Nursing intervention
- Help patient and family identify predisposing factors and eliminate them.

*Available in both the United States and Canada

- Obtain patient's medication history, because the use of certain medications, such as oral contraceptives, may exacerbate problem.
- Teach patient proper use of systemic and topical medications. Also, if patient's taking tetracycline, instruct him to take it with a full glass of water on an empty stomach (1 hour before or 2 hours after meals). He should never take it with milk or an antacid.
- If your patient's using ultraviolet light, warn him to protect his eyes.
- Provide support and encouragement—long-term therapy may be necessary.

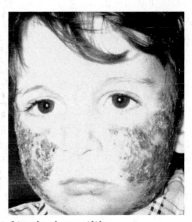

Atopic dermatitis
Recurrent or chronic pruritic skin eruption

Causes
- Allergens, such as pollen, wool, silk, animal dander, ointments, detergents, perfumes, wheat, milk, and eggs
- Temperature and humidity extremes
- Diaphoresis
- Psychological stress

Signs and symptoms
- In children, reddened areas on forehead, cheeks, and extensor surfaces of arms and legs; in adults, at flexion points, antecubital fossa, popliteal space, and neck
- Edema, vesiculation, and scaling during exacerbations, from scratching pruritic areas
- Areas of dryness and scaling (with chronic lesions)

Treatment
- Systemic corticosteroids (but only during exacerbations, because of corticosteroid side effects)
- Preparations with low coal tar content, such as Estar* and Zetar*, and ultraviolet B light therapy to thicken outer epidermal layer (stratum corneum)
- Antihistamines to relieve itching

Nursing intervention
- Help patient identify possible allergens. Prepare him for allergy testing, if necessary. After his allergens are pinpointed, advise him to avoid or eliminate them.
- Teach patient proper use of systemic and topical medications.
- Instruct patient to avoid extreme temperatures.
- Caution patient to avoid rubbing and scratching lesions, which could lead to secondary infection.
- Warn patient that antihistamines may cause drowsiness.
- Instruct patient to limit bathing, according to lesion severity. Have him bathe with a nonfat soap, such as Betadine Skin Cleanser, and tepid water. Caution him to avoid using any soap when lesions are inflamed. Advise him to shampoo frequently. After bathing, he should apply topical corticosteroid cream to affected areas and lubricate unaffected skin with body lotion.

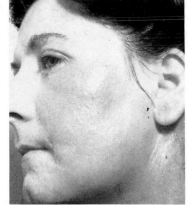

Contact dermatitis
Acute, allergic, inflammatory skin reaction

Causes
- Chronic exposure to mild irritants, such as detergents and solvents
- Strong irritants, such as acids and alkalis
- Sensitization to allergens, such as poison ivy

Signs and symptoms
- With mild irritants and allergens, redness and small vesicles that ooze, scale, and itch
- With strong irritants, blisters and ulcerations
- With classic allergic response, clearly defined lesions at points of contact with allergen
- With severe allergic reaction, marked edema of affected area

Treatment
- Washing immediately after contact with an allergen
- Topical anti-inflammatory agents (including steroids)
- Antihistamines to suppress pruritus
- Cold, wet compresses soaked in Burow's or Epsom salts solution to relieve pruritus
- Systemic corticosteroids to reduce edema and bullae

Nursing intervention
- Teach patient proper use of systemic and topical medications.
- Teach patient how to apply wet compresses.
- Help patient identify allergens. Prepare him for allergy testing, if necessary. After his allergens are pinpointed, instruct him to avoid or eliminate them.
- Encourage patient to wear protective clothing, such as gloves.
- Caution patient to avoid rubbing and scratching, which could lead to secondary infection.
- Warn patient that antihistamines may cause drowsiness.

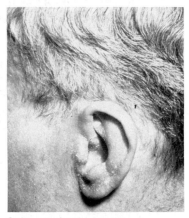

Seborrheic dermatitis
Chronic skin inflammation involving sebaceous glands

Causes
- Unknown
- Predisposing factors include emotional stress, neurologic disorder (such as Parkinson's disease), genetic makeup, poor nutrition, infection.

Signs and symptoms
- Greasy, red, scaly patches in areas with many sebaceous glands (especially the face, scalp, and trunk) and in skin folds; fissures may be present
- Pruritus and inflammation of affected areas

Skin

Nurses' guide to skin disorders continued

Treatment
• Shampooing with selenium sulfide suspension (for example, Selsun*) several times weekly; scalp lotion or mineral oil to help relieve scalp dryness and scaling
• Topical steroid creams to relieve itching

Nursing intervention
• Be aware that treatment addresses symptoms rather than underlying cause.
• Teach patient proper use of shampoo and topical steroid creams.
• Caution patient to avoid rubbing or scratching, which could lead to secondary infection.
• Instruct patient to avoid excessive heat, which can cause diaphoresis.
• Provide emotional support—this condition may be long term.

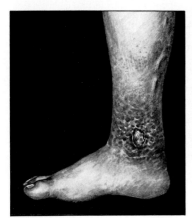

Stasis dermatitis
Inflammatory skin reaction secondary to peripheral vascular disease

Causes
• Peripheral vascular disease, such as chronic venous insufficiency
• Predisposing factors include varicosities, edema, trauma, and irritation.

Signs and symptoms
(Primarily in the lower leg above the internal malleolus)
• Early signs: dusky red spots, with pruritus and induration
• Later signs: edema, redness, and scaling over large area of legs. Crust, fissures, and ulcers may also occur.

Treatment
• Prevention of venous stasis by avoiding prolonged sitting or standing and by using antiembolism stockings.
• For patient who is obese, dieting to lose weight
• Corrective surgery for underlying

*Available in both the United States and Canada

causes
• With decubitus ulcer, rest periods with legs elevated; open, wet dressings; Unna's paste boot (dressing made of zinc oxide, glycerin paste, and gelatin applied with continuous pressure); antibiotics, if necessary, for secondary infection

Nursing intervention
• Teach patient measures to prevent venous stasis.
• If decubitus ulcer appears infected, culture drainage and obtain order for appropriate antibiotic.
• Prepare patient for surgery to correct underlying cause, as necessary.

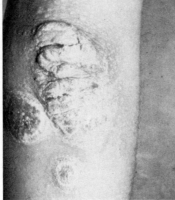

Psoriasis
Chronic skin disease involving epidermal hyperplasia and rapid cell turnover; usually affecting persons between ages 30 and 50

Causes
• Genetically determined
• Predisposing factors include trauma, infection, pregnancy, hormonal change, cold temperature, emotional stress.

Signs and symptoms
• Well-defined plaques, consisting of silver scales covering dull-red lesions, which usually appear on the scalp, elbows, knees, and lower back
• Pruritus
• Occasional pain from cracked, encrusted lesions

Treatment
• Petrolatum to soften scales; then, oatmeal bath for scale removal and relief of pruritus
• Exposure to ultraviolet light to reduce cell growth; may be used with coal tar preparations
• Topical steroid cream applied three or four times daily, after

bathing, to reduce pruritus; at night, application of occlusive dressing (for example, plastic wrap, plastic gloves, vinyl exercise suit)
• Low-dosage antihistamines to suppress pruritus
• Emollients and wet-to-dry compresses to relieve pruritus

Nursing intervention
• Be aware that treatment addresses signs and symptoms rather than underlying cause. Specific treatment depends on type and severity of condition.
• Instruct patient in proper use of petrolatum and oatmeal bath, topical steroid creams, emollients, and ultraviolet light, as appropriate.
• Teach patient how to apply wet-to-dry compresses.
• Caution patient that antihistamines may cause drowsiness.
• Caution patient to avoid rubbing or scratching, which could lead to secondary infection.
• Provide emotional support; this condition may be lifelong. Refer patient to the National Psoriasis Foundation, which can direct him to a local chapter for information and emotional support.

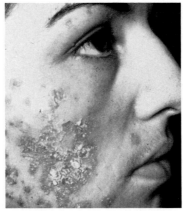

Impetigo
Contagious superficial skin infection; occurring in nonbullous and bullous forms

Causes
• Beta-hemolytic streptococcus (nonbullous impetigo)
• Coagulase-positive *Staphylococcus aureus* (bullous impetigo)
• Predisposing factors include poor hygiene, anemia, malnutrition, warm climate.

Signs and symptoms
Streptococcal impetigo
• Small macules appear on face or other exposed areas and become vesicles within a few hours. Vesicles

break, discharging an exudate that forms a thick, yellow crust. Lesion consists of a clearing encircled by an outer rim.
• Painless pruritus
• Burning and regional lymphadenopathy (uncommon)
Staphylococcal impetigo
• Thin-walled vesicles appear and break, discharging exudate that forms a thin, clear crust. Lesion configuration, sites, and accompanying signs and symptoms are the same as for streptococcal impetigo. Both forms may appear simultaneously and be clinically indistinguishable.

Treatment
• Systemic antibiotics, such as penicillin and erythromycin
• Warm water or normal saline solution compresses to remove exudate; then, washing off crust with mild soap and water
• After washing, applying topical antibiotics

Nursing intervention
• Teach patient proper use of systemic and topical medications.
• Teach patient soaking procedure to remove exudate.
• Urge patient not to scratch lesions. Scratching may cause spread of lesions and lead to secondary infection.
• Instruct family members not to use patient's washcloths, towels, or bed linens. Tell them to soak towels in chlorine bleach or boil them after use.
• Check family members for infection.
• If patient's in school, notify the school nurse of his condition.

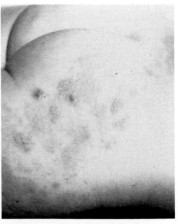

Herpes zoster (shingles)
Acute inflammation of dorsal root ganglia; most prevalent in persons over age 50

Causes
- Herpesvirus varicella (varicella-zoster, V-Z), which also causes chicken pox
- Predisposing factors include history of or exposure to chicken pox, trauma, or cancer.

Signs and symptoms
- Malaise and fever during onset
- Pain, pruritus, and paresthesia or hyperesthesia, usually on trunk along the course of a nerve or group of nerves; occasionally occurs on arms and legs. Pain may be continuous or intermittent and lasts from 1 to 4 weeks.
- Small, red, painful vesicles, occurring within 2 weeks of first symptoms; appear along single nerves or nerve groups (most commonly intercostal nerves) and become purulent, crust, and fall off 1 to 2 weeks after eruption.

Treatment
- Analgesics (aspirin or codeine) for pain relief; should be administered regularly to control neuralgic pain, which can be severe
- Application of compresses moistened with Burow's solution for 20 minutes four times daily to relieve pain and pruritus
- Calamine lotion to relieve pruritus
- For postherpetic neuralgia, systemic corticosteroid, such as cortisone, to reduce inflammation; possibly tranquilizers, sedatives, or tricyclic antidepressants

Nursing intervention
- Teach patient proper use of analgesics.
- Teach patient how to apply compresses and calamine lotion.
- Caution patient to avoid rubbing or scratching, which could lead to secondary infection.
- Encourage family to keep patient as comfortable and pain-free as possible.
- Provide emotional support, especially during severe pain. Reassure patient that pain will subside.
- Be aware that condition seldom recurs.

Herpes simplex I
Recurrent viral infection; most prevalent in children under age 5

Cause
- Herpesvirus hominis (HVH)

Signs and symptoms
- Fever
- Tingling, burning, and pruritus in area before vesicles appear (pro-

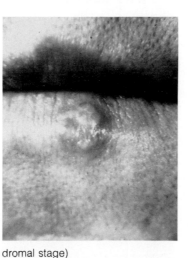

dromal stage)
- Pharyngitis with erythema and edema
- Painful vesicular lesions on erythematous base, which eventually rupture and leave painful ulcers, followed by yellow crusting Vesicles usually form on oral mucosa (especially tongue, gingivae, and cheeks) but also occur on facial skin. Healing begins 7 to 10 days after onset and is complete in 3 weeks.
- In generalized infection, submaxillary lymphadenopathy, salivation, halitosis, anorexia, and fever. Condition usually runs its course in 4 to 10 days.

Treatment
- Cold compresses or ice to relieve pain
- For recurrent infection, tincture of benzoin to toughen skin in prodromal stages; later, petrolatum or other soothing ointment to prevent cracking and discomfort
- Topical antibiotics to help prevent secondary infection
- For generalized infection, antipyretics and analgesics to reduce fever and relieve oral pain

Nursing intervention
- Be aware that treatment addresses symptoms rather than underlying cause; topical antivirals may be expensive and have limited effect.
- Teach patient or family how to apply cold compresses or ice, tincture of benzoin, petrolatum, and topical antibiotics.
- Teach patient or family how to administer antipyretics and analgesics, if necessary.
- Encourage use of cleansing mouthwash for halitosis.
- During acute phase, have patient avoid acidic drinks, such as orange juice, and eat a soft, nonirritating diet to help reduce oral pain.

Coping with athlete's foot

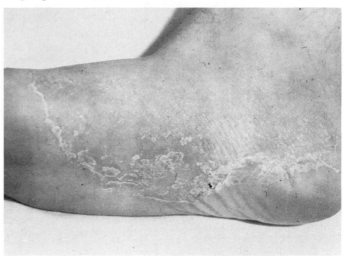

Suppose you're working in a junior high school. Barry Gordon, a 14-year-old student, comes to you complaining that his feet itch "like crazy." When you examine his feet, you see scaling and blisters between his toes and on his soles and note that the skin's beginning to crack.

You suspect he has athlete's foot (tinea pedis), a fungal infection (see photo). *Note:* In addition to Barry's signs and symptoms, severe athlete's foot infection may cause inflammation and pain when he walks.

To help relieve the itching, wash Barry's feet and dry them thoroughly—especially between his toes. Then, apply an antifungal powder, under your working protocol.

Encourage Barry to expose his feet to air as much as possible. Tell him to wear white cotton socks and leather shoes when possible and to wash his feet twice daily. Instruct him to dry his feet thoroughly and apply an antifungal powder.

Also, you may recommend use of the skin toughener, as described below. Refer Barry to his family doctor for further care.

Be sure to send home with Barry information about athlete's foot, so the family can reinforce the program and prevent or control the condition among other family members.

Preventing athlete's foot
You've taken measures to help resolve Barry Gordon's athlete's foot (tinea pedis). Now, you want to prevent the condition from spreading to other students. To do so, you need to understand how it develops.

Until recently, athlete's foot was considered highly contagious, and preventive methods emphasized disinfecting areas thought to harbor infecting fungus spores (such as shower stalls). Today, medical authorities recognize that *lowered skin resistance* plays an important role in the spread of this infection. Because fungus spores thrive on soft, weak skin, doctors recommend that students use a skin toughener, such as Ōnox.

Besides preventing an initial infection, this solution reduces the fungal population in a person already affected, thereby minimizing symptoms.

For best results, daily use is recommended.

To find out how to use Ōnox, read the following photostory.

Skin

Using the Ōnox Super Sprayer

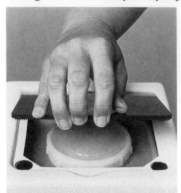

1 To teach Barry Gordon how to use Ōnox solution from a dispenser (Ōnox Super Sprayer), follow these steps. *Note:* Before initiating treatment, determine whether your patient's allergic to any ingredients in Ōnox.

Begin by having him fill the dispenser. First, ask him to open the Plexiglas door on the top of it.

2 Then, tell him to unscrew the cap on the solution holding tank.

3 Next, have him fill the tank with Ōnox solution. (The tank holds 1 gal, or 3.7 liters.) Then, have him replace the cap.

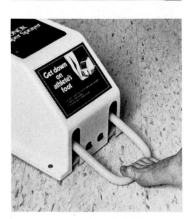

4 Now, the Ōnox dispenser's ready for use. Instruct Barry to depress the dispenser bar with his bare foot for a few seconds. When he does this, a mist of Ōnox will envelop his foot. Have him repeat the procedure with his other foot.

Instruct Barry to use this dispenser after every shower.

Tell him to clean the dispenser daily by wiping it with a damp rag or rinsing it under lukewarm water.

Document your teaching.

Learning about lice

By working in the community, you're in a good position to detect, manage, and prevent louse infestation (pediculosis). But how much do you know about lice? Do you know how they spread? Or where they live? Read the information below to familiarize yourself with these parasites.

Three types of louse affect humans:
• Head louse (*Pediculus humanus capitis*)
• Body louse (*Pediculus humanus corporis*)
• Pubic, or crab, louse (*Phthirus pubis*).

Lice range in size from about 0.8 mm to 4 mm, with the

Head louse (*Pediculus humanus capitis*)

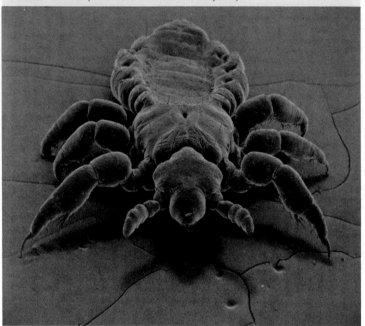

Primarily infests human hair

Signs and symptoms
• Pruritus
• Red papules or louse bites on scalp, back of head and neck, and behind ears
• Excoriation
• Oval, gray-white nits on hair shafts
• Rash on trunk (possibly from sensitization to louse toxin)
• In severe cases, matted, foul-smelling, and lusterless hair; occipital and cervical lymphadenopathy; scalp scarring, induration, pigmentation, and ulceration

Transmission
By direct contact with infested person's head or body hair or by contact with such personal items as hats, hairbrushes, combs, or bedding; usually spreads rapidly

Nursing considerations
• Wash affected areas with a shampoo containing gamma benzene hexachloride (lindane), such as Kwell. Or, apply Kwell cream or lotion and leave it on for 8 to 12 hours, followed by thorough washing. If necessary, repeat Kwell application in 8 to 10 days.
• After rinsing out lotion or shampoo, remove nits and lice with a fine-tooth comb that has been dipped in vinegar.
• Wash all clothing and linens in hot water or have them dry-cleaned (see page 71.)
• Instruct patient and family not to share hats, clothing, combs, or hairbrushes.

pubic louse being the smallest. They live outside the host's body and are dependent on human blood for nourishment. When they feed, they inject a toxin that causes pruritus and possibly fever or an allergic reaction.

Female lice lay eggs (nits) on the hair shafts close to the skin. Because nits only hatch at temperatures above 71.6° F. (22° C.), they must remain close to the skin to survive. To secure the nits, the female louse secretes a cementlike substance over the hair shaft. About 24 hours after hatching, the young louse requires its first blood meal. A louse lives in a favorrable climate for approximately 30 to 35 days.

What conditions are favorable for lice? Although more prevalent where hygiene is poor, louse infestation is not restricted to any socioeconomic group. Lice can infest anyone who comes in contact with a carrier. Infestation is more common in females than in males and in children than in adults. You'll see head lice most often in preschool children. Pubic lice occur most frequently in young, unmarried persons.

For the information you need to distinguish lice types and provide appropriate care, read the chart below.

Body louse (*Pediculus humanus corporis*)

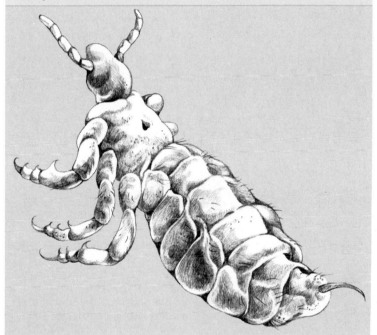

Clings to clothing (especially seams) next to skin, only moving onto body for feeding

Signs and symptoms
- Excoriation from scratching trunk and neck
- Louse bites on body parts that come in contact with clothing, especially the shoulders, axillae, between the shoulder blades, and around the waist
- Small, red papules on shoulders, trunk, and buttocks, which may change to hives from scratching
- If infestation goes untreated, dry, discolored, thickly encrusted, scaly skin, with bacterial infection and scarring
- Headache, fever, and malaise (in severe cases)

Transmission
By direct contact with infested persons, clothing, or bedding

Nursing considerations
- Have patient bathe with soap and water. (Only use gamma benzene hexachloride preparation to treat severe cases.)
- Wash all clothing and linens in hot water, or have them dry-cleaned. When pressing, give special attention to seams.
- Teach parents and children proper hygiene, including changing clothing daily and bathing frequently.
- Be aware that body lice may indicate the existence of other disorders, such as nutritional disturbances. Also, they may transmit such diseases as louse typhus, relapsing fever, and trench fever. Refer patient for more complete examination.

Pubic louse (*Phthirus pubis*)

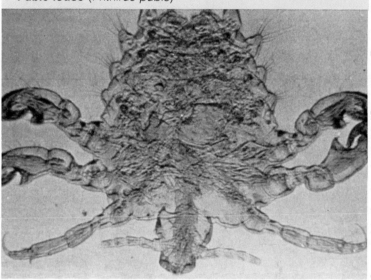

Courtesy of the American Academy of Dermatology, Evanston, Ill.

Primarily infests pubic hair but may also occur in eyebrows, eyelashes, and axillary or body hair; in children, occurs primarily in eyebrows and eyelashes, from close contact with infested persons

Signs and symptoms
- Pruritus, especially at night
- Excoriation from scratching in pubic region
- Louse bites in genital area, on abdomen and lower thighs, and, occasionally, in axillae
- Nits and rust-colored lice attached to hair in affected areas; pubic hairs feel grainy
- Gray-blue macules on thighs and upper body
- Inflamed eyelids, if eyelashes are infested
- In severe cases, febrile episodes and lymphadenopathy

Transmission
- By close physical contact (particularly during sexual intercourse); less frequently, through clothing, bedding, and toilet seats; usually spread rapidly

Nursing considerations
- To treat, apply gamma benzene hexachloride shampoo or cream, as for head lice. A second application in 1 week may be necessary.
- After treatment, have patient use freshly laundered underclothing, pajamas, sheets, and pillowcases.
- Wash clothes and linens in hot water or have them dry-cleaned, as necessary.
- If possible, obtain a list of the patient's sexual contacts, so they can receive treatment also.
- Be aware that pubic lice infestation may be present concurrently with other sexually transmitted diseases, such as gonorrhea, trichomonas, candidiasis (moniliasis), and syphilis. Refer patient for more complete examination.

Skin

Assessing a child for head lice

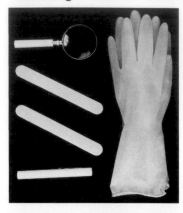

1 Let's say you're working in an elementary school when you're asked to examine 7-year-old Jimmy Bowen. His teacher tells you Jimmy constantly scratches his head; from her description, you suspect he has lice. Read this photostory to learn how to confirm your suspicion.

First, obtain disposable wooden applicator sticks, disposable gloves, a penlight (or high-intensity lamp), and a magnifying glass.

2 Then, carefully part his hair with the wooden applicator sticks, as shown. Look for bite marks and redness on his skin, and for tiny, white oval specks (nits) and lice on the hair shaft about ¼" (0.6 cm) from his scalp.

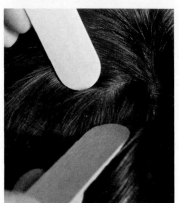

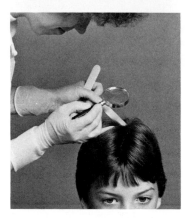

3 If you see small, white specks, try to move them with the applicator stick. Look at them closely with a magnifying glass. Unlike dandruff, nits won't move easily. If you positively identify the specks as nits, you'll need to distinguish active from inactive infestation. Keep in mind that inactive infestation is indicated by empty nit cases located higher on the hair shaft, away from the scalp.

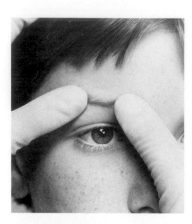

4 Don't forget to examine Jimmy's eyebrows and eyelashes for nits (see photo).

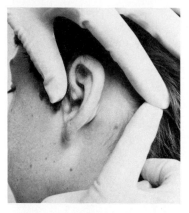

5 Examine the skin behind his ears, where louse bites are easy to detect.

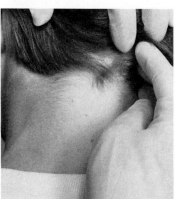

6 Also check the back of his head, as shown here.

Suppose you determine that Jimmy has an active louse infestation. Reassure him that his problem can be easily treated. Immediately find out whether other children in the school are infested. Examine all the children in his classes. If you find a number of cases of louse infestation, enlist volunteers to help examine all the children in the school, as well as all staff members.

Managing a louse infestation problem

After you've established that a child in your school has lice, prepare an information sheet to send home with him.

Chances are, your patient's family doctor will prescribe a medication containing gamma benzene hexachloride (lindane). Or, the family can purchase over-the-counter medication. Because excessive use of medication containing lindane can cause such adverse effects as seizures, caution the family to use this medication *exactly* as prescribed.

After you send your patient home, be sure to contact the local community health nurse. She'll monitor and follow up on treatment in the family.

When a child with head lice returns to school, examine him before readmission. If you see active nits or lice on him, he'll need additional treatments. In such a case, refuse readmission and send the child home with another letter to his parents, requesting retreatment. But if you observe only empty nit cases or dead lice, readmit the child to school. Remember: Nit cases and dead lice are easily removed from the hair shafts.

To help control the spread of lice and prevent further outbreaks in the classroom, make sure each child's hat and coat are hung separately. To do this, assign each student an individual locker or a wall hook spaced at least 12" (30.5 cm) from other wall hooks or allow each student to hang his coat on the back of his chair—whichever is most feasible.

Dealing with head lice

Suppose you discover that a child in your school has head lice. To prevent spreading the condition to other schoolchildren, ask his parents to treat the child *immediately*. Also, urge them to check everyone living in or visiting their home. Tell them to part the person's hair and check for lice or eggs. Every person with lice will have to be treated.

To ensure proper treatment of lice, explain the following guidelines to parents:

• Buy a nonprescription medicated shampoo—for example, R & C shampoo—that kills lice and destroys their eggs. You can find this shampoo at your local drugstore. Or, ask your family doctor to give you a prescription for medicated shampoo.

Important: Be sure to use this shampoo only as the label on the bottle instructs or the doctor tells you.

• Before you apply the shampoo, have your child undress.

• Pour a small amount of shampoo on his head. Using your fingertips, work the shampoo into his scalp. While you're washing his head, have your child hold a towel over his eyes to keep out the shampoo. If it does get in his eyes, rinse it out with water.

• After shampooing, rinse your child's head thoroughly. Make sure you rinse out *all* the shampoo.

• Dry his hair with a clean towel.

• Use a fine-tooth comb soaked in vinegar to comb his hair. This will remove any remaining lice and eggs.

• Now, have your child put on freshly washed or dry-cleaned clothing.

• Remove all linens from the bed (sheets, pillowcases, mattress pads, blankets, and bedspread) and clean them immediately. Wash all clothing, sheets, blankets, pillowcases, mattress pads, and towels in very hot water. Use a washing machine, if possible. Either machine-dry them on a hot cycle or line-dry them and then press with a hot iron.

• Dry-clean unwashable articles, if possible. Or, a less expensive way to clean them is to place clothing or bedding articles in a plastic bag, which you've checked first for holes. Keep it sealed for 30 to 35 days to kill all lice.

• To keep lice from spreading, make sure family members don't share any articles that come in contact with the head, neck, or shoulders; for example, combs, brushes, hats, and towels.

Learning about scabies

Besides the louse, another parasite that commonly infests humans is the itch mite (*Sarcoptes scabiei* var. *hominis*). Transmitted through close physical contact with an infected person, scabies can affect anyone but occurs more frequently in persons under age 30 living in a crowded, unsanitary environment. The condition is highly contagious.

Unlike the louse, which lives *on* the host, the itch mite lives within the host's skin. The female mite burrows into the skin to deposit her eggs. When the larvae hatch, they emerge from the skin to copulate and then burrow into it again.

The mites' burrowing, feeding, and excretion causes intense, localized pruritus, especially at night. The burrows appear as gray-white, elevated, threadlike lesions about ⅜″ (9.5 mm) long. Usually, the lesions are excoriated and may appear as reddened nodules. The end of the burrow, where the mite lives, may be capped by a small vesicle. Prolonged scratching may cause severe excoriation and secondary bacterial infection. Also, if the host becomes sensitized to the mite, pruritus may become generalized.

Which are the most common lesion sites? Wrists, extensor surfaces of elbows and knees, webs of fingers (see photo), axillae, waistline, genitalia, buttocks, nipples (in females), and outer edges of the feet. Infants may have burrows in the head area.

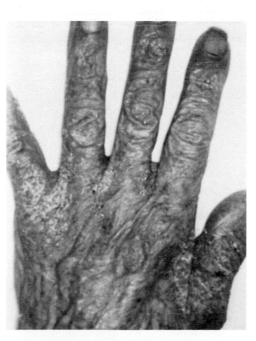

You may be able to detect the itch mite visually through close examination. If not, you'll need to obtain a skin sample (see page 72). Then, have a doctor confirm your findings. However, this test isn't always conclusive. Sometimes the only way you're sure the patient's had scabies is because he's responded to treatment for it.

Whether you've actually detected scabies or merely suspect it, be sure to check family members or other close personal contacts for signs and symptoms.

Treatment

Usually, the doctor prescribes gamma benzene hexachloride (lindane) lotion or cream; for example, Kwell. For treatment, have the patient follow these steps:

• First, bathe with soap and warm water, which helps soften crusted lesions.

• Then, allow the skin to air-dry and cool.

• Next, apply a thin layer of lotion or cream to the entire body; from the neck down. Rub in the lotion or cream thoroughly.

• Leave it on for 12 to 24 hours. Then, remove it by thorough washing.

In most cases, scabies is cured with a single application. If it's not cured, your patient may repeat the application in 1 week.

Note: If pruritus persists after treatment, it may mean the patient's developed mite sensitization. Tell your patient to report continuing itching. Then, check the treated area for lesions to be sure the mites are dead.

After treatment, have the patient put on freshly laundered or dry-cleaned clothing and use clean bed linen.

Instruct him to wash all his clothing, towels, and bed linens in hot water, machine-dry them, or press with a hot iron. Also, encourage him to have nonwashable items dry-cleaned or to seal them in a plastic bag for 10 days.

Skin

How to take a skin sample to test for scabies

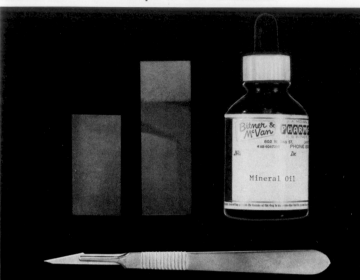

Does your patient have signs or symptoms of scabies? If he does but you can't see any evidence of the mite itself, use the skin-sampling procedure described below to help confirm your suspicions.

First, gather the following equipment: mineral oil in a dropper bottle, scalpel and scalpel blade #15, glass slide and a coverslip.

Remember to wash your hands thoroughly. Also, explain the procedure and its purpose to your patient.

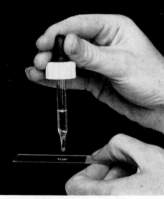

1 To begin, place a small drop of mineral oil in the middle of a glass slide.

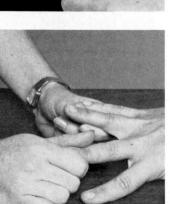

2 Now, inspect the skin on your patient's lower abdomen, pubic area, axillae, legs, arms, and between his fingers. Look for an unexcoriated burrow, from which you can take a sample. Such a burrow will contain a female itch mite, eggs, and fecal deposits.

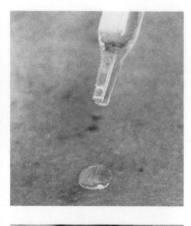

3 Next, drop a small amount of mineral oil on the burrow you select, as the nurse is doing here. The mineral oil holds the specimen together and causes it to float, so you can see it better.

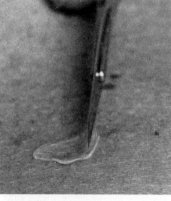

4 Now, carefully scrape the involved skin with a scalpel blade.

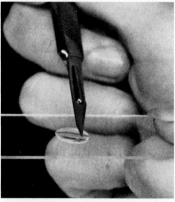

5 Transfer the scrapings to the prepared glass slide and apply a coverslip.

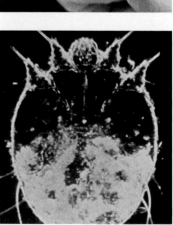

6 Finally, send the specimen to the lab for analysis. This photo shows a microscopic view of a mite.

Document your findings. Treat the patient as instructed above or give him instructions for self-treatment.

Reviewing skin trauma

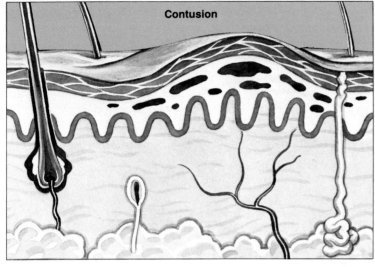

Contusion

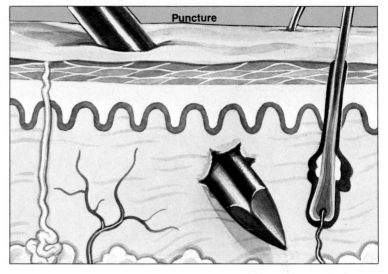

Puncture

Contusion
Injury or bruise caused by blunt trauma that doesn't penetrate the skin. The affected area appears ecchymotic and swollen.

Nursing management
● Clean the affected area with mild soap and water.
● Apply cold packs.
● Assess neurovascular function.
● Elevate the affected extremity.
● Administer mild analgesics, if indicated.
● Monitor edema by measuring affected extremity distal to injury site, if indicated.
● Assess your patient for other injuries, such as a fracture.
● Teach the patient and his family how to apply cold packs, assess circulation, and elevate an extremity correctly. Emphasize the importance of elevating an affected extremity to prevent edema. Also have them check the patient's skin temperature and color and monitor his pulse rate distal to the injury.

Abrasion
Superficial open wound caused by shearing or friction that involves loss of epidermis and, occasionally, dermis. The wound bleeds only slightly but usually exudes serosanguinous fluid. Because the epidermal layer's removed, infection is possible. Also, many nerve endings are exposed, causing pain. Scratches, red welts, and ecchymotic areas may be present.

Nursing management
● Gently clean the wound with a sterile 4"x4" gauze pad or soft brush and sterile normal saline

solution. *Caution:* Vigorous scrubbing increases tissue damage and pain.
● Before removing any embedded foreign objects, irrigate the wound liberally with saline solution.
● Anesthetize the area, if necessary, using lidocaine jelly applied directly to the wound (or with a gauze pad). Or, inject the area with 1% lidocaine solution. Then, use tissue forceps to remove the object.
● Apply a thin layer of antimicrobial ointment (such as povidone-iodine) or sterile petrolatum gauze to prevent crusting.
● Leave the wound exposed to air, if possible. Apply a sterile dressing only if the wound's large or if it's on a body part where friction's expected. Avoid applying tape directly over the wound; apply it toward the dressing margins instead. But make sure you leave the dressing loose enough to allow air

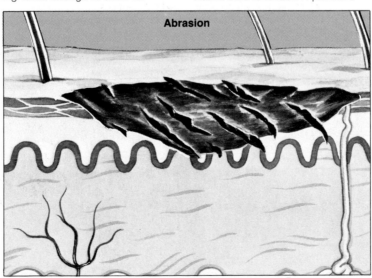

Abrasion

circulation.
● Administer tetanus toxoid prophylaxis, if necessary.
● Instruct the patient and his family to observe for such signs and symptoms of infection as redness, warmth, swelling, wound drainage, pain, and fever. If the wound's uncovered, teach them how to clean it and apply an antimicrobial ointment. Tell them they'll have to do this every day or as directed by the doctor. If the wound's covered with a dressing, the dressing should be changed only as ordered.

Puncture
Small wound caused by a sharp, pointed object (such as teeth or a nail) that penetrates the skin. The wound doesn't bleed readily and may be covered with a small skin flap or have ragged edges. The wound area is tender. A puncture

wound usually has a small opening and no exit site, making it difficult to clean and irrigate; infections commonly result from foreign matter retained in the wound.

Nursing management
● Obtain a history of the injury, including how forcefully the penetrating object entered.
● Assess the extent of injury.
● If the foreign object's still in the wound, remove it *only* after thorough evaluation.
● Obtain X-rays to find out if the object's retained deep within the wound.
● Thoroughly clean the wound with soap and water. Then, irrigate the wound with large amounts of sterile normal saline solution. *Note:* Remove any wood splinters *before cleaning.* Once wet, they'll be more difficult to remove.
● Teach the patient and his family to observe the wound for signs and symptoms of infection, such as redness, swelling, warmth, purulent or bloody drainage, and increased pain. Teach them how to apply warm, wet compresses or to soak the affected area, as ordered. Arrange for the patient to return for follow-up care.
● Administer tetanus toxoid prophylaxis if necessary. Teach patient and family about possible side effects.
● If wound is the result of a wild animal bite, report to appropriate authorities.
● Deep wounds that result in damage to underlying tissues may necessitate exploratory surgery or surgical debridement. Prepare the patient and family for surgery, as indicated.

Skin

Reviewing skin trauma continued

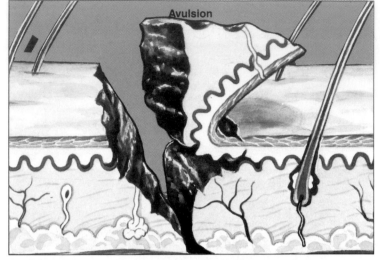

Avulsion

Avulsion
Complete or partial removal of tissue or a body part due to trauma. May result from a cutting, gouging, tearing, or crushing injury. The wound bleeds freely and is usually painful.

Nursing management
• Check the patient's history for bleeding tendencies and use of anticoagulant.
• Record time of injury. Doing so helps determine whether avulsed tissue can be reimplanted.
• Control hemorrhaging with direct pressure, absorbable gelatin sponge, or topical thrombin.
• Save all avulsed tissue. If you're at the accident scene, roll up the tissue so the subcutaneous tissue is on the inside and protected from drying out. Then, place the tissue in an airtight container. If you're at a clinic or other medical facility, place the tissue in normal saline solution. Keep it cool or refrigerate it. *Caution:* Never place an amputated part in ice, water, or other nonisotonic solution, because this may cause further cell damage.
• Clean the wound gently and irrigate it with normal saline solution.
• Debride the wound, if necessary.
• Cover the wound with a bulky dressing.
• Administer analgesics and tetanus toxoid prophylaxis, if necessary.
• If the injury is severe or requires further treatment, send the patient to the local hospital's emergency department or to a doctor.
• Instruct the patient to leave the dressing in place. Tell him to keep it dry and to watch for signs and symptoms of infection, such as fever, warmth, swelling, redness, drainage, and increased pain.

Laceration
Open wound that may extend deep into the epithelium. Usually results from penetration with a sharp object, such as a knife or piece of glass, or from a severe blow with a blunt object. Usually, the wound is painful and bleeds freely.

Nursing management
• Check the patient's history for diabetes, bleeding tendencies, and use of anticoagulant.
• Determine the approximate time of injury and estimate blood loss.
• Assess for neuromuscular, tendon, and circulatory damage.
• Administer tetanus toxoid prophylaxis, as necessary.
• If the area around the sutures becomes infected, culture the infection site and scrub it with surgical soap preparation. Then, remove some or all sutures, depending on extent of infection. Administer broad-spectrum antibiotics, as ordered. Instruct the patient to soak his wound in the prescribed

solution for 15 minutes, three times daily, and to return for follow-up care every 2 or 3 days, until the wound heals.
• If the injury is from an assault, report it to the police department, as soon as possible.
• Stress the need for follow-up care and suture removal.
For a laceration less than 8 hours old, a facial laceration, and a laceration to an area that's over a joint, such as the elbow and knee:
• Apply pressure and elevate the injured extremity to control hemorrhaging.
• Clean the wound gently with mild soap and sterile water. Then, irrigate it with normal saline solution.
• Debride necrotic tissue, as necessary.
• Close the wound, using sutures or strips of tape.
• Be aware that a severe laceration with underlying structural damage necessitates surgery. Prepare the patient and family, as necessary.
For a grossly contaminated laceration or a laceration more than 8 hours old:
• Administer a broad-spectrum antibiotic, such as tetracycline, for at least 5 days after the injury occurs, as ordered.
• Instruct the patient to elevate the injured extremity for 24 hours to reduce swelling.
• After 5 to 7 days, if the wound doesn't appear infected and contains healthy, granulated tissue, close it with sutures or butterfly strip, as ordered.
• Apply a sterile dressing. Splint the area, if necessary.
• Tell the patient to keep the dressing clean and dry and to watch for signs and symptoms of infection, such as redness, fever, warmth, swelling, drainage, and increased pain.

Wound closure: Two techniques
Wound closure helps control bleeding, prevents bacterial entry, and allows tissues to heal properly, with the least amount of scarring.

Whenever possible, use a noninvasive closure technique, which is usually adequate for shallow lacerations. Noninvasive measures include adhesive bandage strips, nylon-reinforced adhesive bandage strips (Steri-Strips), butterfly strips, and nonallergenic tape strips notched to provide tighter closure.

Use whichever type of noninvasive strip you have on hand. But remember, when applying the strips, pull the wound edges together evenly.

Suturing
As you probably know, suturing involves stitching the wound with a material the body can absorb (such as catgut) or a nonabsorbable material (such as silk), which you'll need to remove later. Use this technique for long, deep, and irregular wounds.

Consult your working protocol to determine whether or not you're permitted to suture. Also, in deciding whether to do the suturing yourself, consider the condition of the wound. Refer a patient with a wound involving arterial bleeding or muscle or tendon laceration to a doctor for suturing. And remember, for cosmetic reasons, you may want to have a plastic surgeon suture certain facial lacerations.

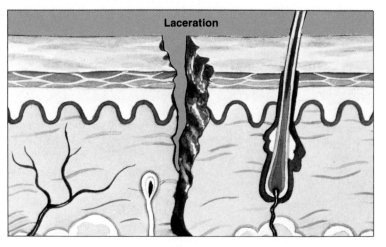

Laceration

Using adhesive tape strips to close a wound

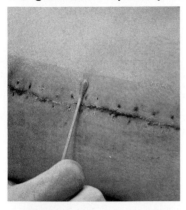

1 Suppose you're using adhesive tape strips to close a wound. (In this photostory, we'll use Steri-Strips.) Begin by cleaning the wound with alcohol. Remove any debris (such as dried blood) with hydrogen peroxide solution. Dry the area with a sterile gauze pad.

Next, using a cotton-tipped applicator, apply tincture of benzoin around—but not on—the wound, as shown here. Doing so improves tape strip adhesion.

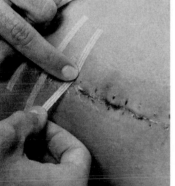

2 Now, press one end of the tape strip to the skin on one side of the wound.

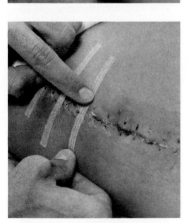

3 Then, applying gentle tension on the tape strip, draw the wound edges together, making sure you approximate the edges.

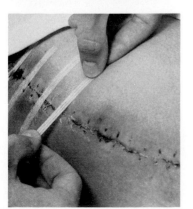

4 Secure the tape to the opposite side of the wound. *Caution:* Avoid inverting the wound edges as you apply the strip.

Use as many strips as necessary to prevent wound edges from gapping.

📨 *Nursing tip:* To reinforce the tape, apply tape strips ¼" (0.5 cm) from the wound and parallel to it.

Document the procedure.

Learning about local anesthetics

Administration of a local anesthetic's almost always necessary to suture a wound. Sometimes it's needed before suturing, to perform thorough cleansing without inflicting severe pain. Consult your working protocol to determine whether you're responsible for administering a local anesthetic.

How does a local anesthetic work? A local anesthetic blocks conduction of impulses along a peripheral nerve, so pain impulses don't reach the brain. *Note:* Because peripheral nerves contain motor and sensory fibers, alone or in combination, anesthetizing the peripheral nerve pathway may cause motor as well as sensory loss distal to the injection point.

Administration techniques

Administer a local anesthetic in any one of three ways:
• *Local infiltration:* injecting an anesthetic directly in the wound or proposed incision line. This method, which produces an immediate effect, should be used primarily when draining abscesses. Avoid using local infiltration with an incised or open wound that requires accurate approximation of wound edges. Why? Because during injection, the anesthetic may distort the tissues or introduce contaminated material into the wound.
• *Field block:* injecting an anesthetic in normal tissues around and beneath the wound but not in the wound itself. Because this method causes little or no tissue distortion, it's most commonly used for wound closure. The anesthetic begins to act in several minutes.
• *Nerve block:* injecting an anesthetic in a specific peripheral nerve at a point between the wound and the spinal cord. This technique, usually performed by the doctor, anesthetizes the nerve, distal to the block. Generally, a nerve block necessitates the least amount of anesthetic and anesthetizes a wider area than local infiltration or a field block. It takes several minutes to work.

Of course, effective administration of a local anesthetic depends on a number of factors. Generally, the larger the nerve's diameter, the higher the concentration of anesthetic needed.

You'll also need to assess local tissue. For example, tissue vascularity affects anesthetic diffusion and absorption; local tissue fluid may dilute the anesthetic and impair or delay its effect; and acidic tissue (such as infected tissue) reduces the anesthetic's effectiveness. In these situations, you may need to increase the dose or use a higher concentration.

Anesthetic agents

A number of medications are available for use as anesthetics. Commonly used medications include procaine hydrochloride (Novocain*), lidocaine hydrochloride (Xylocaine Hydrochloride*), and bupivacaine hydrochloride (Marcaine*).

When administering an anesthetic, give the minimum dose needed to achieve maximum effectiveness. Assess each patient individually in terms of pain tolerance, size of wound, body weight, and tissue condition. If your patient is debilitated, elderly, acutely ill, or a child, he should be given reduced doses commensurate with age, weight, and physical status.

When to use epinephrine

Administering a field block in a highly vascular area, such as the scalp? Use epinephrine in combination with an anesthetic (available in premixed solution). Because epinephrine has a vasoconstrictive effect, it'll help reduce bleeding. Be aware that epinephrine delays anesthetic absorption, thereby prolonging onset of anesthesia and extending its duration.

For details on local anesthetics, see DRUGS in the NURSE'S REFERENCE LIBRARY™.

*Available in both the United States and Canada

Skin

Administering a field block

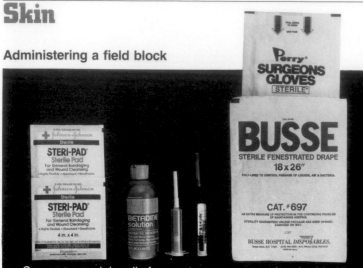

Suppose your job calls for you to remove gravel embedded in your patient's lacerated arm. Before you can proceed, you must administer a field block to anesthetize the wound area.

To do so, gather the following sterile equipment: 5- or 10-cc syringes, depending on wound size; 25G ⅝″ needle; 22G 1½″ needle; 4″x4″ gauze pads; precut drape; and sterile gloves.

Also obtain a prefilled syringe of lidocaine hydrochloride (Xylocaine Hydrochloride), such as the Abboject® single-dose vial, and an antimicrobial agent, such as povidone-iodine solution.*

Important: *For a wound deeper than 1½″ (3.8 cm), you may need to use a larger needle, such as a 22G 3½″ needle. But to reduce patient discomfort, always use the smallest-gauge needle possible.*

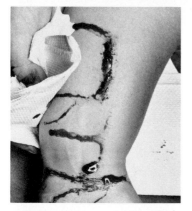

1 Now, wash your hands. Explain the procedure and its purpose to your patient. Position him comfortably, with his arm extended on a firm surface. *Note:* If the wound has hair around it, shave the surrounding area. Don't shave an eyebrow, however, which may not grow back.

2 Next, open all sterile supplies, following aseptic technique. Put on sterile gloves, and remove the safety caps from the syringe and vial. Then, screw the vial into the syringe, as the nurse is doing here.

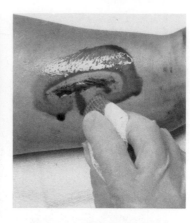

3 Using a gauze pad soaked in povidone-iodine solution, clean an area 3″ (7.6 cm) in diameter around the wound, moving from the center outward in a circular motion.

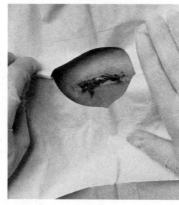

4 Next, position the precut drap over the wound. Then, mentally draw a diamond around the wound.

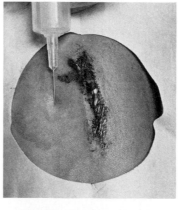

5 Now, using the 25G needle with the lidocaine-filled syringe attached, insert the needle into the dermis, using a quick, darting motion, as shown here.

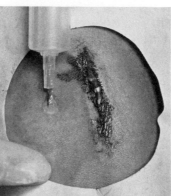

6 Keeping the needle as parallel to the surface of the skin as possible, inject 0.2 to 0.3 ml of anesthetic until the skin blanches and a small wheal appears, about ⅜″ (1 cm) in diameter.

Note: If your patient feels intense burning, reassure him that the sensation's only temporary.

*Available in both the United States and Canada

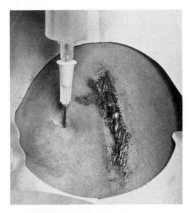

7 After raising the wheals, replace the 25G needle with the 22G needle.

Introduce the needle into one wheal. Insert it in the subcutaneous tissue at a 45° angle. Aspirate in two planes, to make sure you haven't pierced a blood vessel. If no blood enters the syringe, inject a small amount (0.5 ml) of anesthetic solution.

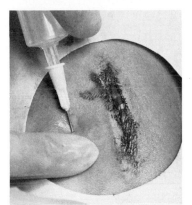

8 Continue to advance the needle deeper, in the direction of an adjacent wheal, alternately aspirating and injecting solution along this line, until you reach the next wheal.

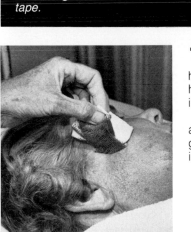

9 As you inject the anesthetic, palpate the skin overlying the needle tip to make sure the solution's in the subcutaneous tissue surrounding the wound.

When you've finished filling in the diamond outline, direct the needle to tissues deep under the wound. After aspiration, inject a small amount of anesthetic solution.

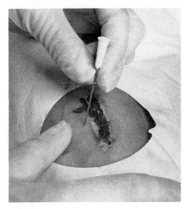

10 Now test the skin within the diamond for effectiveness. To do so, use the needle's point. When the patient no longer responds to the needle (usually in 3 to 5 minutes), you're ready to remove the gravel. After doing so, suture the laceration as described at right. Document the procedure in your nurses' notes.

How to suture a wound

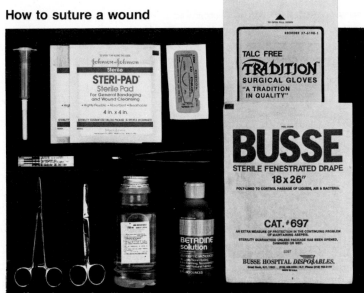

If you're not familiar with suturing, read this photostory. We show you how to suture a wound after cyst removal.

Note: Consult your working protocol to determine whether suturing is one of your responsibilities.

To begin, obtain the following sterile equipment: skin forceps, scissors, needle holder, precut drape, gloves, 4"x4" gauze pads, curve suturing needle with suture material, povidone-iodine solution, normal saline solution, and prefilled syringe containing local anesthetic. You'll also need nonallergenic tape.

1 Explain the procedure to your patient. Then, place her in supine position, with her head turned to expose the incision site. Wash your hands.

Now, thoroughly clean the area to be incised, using a gauze pad soaked in povidone-iodine solution.

2 Wash your hands again. Using strict aseptic technique, open all the sterile supplies. Next, open the suture material package and allow the contents to fall onto the sterile field. Put on your gloves, and place the precut sterile drape on the patient's face so the opening's over the incision site.

To perform a field block, inject the anesthetic solution in a diamond shape around the cyst, as shown.

Skin

How to suture a wound continued

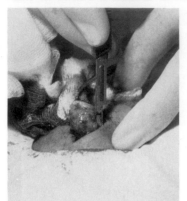

3 After the anesthetic has taken effect, the doctor removes the cyst.

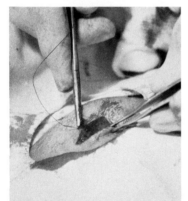

4 When he has completed this part of the procedure, begin suturing. To do so, use the interrupted stitch technique, as shown in the illustration. Because each stitch binds the wound independently, the wound won't open if a stitch loosens or breaks.

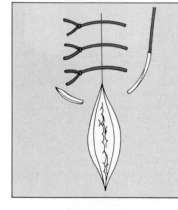

5 Anchor the skin as you push the needle through by grasping the wound margin gently with the skin forceps. Then, using the needle holder, grasp the needle at the middle of its curve. Insert the needle into the skin, as shown.

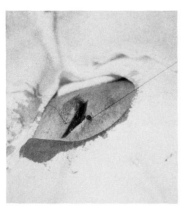

6 Gently push the needle through the tissues, and pull the suture material through the opposite wound margin. Make each suture as deep as it is wide.

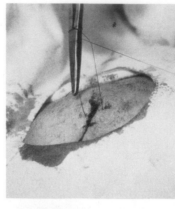

7 Secure the suture with a square knot, but be careful not to tie the knot too tightly because this will cause edema.
To tie the knot, loop one end of the suture material around the needle holder, as shown here. Then, pull the opposite end through the loop.

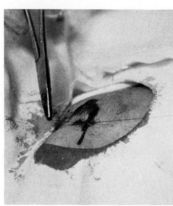

8 Tighten the knot by pulling the thread ends in opposite directions.

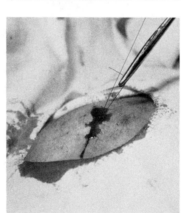

9 Now, repeat the procedure on the opposite sides of the suture. First, make a loop around the needle holder. Then, pull the other end of the thread through the loop.

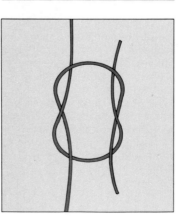

10 Tighten the ends to make a square knot, as illustrated.

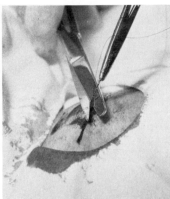

11 To cut the suture, hold the suture ends taut in one hand, at approximately a right angle to the skin. Hold the scissors almost closed in your other hand, parallel to the skin. This gives you more control, so you won't cut the skin.

Now, slide the scissors along the suture material. Snip the stitch, leaving ¼" (0.6-cm) tails extending from the knot, as shown. Leaving tails this long helps keep the knot from becoming untied.

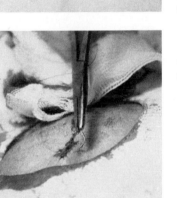

12 Continue making the number of stitches necessary to close the wound, spacing the sutures evenly.

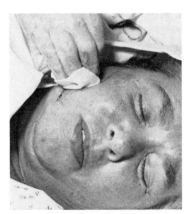

13 When you've finished, clean the suture line with a gauze pad moistened with normal saline solution.

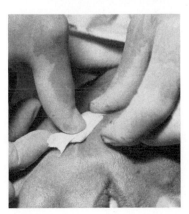

14 Apply a dry, sterile dressing, using a piece of nonadhering dressing, if necessary, for the first layer. Cover it with a gauze pad. Secure the dressing with nonallergenic tape, as shown.

Teach your patient how to care for the wound and how to observe for complications. Tell her when to return for suture removal. Then, document the procedure, how well your patient tolerated it, and your patient teaching.

Removing sutures

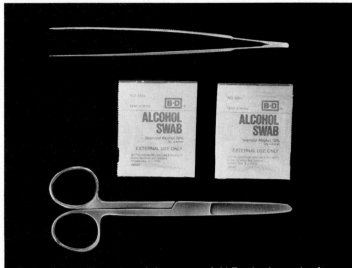

Because you've sutured the nape of Al Becker's neck after a cyst removal, he'll be returning to you to have the sutures taken out. To do this without contaminating the wound, take these steps. Note: *Depending on your working protocol, the doctor may perform this procedure.*

First, obtain a sterile suture-removal kit containing skin forceps and scissors. Also obtain alcohol swabs to clean the suture line.

Explain the procedure to your patient and position him comfortably. Then, wash your hands.

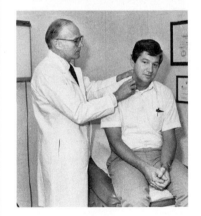

1 Assess how the wound is healing. To do so, remove the dressing and inspect the wound. Check for signs and symptoms of infection, such as redness, swelling, tenderness, and purulent drainage.

Check to see if the wound margins have closed properly. If they haven't, remove only *every other* suture, following instructions in steps 2 to 6.

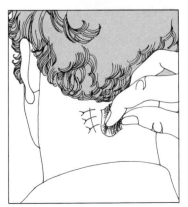

2 Clean the wound with an alcohol swab or a gauze pad soaked in povidone-iodine solution.

☞ *Nursing tip:* If blood has caked in the suture area, remove it with hydrogen peroxide solution.

Skin

Removing sutures continued

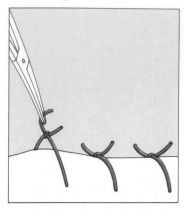

3 Now, use the skin forceps to grasp the first suture knot. Gently pull upward, lifting the suture away from the skin.

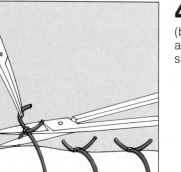

4 Use the scissors to cut the short end of the suture (between the knot and the skin) as close as possible to the skin.

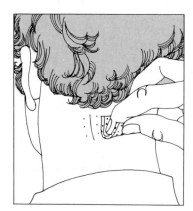

5 Gently pull the suture out of the skin. Take care not to pull the part of the suture that was above skin level through the healing wound. Doing so may contaminate the wound, causing infection.

Repeat until all sutures are removed.

6 Clean the skin again with a povidone-iodine–soaked gauze pad. Then, leave the wound uncovered (in most cases). Instruct your patient to return for follow-up care if drainage occurs.

After giving care, be sure to wash your hands. Document the procedure, including wound appearance and how well your patient tolerated the procedure.

Removing skin staples

Debbie Gehman, a 20-year-old college student, had an open reduction of her right femur after an automobile accident. To close the incision after surgery, her doctor used skin staples. The staples are to be removed today.

As a community nurse, you may be asked to remove the skin staples from Debbie's leg. Do you know how?

Begin by obtaining the necessary equipment for the procedure: alcohol swabs, hydrogen peroxide solution, sterile 4"x4" gauze pads, and a sterile skin-staple remover. Open the staple remover's package. Then, explain the procedure to your patient and answer any questions she may have. Wash your hands and dry them thoroughly.

Clean the incision line on Debbie's leg with alcohol swabs. If blood has dried around the incision, remove it with sterile gauze pads soaked in hydrogen peroxide solution.

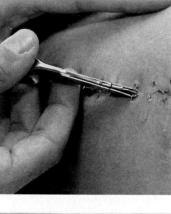

1 Now, using aseptic technique, lift the staple remover from its package and slide its lower tips firmly under the first staple.

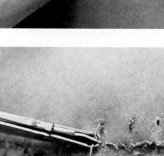

2 Squeeze together the handles of the staple remover, as shown in this photo. This action puts a notch in the staple, which makes the staple easier to remove.

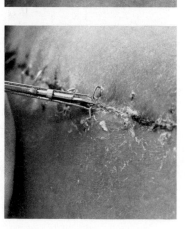

3 To remove the staple from the skin, lift straight up on the staple remover, as the nurse is doing here. Set this staple to one side; then, remove the others, following the same procedure.

Document everything you've done—as well as your observations about your patient's incision—on the appropriate form.

Removing a ring from a finger

Almost everyone's had the experience of trying on a ring and then being unable to get it off immediately. Usually, a moment's twisting makes it easy to remove. But suppose your patient's jammed or bruised his finger while wearing a ring. His finger swells, making ring removal difficult.

Several techniques are recommended for ring removal. If your patient's finger isn't injured, lubricate it or use umbilical tape, as we explain in the following steps. But if his finger has been injured, your primary concern must be to prevent further injury. Use a ring cutter, as shown in the photostory following this one. Also use a ring cutter if the ring has sharp edges or cuts into adjacent skin.

Are you concerned about damaging the ring permanently? Don't cut the band near the ring's setting. Instead, cut at a point opposite the setting, where the ring can be easily repaired.

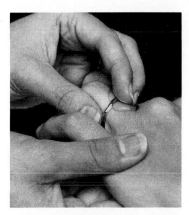

1 Let's assume your patient has an arm injury, necessitating ring removal. To remove his ring, lubricate the finger with soap or water-soluble jelly.

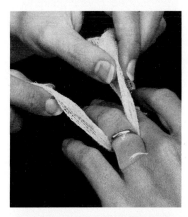

2 Then, loop dry gauze through the ring. Pull on the ends gently to remove the ring.

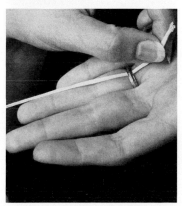

3 Suppose this method fails. Try wrapping the finger with umbilical tape. To do this, slip one end of the umbilical tape under the ring from the distal side. Draw through 1½" to 2" (3.8 to 5 cm) of tape, as shown here.

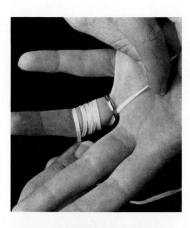

4 Grasp this end of the tape with one hand as you wrap the longer end around the patient's distal finger, to a point beyond the proximal interphalangeal joint.

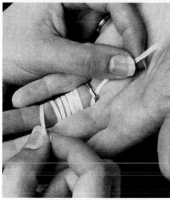

5 Now, hold *this* end of the tape in place.

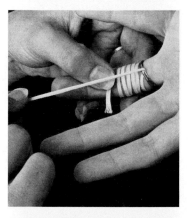

6 Pull the short proximal end of the tape *over* the ring and unwind it toward the distal end of the finger, as the nurse is doing here.

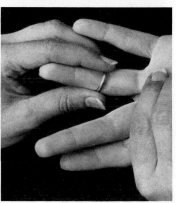

7 As the tape unwinds, the ring will begin to slide off the finger, distally. After the ring passes over the proximal interphalangeal joint, you should be able to slip it off easily.

Skin

Using a ring cutter

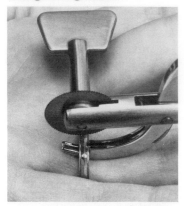

1 To remove a ring with a ring cutter, begin by selecting a site for cutting, preferably opposite the ring's setting. Rotate this part of the ring to the palmar aspect of the finger, unless this would position the cutting site closer to the patient's injury.

Now, slip the ring cutter's curved tip under the ring at the chosen site.

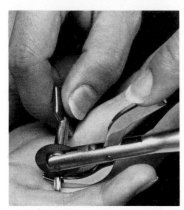

2 Rotate the cutting wheel until you've cut through the metal.

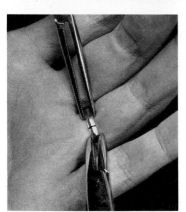

3 Using hemostats, spread the opening you've made just enough to slip the ring off the finger. Then lubricate the finger.

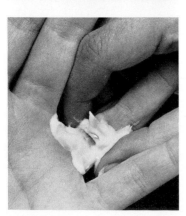

4 Finally, slide the ring off. Remember to document the procedure. Provide further assessment and care, as needed.

Removing a foreign object from the skin

You've probably removed small foreign objects from the skin so many times you find it easy to do. But to minimize your patient's pain and reduce the risk of infection, review this information.

Before you proceed, decide whether to remove a foreign object yourself or refer your patient to a doctor. To make this decision, you need to find out how the foreign object became embedded in your patient's skin, how long it's been embedded in the skin, and its nature and size. Also, try to estimate how deeply the foreign object's penetrated the skin.

Usually, you can remove a superficial foreign object, such as a splinter, with a pointed forceps and a magnifying glass. No anesthetic should be necessary. Work gently, however, and reassure your patient frequently throughout the procedure.

Be sure to ask him about any unusual bleeding tendencies, allergies, and any other medical problems, such as diabetes, as well as about any medications he's currently taking. If the object's small enough, consider allowing it to work itself out. Tissues tend to force out small objects.

If the foreign object's a complication of a laceration or other wound, you may need to refer the patient to a doctor. He'll administer a local anesthetic, probe to locate the foreign object, and remove it by debridement and excision.

Important: Consider all foreign objects contaminated; administer tetanus toxoid prophylaxis, as indicated.

Suppose you note a small entrance wound but can't see the foreign body. Consider the possibility that high-velocity fragments may have entered your patient's skin. In such a case, arrange for X-rays to be taken to detect the object and determine its depth and location.

Do you suspect a radiopaque foreign object, such as metal, stone, or safety glass, is embedded in your patient's skin? You'll need to arrange for an X-ray. But first tape metal markers to the skin's surface in the suspected area. Then, have the area X-rayed from several angles. This way you use the markers as guides in locating the object.

Wondering how to remove a foreign object that's been located by X-ray? After anesthetizing the area, as needed, the doctor may follow one of these two methods:
• use the X-ray view to insert needles around the object and using these as a guide, perform a cutdown procedure
• use forceps to remove the object under fluoroscopy and image intensification.

To remove other types of foreign objects, consider the following suggestions. *Note:* Check your clinic's protocol; the doctor may perform these procedures.
• *Sewing needle.* Arrange for X-ray, to determine location. Remove with a hemostatic forceps through an incision over the end closest to the skin. If the needle has penetrated bone, the doctor will use a sterile pliers to remove the splinter.
• *Subungual splinter.* Anesthetize the area, if necessary. Make a small notch in the nail over the splinter, and remove the splinter with a small forceps.
• *Radiolucent material* (such as wood). Inject a local anesthetic into the area, as needed. Remove material with a pointed forceps. Take care not to soak the affected area before removal. Doing so may make removal more difficult.
• *Earth or gravel particles from abrasion injury* (if irrigation has been unsuccessful). Gently rub affected area with a stiff brush to loosen foreign object. Allow area to heal; excise healed area later, as needed.
• *Nail or spike.* Remove by pulling out of puncture wound. Be alert for retained matter, which may lead to infection.

Removing a superficial splinter

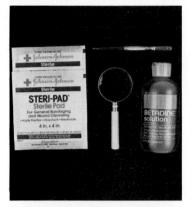

1 Your patient has a superficial splinter in his finger. To remove the splinter correctly, follow these steps:

Begin by gathering the equipment you'll need: pointed forceps, magnifying glass, sterile 4"x4" gauze pads, and povidone-iodine solution.

Tell your patient what you're going to do. Position him with his hand resting on a firm, flat surface. Then, wash your hands.

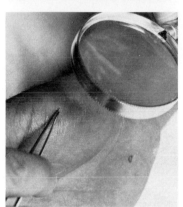

2 Moisten a gauze pad with povidone-iodine solution. Starting at the splinter's entry site, gently wipe outward, in a circular motion. Allow the area to dry.

Grasp the forceps with one hand and hold the magnifying glass with the other hand. Looking through the glass, use the forceps to gently withdraw the splinter at the angle of entry, as the nurse is doing here.

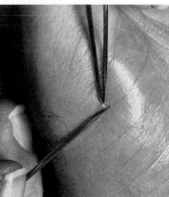

3 Is the splinter embedded below the skin surface, between the epidermal and dermal layers? Position the bevel of a 26G needle against the patient's skin, about ½" (1.3 cm) from the splinter's entry point.

Without piercing the skin, gently draw the needle across the skin toward the entry point, as shown here. Repeat the procedure until you see the splinter's edge. Then, grasp the splinter with the forceps and withdraw it at the same angle.

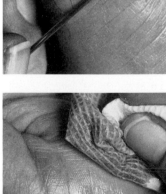

4 After the splinter's removed, wipe the area with a clean gauze pad moistened in povidone-iodine solution. Allow the area to dry. Administer tetanus toxoid prophylaxis, if needed.

Finally, instruct your patient to keep the area clean and to watch for signs of infection, such as redness, pain, swelling, and drainage. Tell him to notify you immediately if any of these occur.

Removing a splinter from under the fingernail

John Carroway, a 13-year-old student, comes to your clinic with a splinter under his fingernail. "I tried to pull it out," he says in dismay, "but it just wouldn't work."

A splinter under a fingernail can be particularly painful if the bacteria on the splinter becomes trapped, causing infection.

Your first step in removing the splinter is to assess the fingernail. Take an accurate history and examine the nail. If you can reach the splinter with a forceps, you may be able to withdraw it.

If the splinter's deeply embedded in the nail bed, you may need to anesthetize the finger and cut a small wedge in the nail to gain access to the splinter's proximal end. Doing so also helps prevent infection by opening up the area so bacteria can't multiply.

Before beginning, obtain a prefilled syringe of anesthetic, a scalpel and blade, and a sharp forceps.

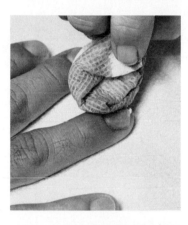

1 Explain the procedure to your patient. Position him comfortably, with his hand resting palm down on a firm surface. Wash your hands.

Now, clean your patient's finger with a gauze pad soaked in povidone-iodine.

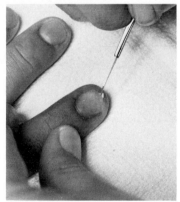

2 Administer the anesthetic. Then, test your patient's finger with the end of the needle to determine whether the anesthetic's taken effect. When it has, use the scalpel to cut as small a wedge in the nail as possible, as the nurse is doing here.

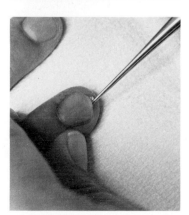

3 Then, grasp the splinter with the forceps and pull it straight out from under the nail. Administer tetanus toxoid prophylaxis, if necessary.

Instruct your patient to soak the wound three times a day, and observe it for signs and symptoms of infection. Have him return for a follow-up evaluation in 2 days.

On the appropriate form, document the procedure, how your patient tolerated it, and your teaching.

Skin

Removing a barbed fishhook

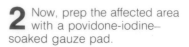

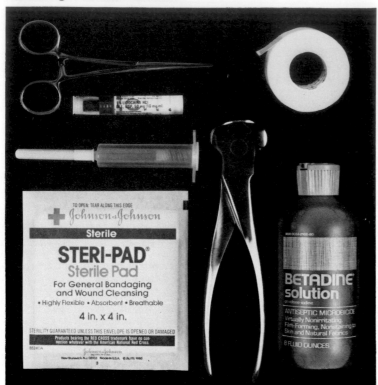

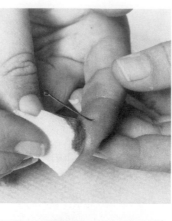
2 Now, prep the affected area with a povidone-iodine–soaked gauze pad.

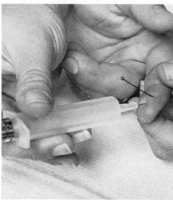
3 Next, anesthetize the area, using the lidocaine-filled syringe.

George Horchner, a 20-year-old bus driver, walks into the community health center where you work. "I was sorting out my fishing tackle," he says, "when I got this barbed fishhook embedded in my finger. I thought about trying to get it out myself, but I didn't know whether to push or pull it."

George has raised the key question in dealing with fishhook removal. If the hook has a barb, pulling it back through the entry point can cause severe tissue damage. Your patient will suffer less damage if you push the hook forward through the skin, cut it in two pieces, and remove each segment separately. To reduce his pain as you do this, administer a local anesthetic. Follow the procedure outlined here.

First, obtain a prefilled syringe containing 1% lidocaine hydrochloride, a wire cutter, a small hemostat, sterile 4″ × 4″ gauze pads saturated with povidone-iodine solution, and nonallergenic tape. You'll also need povidone-iodine ointment and a roll of sterile gauze.

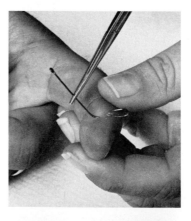
4 Then, use the hemostat to advance the hook so the barbed end protrudes through the skin.

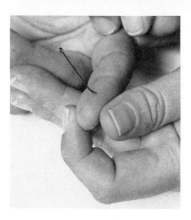
1 Be sure to wash your hands. Then, explain to your patient the procedure and its purpose.

Position your patient comfortably, holding his affected hand palm up in your nonworking hand. Be sure the fishhook is within easy reach.

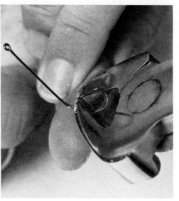
5 Now, cut off the barbed end of the hook with the wire cutter.

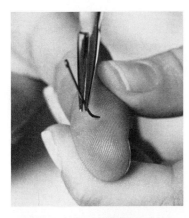

6 Using the hemostat, withdraw the remainder of the cut hook, pulling it back through the entry point.

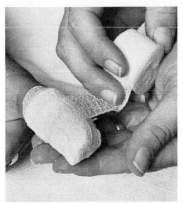

7 Then, apply povidone-iodine ointment and a sterile dressing, securing it with nonallergenic tape. Administer tetanus toxoid prophylaxis, if necessary. Instruct your patient to return in 2 days, reminding him to immediately report any signs and symptoms of infection.

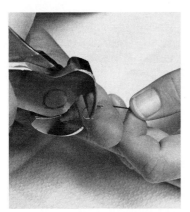

8 Suppose the hook protrudes *through* your patient's finger. Clean and anesthetize the area as in steps 2 and 3. Then, cut the fishhook flush with the skin.

9 Now, grasp the other end with a small hemostat and draw this fragment from the tissue.

Remember to document the procedure.

Learning about paronychia

Most patients who bite their nails know that nail-biting is a bad habit. But few realize that it could lead to infection of the skin around the cuticle. This common problem, *paronychia,* occurs at the skin fold of the nail periphery as a painful, swollen, reddened area with a pocket of yellow, purulent drainage.

Usually, the infection's caused by a gram-positive organism, such as *Staphylococcus aureus;* however, *Pseudomonas* or other gram-negative organisms may be responsible.

Besides nail-biting and other minor trauma to the cuticle, predisposing factors include emotional stress, continually wet hands (found in some occupations), diabetes, alcoholism, peripheral arterial disease, decreased immune response (from corticosteroids, immunosuppressives, and antibiotics), allergies, and diaphoresis. Also, a benign tumor (for example, a wart or mucous cyst) or a malignant tumor (for example, a melanoma or squamous cell carcinoma) of the nail edge may be associated with paronychia.

Note: Before caring for a patient with paronychia, find out if he's a diabetic. If so, refer him to a doctor for treatment.

Keep in mind that early-stage paronychia treatment—including intermittent warm soaks and antibiotics, as needed—is aimed at relieving acute cellulitis of the soft tissue of the eponychial fold, as shown in the top illustration. If untreated, paronychia progresses from the early stage to an intradermal or subdermal abscess, causing throbbing pain and localized tenderness (see middle illustration).

Failure to treat the *abscess* may result in periungual extension, as shown in the bottom illustration. Two complications occur at this stage: the nail acts as a foreign body, perpetuating the infection; and it softens, becoming vulnerable to invading microorganisms. Even the extensor tendon controlling the distal interphalangeal joint may become involved, causing finger drop or mallet finger.

A patient with second- or third-stage paronychia needs to have the paronychia incised and drained.

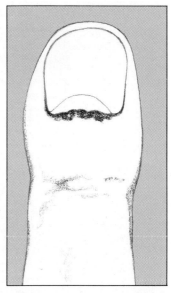

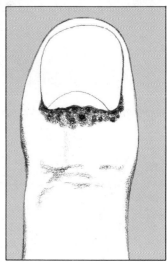

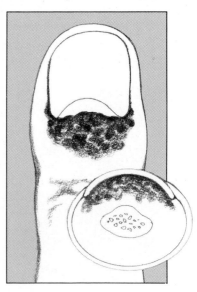

Skin

Managing acute paronychia

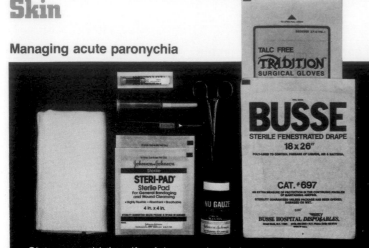

Sixty-year-old Jennifer Adams, a local dressmaker, comes to your clinic in tears. Her right index finger is red, swollen, painful, and throbbing. "I'm always sticking it accidentally with my sewing needle," she sobs.

You assess Ms. Adams' finger and conclude that she has acute paronychia. To treat it, you will have to incise and drain it—after the doctor anesthetizes the area with a local anesthetic. Do you know how to perform your part of the procedure?

First, obtain the following sterile equipment: a 5-cc prefilled syringe containing 1% lidocaine hydrochloride, gloves, a drape with an opening, a towel, 4"x4" gauze pads, a scalpel and blade, ½" iodoform gauze packing, and a hemostat. You'll also need povidone-iodine solution, a Culturette, and tube gauze.

Seat your patient comfortably and rest her wrist and hand on a firm, flat surface. Reassure her as you explain the procedure. Then, wash and dry your hands thoroughly.

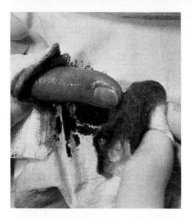

1 Using strict aseptic technique, open the sterile supplies. Put on your gloves, and place the sterile towel under Ms. Adams' hand. Then, position the drape with the opening over her affected finger. Clean the area with povidone-iodine solution, as shown. Prepare the syringe.

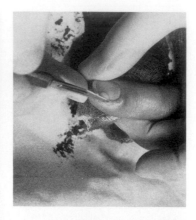

3 Working carefully, pass the tip of the scalpel blade along Ms. Adams' fingernail where the pain is most severe. Doing so will drain the infection site.

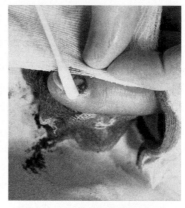

4 Collect a sample of the drainage, as shown here, for culture and sensitivity testing.

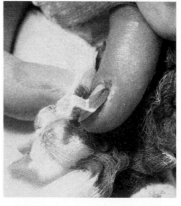

5 Now, using the hemostat, insert iodoform gauze packing under the cuticle at the infection site to promote drainage.

2 Next, the doctor anesthetizes your patient's finger. As soon as the area numbs, you can incise and drain the paronychia.

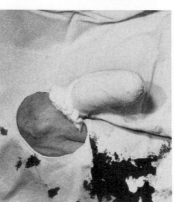

6 Apply a 4"x4" gauze pad to the finger and cover it with tube gauze, as shown.

Instruct Ms. Adams to keep her finger clean and dry until she returns to the clinic the next day to have the dressing changed.

Administer an antibiotic, as ordered. Document the procedure and any patient teaching.

Draining a subungual hematoma

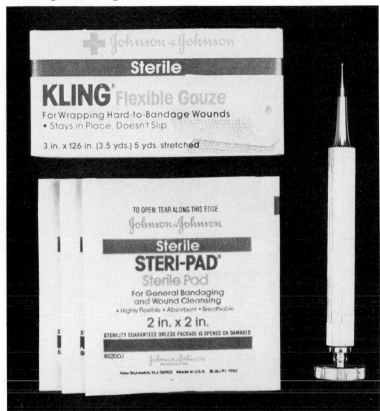

Slamming a door on your finger can be painful, as many of us know. But when a person develops a subungual hematoma (an accumulation of blood under the fingernail), his pain may become severe. You can provide immediate relief by draining the hematoma. Here we show you how to drain a hematoma located in the proximal portion of the nail bed.

First, obtain a hand drill (or battery-operated drill with a dental drill tip), sterile 2"x2" gauze pads, and roller bandage. You'll also need povidone-iodine solution and nonallergenic tape.

Note: Your patient won't require an anesthetic for this procedure.

Explain to your patient the procedure and its purpose. Then, seat him comfortably and extend his finger on a firm surface. Wash your hands.

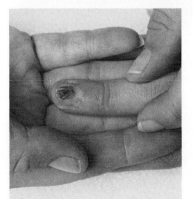

1 Now, examine your patient's fingernail. The hematoma appears as a dark blue, discolored area under the fingernail.

Important: To rule out a terminal phalanx fracture, arrange for an X-ray.

As you assess the wound, check for blood oozing from underneath the fingernail. If you see any, gently press on the nail to help the blood drain. If enough blood drains spontaneously, you may not need to drill a hole.

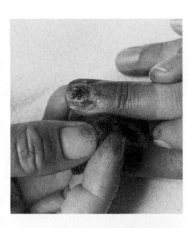

2 Now, prep the patient's finger with the povidone-iodine solution, as the nurse is doing here. Then, using the drill tip, apply firm, gentle pressure to the nail over the hematoma. *Note:* As the drill moves through the nail, decrease pressure on it to avoid penetrating the nail bed.

As soon as you perforate the nail, withdraw the drill. Trapped blood should flow out through the drill hole.

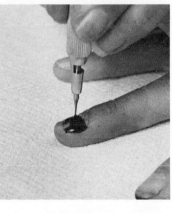

3 Drill two or three holes to allow for complete drainage. Doing so helps ensure that the hematoma won't form again.

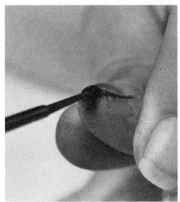

4 Suppose your patient's hematoma occurs close to his fingertip. Insert a scalpel blade directly into the hematoma, under the fingernail. As you do, keep the blade in contact with the nail's undersurface. Drain the hematoma.

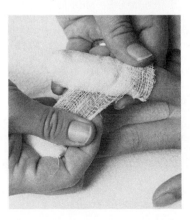

5 Finally, cover the nail with a sterile dressing.

Assure your patient that although his nail may fall off eventually, a new nail will grow. Also, tell him to keep his finger dry and to return to the clinic in 2 days. If swelling, increased redness, severe pain, drainage or bleeding, or a fever occur, have him notify his doctor.

Muscle and bone

Do you know that muscle and bone disorders account for pain and joint stiffness in persons of all ages? As an ambulatory-care nurse, you may see many patients with muscle and bone problems. Do you know all that's necessary to give quality nursing care?

On the following pages we provide this information. For instance, we tell you:
• how to identify musculoskeletal trauma
• how to manage soft-tissue injuries
• how to assess neurovascular impairment
• how to detect low back pain
• how to set up a scoliosis screening.

We also provide important information on common musculoskeletal disorders, including osteoarthritis and fractures.

Read these pages carefully.

Taking a muscle and bone history

When caring for a patient with a muscle or bone disorder, try to get a sense of how he perceives his problem and the effect it may have on his life. Remember that the problem may interfere with his ability to perform his job, with his social life, or with both. If your assessment and treatment don't help his problem, he faces the possibility of reduced capability of earning a living and of interacting with family and friends.

Do you know what assessment questions to ask your patient about his disorder? If not, use the samples below as a guide.
• Do you have pain? If so, describe it. Point to the pain's exact location.
• Have you fallen recently or otherwise injured yourself? Describe what happened.
• Have you noted any swelling?
• Were you born with any physical deformities? Has your condition been treated?
• Has the muscle or bone problem interfered with your day-to-day activities?
• Have you experienced muscle weakness in your arms or legs?
• Have you had any major bone or muscle disorders, such as fractures or dislocations?
• How active are you?

Learning about hot and cold treatments

"My little boy hurt his ankle. Should I put ice or a heating pad on it?" How many times has a concerned parent asked you a question like this? You know that hot and cold treatments have pronounced effects on blood flow, which, in turn, affect swelling, bleeding, and inflammation. But do you know why these treatments work?

Consider the principles of vasoconstriction and vasodilation. When cold is applied to a soft-tissue injury, vasoconstriction occurs. Cold decreases bleeding from torn blood vessels and fluid from injured tissues (see top illustration). And because cold also decreases muscle spasms, slows nerve impulses, and reduces inflammation and swelling, the patient experiences less pain. By applying cold to your patient's injury, you decrease the amount of damage your patient may suffer from the injury.

When heat's applied to a soft-tissue injury, vasodilation occurs. Because heat stimulates blood flow to the injured area, it also increases the availability of nutrients and repair agents, such as scar-tissue cells and white blood cells, to the area (see bottom illustration). In addition, heat stimulates metabolic activity, relaxes tense muscles, and inhibits muscle cramps and spasms.

Special considerations

When applying hot or cold treatments to an injury, consider the patient's age. For example, very young or old patients are more vulnerable to burns and other problems associated with temperature extremes. Take care to assess your patient's vital signs every 20 to 30 minutes. Be alert for signs of increased internal bleeding, such as tachycardia and decreased blood pressure. If present, notify the doctor immediately. Also instruct your patient to tell you if the treatment is too hot or too cold on his skin. Keep in mind that prolonged application of cold treatments may cause vasodilation elsewhere in the body.

Applying a cold treatment

Immediately apply cold to a patient's injury, using an ice bag, cold compress, or chemical cold pack. In an emergency, consider using a bag of ice cubes or even a cold can of soda. *Caution:* Never apply ice directly to the injury. Doing so may cause a thermal burn.

Apply the cold treatment to the injury and let it remain there for 20 to 30 minutes. Remove the cold

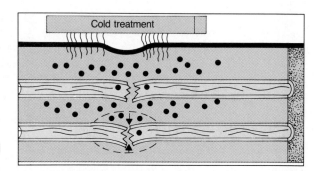

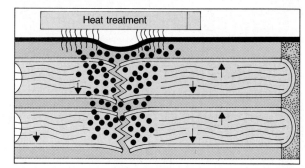

for 10 minutes and then reapply. Continue to apply the cold treatment for the next 24 to 72 hours.

Important: If you're switching from cold to heat treatment, wait at least 6 to 10 hours after the last cold treatment. An abrupt switch may cause resumption of minor internal bleeding stopped by the cold treatment.

Applying a hot treatment

After 24 hours, or as ordered by the doctor, administer heat to a patient's injury. To do this, use a hot-water bag; a warm, moist compress; or a commercial hot pack or immerse the injured body part in warm water. *Caution:* Never use a hot-water bag, a heating pad, or a hot foot-soak if your patient is in shock or has a history of vascular disease. Apply the heat treatment for 20 to 30 minutes every 2 to 3 hours.

If your patient or his family will be applying hot or cold treatments at home, instruct them to notify the doctor or go to the hospital's emergency department if the treatment causes a return of pain or redness or if the pain and swelling don't subside after about 24 hours.

Assessing musculoskeletal trauma

After you take a quick but complete musculoskeletal history, begin assessing your patient's injury. Closely observe the injury site and surrounding area for these signs and symptoms:
• *Swelling:* appears as a soft, compressible area 15 to 30 minutes after the injury occurs
• *Ecchymosis:* indicates subcutaneous bleeding and may appear immediately or be delayed for several hours or days. How rapidly ecchymosis appears depends on the depth and extent of the injury. If ecchymosis is present, suspect major tissue damage or possibly a fracture.
• *Crepitation:* grating sound and sensation from two ends of bone rubbing against each other; may indicate a fracture.
• *Instability:* the unnatural or impaired motion of an injured extremity may indicate a fracture or a significant ligament rupture. If swelling and ecchymosis are present, the doctor will move the injured extremity gently to detect instability.
• *Neurovascular damage:* may appear as circulatory impairment or as sensory or motor loss and occur immediately as a result of the injury or later as a result of treatment, such as wrapping.

Treatment

When caring for a patient with a suspected musculoskeletal injury, elevate the affected extremity above heart level, if possible. If the extremity's unstable, temporarily splint it until the patient can receive more complete care. Administer medication for pain relief, as indicated, and apply cold or hot treatments, as ordered.

Identifying neurovascular impairment

You've put in a full day at the ambulatory-care clinic where you work when 35-year-old Clark Matheson hobbles in the door. With a sigh of frustration, he tells you he thinks he injured his knee while playing football with the boys. He confesses that his knee is "throbbing."

When you've completed your musculoskeletal assessment of Mr. Matheson's knee, you'll want to check for associated nerve and vascular damage. Do you know how to perform a neurovascular assessment? If you're unsure, review the following guidelines carefully.

Note: *If your assessment indicates that your patient's suffered impairment, elevate the injured extremity above heart level; assess his vital signs; check his dressing, cast, or splint (if any) to be sure it's not too tight; and arrange for X-rays (if you've noted paralysis or paresthesia).*

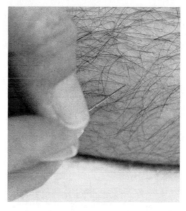

3 To assess Mr. Matheson's sensory ability, use a pin to prick lightly areas distal and proximal to the injury site, as shown here. Ask him to tell you if he notices any increase or decrease in sensation, lack of sensation, numbness, or tingling. Then, ask him about the same area on his unaffected side. Compare your findings. If he's experiencing paresthesias, suspect local, cerebral, or spinal injury.

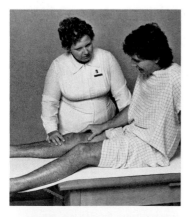

1 Begin by explaining the assessment procedure. Find out if the pain is subsiding or becoming more intense.
   If your patient's unconscious, palpate the suspected injury site and note any response, such as twitching, jerking, or grimacing. Perform neurochecks, as ordered. *Remember:* Pain worsens with increased edema.

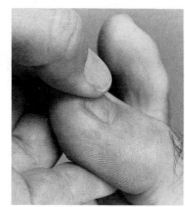

4 Next, check the skin color and the temperature of Mr. Matheson's knee. Note where cyanosis and pallor occur with respect to the injury.
   Compress the nail bed of his great toe for a moment and observe how quickly the blood returns (capillaries usually refill in 3 to 5 seconds). Now, check his unaffected side and compare your findings.

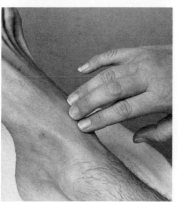

2 Next, check Mr. Matheson's pulse distal to the injury site, as the nurse is doing here. Be sure to compare bilateral pulses at the same time to detect discrepancies between them. *Note:* Many patients have a congenital or bilateral lack of the dorsalis pedis pulse. Ask your patient if he's been told that he lacks a pulse in his feet or check his history.

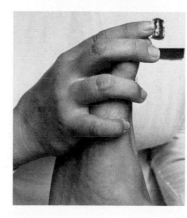

5 To detect paralysis, the nurse in this photo is assessing mobility in the first joint distal to Mr. Matheson's injured knee. If the patient's arm or leg is wrapped or already in a cast, check his fingers or toes for mobility. Be sure to assess his unaffected side as well. If paralysis is present, suspect peripheral nerve, spinal cord, or brain injury. Perform neurochecks as ordered.
   Document your assessment.

Muscle and bone

Nurses' guide to musculoskeletal disorders

Osteoporosis

Chief complaint
- *Sudden pain:* in lower back after bending, followed by a snapping sound; symptom of fracture or vertebral collapse; aggravated by movement
- *Deformity and immobility:* fractures of involved vertebrae; increasing kyphosis or dowager's hump possible

History
- Predisposing factors include endocrine disorders, chronic low dietary calcium intake, malabsorption, prolonged immobility, excessive cigarette smoking.
- Most common in elderly women

Physical findings
- Evidence of healed fracture; loss of height; wedging of dorsal vertebrae or anterior vertebrae
- Diagnostic studies include X-rays, bone biopsy, and densitometry measurements. (Results may show a parathyroid hormone elevation.)

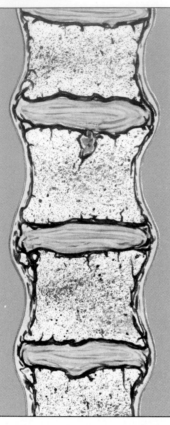

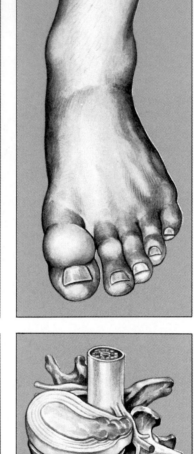

Gout

Chief complaint
- *Pain:* present, severe; worse after high purine food ingestion; frequently nocturnal; onset usually sudden
- *Joint stiffness:* joint immobility caused by pain and swelling
- *Swelling and redness:* red or cyanotic tense, hot skin over affected swollen joint
- *Deformity and immobility:* painless tophi (urate deposits) in external ears, hands, elbows, and knees; can't bear weight on affected limb

History
- Predisposing factors include renal disease, family history of gout, disorders that cause alterations in purine metabolism or decreased renal clearance of uric acid.

Physical findings
- Altered bone contour; elevated blood pressure; tachycardia; fever; nephrolithiasis; renal failure; thickened, wrinkled, desquamated skin
- Diagnostic studies include X-rays of involved joint, uric acid levels, complete blood count, synovial fluid analysis, and arthroscopy.

Osteoarthritis

Chief complaint
- *Pain:* during inclement or changing weather; worse after exposure to cold, exercise, or weight-bearing; relieved by rest
- *Joint stiffness:* transient stiffness worse in morning or after inactivity; affects weight-bearing joints
- *Swelling and redness:* joints swollen and tender but not red or hot
- *Deformity and immobility:* Heberden's nodes in distal joints; Bouchard's nodes in proximal joints; flexion contracture possible

History
- Onset usually after age 55
- Moderate to severe disease most common in postmenopausal women
- Predisposing factors include joint damage from trauma, infection, or stress; dietary calcium deficiency; history of arthritis in one or both parents; occupation.

Physical findings
- Decreased range of motion; altered bone contour; bony enlargement; malaligned joints; no systemic manifestations; crepitation on motion
- Diagnostic studies include X-rays of affected joints.

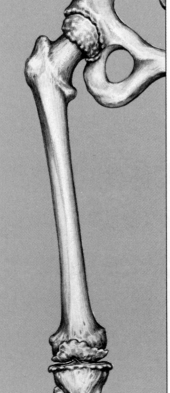

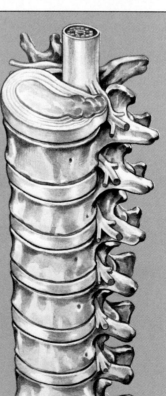

Herniated lumbosacral disk

Chief complaint
- *Pain:* present in low back; radiates to buttocks and legs; intensifies with Valsalva's maneuver, coughing, sneezing, bending, and lifting; may be accompanied by muscle spasms; occurs over dermatome for that specific disk; usually unilateral.
- *Joint stiffness:* inflexible spine
- *Deformity and immobility:* muscle atrophy of affected extremities
- *Sensory changes:* decreased sensation, paresthesias; muscle weakness; absent reflexes; voiding or defecating difficulties

History
- Predisposing factors include congenital small lumbar spinal canal, recent spinal trauma, occupational stress on back, lack of exercise, obesity, degenerative changes.

Physical findings
- Decreased spinal range of motion; unequal limb circumferences; abnormal posture; scoliosis; loss of ankle or knee jerk reflex; positive straight-leg–raising test; posterior leg (sciatic) pain without back pain
- Diagnostic studies include X-rays, myelography, and computerized tomography.

Kyphosis

Chief complaint
- *Pain:* present in back, at apex of curve; radiates to legs
- *Joint stiffness:* in involved area or along entire spine
- *Deformity and immobility:* humpback in thoracic region; lordotic curve; hamstring-tendon tightness
- *Sensory changes:* decreased sensation in lower legs

History
- Compression fracture of thoracic vertebrae is a predisposing factor.
- Excessive physical activity
- Recent spinal trauma, osteoporosis, chronic arthritis, tuberculosis

Physical findings
- Prominent vertebral spinous processes at the lower dorsal and upper lumbar levels, with compensatory increased lumbar lordosis
- Limited spinal range of motion; decreased pulmonary function
- Diagnostic studies include X-rays.

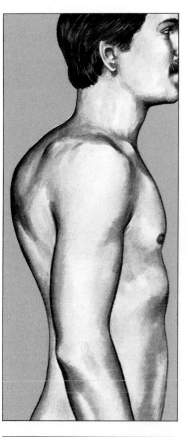

Fracture

Chief complaint
- *Pain:* intensity increases until fragments are set
- *Joint stiffness:* may be present with fracture near joint; crepitation
- *Swelling and redness:* varying degrees of swelling and bleeding into tissues
- *Deformity and immobility:* bone deformity; bone may project through skin; lost or diminished function of fractured part
- *Sensory changes:* if nerves severed, bleeding and swelling cause pressure on nerves; if large vessel severed, blood loss to fractured part

History
- Direct trauma
- Indirect trauma above or below injury site
- Predisposing factors include repeated stress, osteogenic sarcoma, osteoporosis, Paget's disease, hematopoietic diseases, nutritional deficiencies

Physical findings
- Bone contour defect, abnormal bone motion, possibly shock
- Diagnostic studies include X-rays.

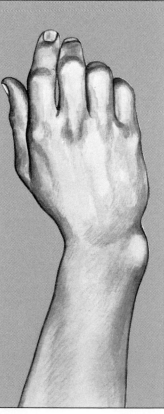

Bursitis

Chief complaint
- *Pain:* sudden or gradual; in chronic form, nagging, intermittent pain
- *Joint stiffness:* inflammation of bursae and calcific deposits in subdeltoid, olecranon (miners' elbow), trochanteric, or prepatellar bursae (housemaid's knee)
- *Swelling and redness:* over affected joint
- *Deformity and immobility:* limited mobility

History
- Predisposing factors include recurring trauma that stresses or presses a joint, occupational stress to joint, and inflammatory joint disease, such as rheumatoid arthritis, gout, and infection.

Physical findings
- Decreased range of motion in affected joint
- Diagnostic studies may include X-rays to identify calcific bursitis.

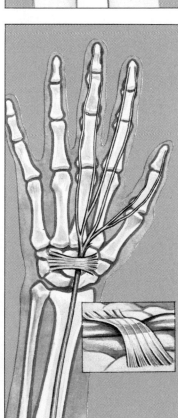

Carpal tunnel syndrome

Chief complaint
- *Pain:* intermittent or constant; intensity increases after manual activity or in the morning and night; radiates up arm, reaching shoulder
- *Swelling and redness:* soft-tissue swelling possible
- *Deformity and immobility:* inability to oppose thumb and little finger and make a fist
- *Sensory changes:* numbness, burning, or tingling in one or both hands; paresthesia affecting thumb and index and middle fingers

History
- Predisposing factors include trauma or injury to wrist, rheumatoid arthritis, gout, myxedema, renal failure, diabetes mellitus, leukemia, edema, nerve compression, Colles' fracture, Reynaud's disease, tuberculosis, and pregnancy.

Physical findings
- Thenar muscle atrophy; positive Tinel's sign; positive Phalen's sign; muscle weakness; dryness of skin over thumb and first two fingers
- Inability to make a fist or oppose thumb and little finger; decreased sensation to touch in affected fingers
- Diagnostic studies may include X-ray and electromyography.

Muscle and bone

Nurses' guide to musculoskeletal disorders continued

Sprain

Chief complaint
- *Pain:* localized and occurring in varying degrees over involved joint, especially during movement
- *Joint stiffness:* present
- *Swelling and redness:* soft-tissue swelling; superficial bruise
- *Deformity and immobility:* limited range of motion
- *Sensory changes:* can be seen in cervical sprain

History
- Sudden twisting injury
- Chronic overuse

Physical findings
- Edema and discoloration around joint; no X-ray changes except soft-tissue swelling; tenderness over joint
- Diagnostic studies include X-ray to rule out a fracture.

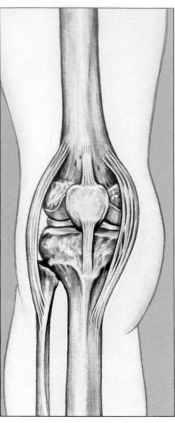

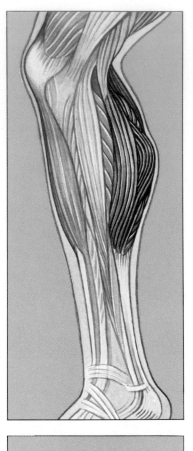

Muscle cramp

Chief complaint
- *Pain:* present; cause unknown
- *Deformity and immobility:* immobility during cramp; deformity also present

History
- Common during pregnancy and in athletes
- Usually occurs at night after strenuous activity

Physical findings
- Muscle is visibly and palpably tight; fasciculations; excessive sweating
- Diagnostic studies include electromyography.

Tenosynovitis

Chief complaint
- *Pain:* insidious or precipitated by strenuous activity; extreme tenderness; may radiate
- *Joint stiffness:* joint locking possible; inflammation common
- *Swelling and redness:* local swelling
- *Deformity and immobility:* deformity increases and immobility decreases with pain

History
- Predisposing factors include calcium deposit of tendon and injury or surgery of involved joint.
- Most common in women in early 40s

Physical findings
- Decreased range of motion; pain on palpation
- Cracking sound with motion; tendons may be swollen
- Diagnostic studies may include X-rays to identify calcium deposits.

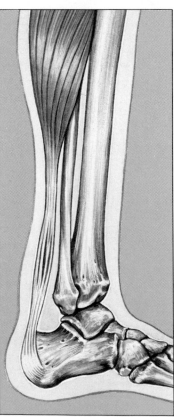

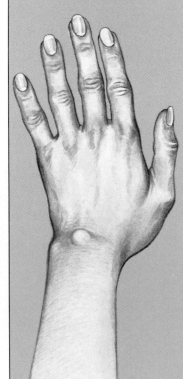

Ganglion

Chief complaint
- *Pain:* continuous aching aggravated by joint motion
- *Joint stiffness:* present
- *Swelling and redness:* gradual swelling over joint; increases with extensive use of affected extremity; tense or fluctuant; rounded; nontender
- *Deformity and immobility:* nodule over joint; weak fingers and joint next to ganglion, if connected to tendon sheath

History
- May occur after trauma, weight gain, compression
- Disappears and recurs
- Onset between adolescence and age 50
- Most common in women

Physical findings
- Limited range of motion of affected joint; palpable nodule more prominent on flexion, less prominent on extension

Meniscal tear

Chief complaint
- *Pain:* acute pain or localized tenderness
- *Swelling and redness:* local swelling
- *Deformity and immobility:* muscle atrophy of quadriceps muscle above knee; inability to straighten knee

History
- Predisposing factors include twisting injury or direct blow to knee and repeated squatting or kneeling.
- Most common in athletes

Physical findings
- Unequal knee contour; positive McMurray sign; blood in joint space
- Diagnostic studies include X-rays and arthroscopy.

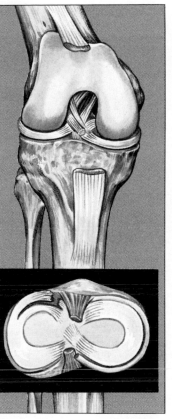

Ligamental tear

Chief complaint
- *Pain:* at joint; tenderness on palpation
- *Joint stiffness:* sensation of slight catching
- *Swelling and redness:* fluid around joint; swelling; ecchymosis
- *Deformity and immobility:* excessive motion at joint
- *Sensory changes:* weakness, instability

History
- Popping sound heard when injury occurred; trauma to joint
- Most common in athletes

Physical findings
- Unstable joint; abnormal range of motion; localized tenderness; changed joint contour

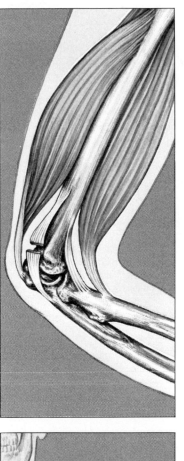

Lower back strain

Chief complaint
- *Pain:* localized, especially with movement; acute and severe, or chronic pain less severe and aching; may radiate down legs along sciatic nerve
- *Joint stiffness:* may be present
- *Swelling and redness:* swelling caused by hemorrhage into surrounding tissues
- *Deformity and immobility:* limited movement

History
- Muscle suddenly forced beyond capacity; trauma; degenerative disk disease; congenital defects of the low lumbar and upper sacral spines (spina bifida occulta) of the lumbosacral area; continued mechanical strain; pregnancy
- Incidence increases with age.
- Obesity

Physical findings
- Tenderness with firm pressure; bruise; muscle spasm; inflammation; decreased range of motion
- Diagnostic studies include X-rays of intervertebral facet joints.

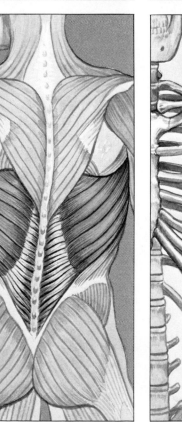

Dislocation (subluxation) of the shoulder

Chief complaint
- *Pain:* localized around involved joint; if from trauma, extreme pain may be accompanied by joint surface fracture
- *Joint stiffness:* present; torn ligaments
- *Swelling and redness:* soft-tissue swelling
- *Deformity and immobility:* displaced bones at joint; muscle atrophy

History
- Traumatic injury
- Predisposing factors include congenital changes in skeletal contour, weakness of dislocation.
- May reduce itself or recur
- Most common in young adults, athletes

Physical findings
- Decreased range of motion; altered joint configuration; changed extremity length
- Diagnostic studies include X-rays of involved joint.

Muscle and bone

Assessing low back pain

You're an occupational health nurse for a company that manufactures auto parts. Roger Storz, a 30-year-old container handler who works in the warehouse, comes to you complaining of low back pain. "It's not too bad when I first get to work," he says, "but by the end of the day, after I've lifted cartons, my back is killing me." Mr. Storz explains that he's had the pain for about a month but thought it might go away.

The guidelines that follow will show you how to perform a thorough low-back–pain assessment.

Explain the procedure to your patient and answer any questions he may have. Ask him to describe the pain. Tell him if he notices numbness, pain, or tingling during your assessment to let you know when and where he's experiencing it. Then, ask him to remove all his clothes, except for his briefs. As he does, note any obvious limitations of movement.

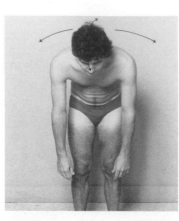

4 Instruct your patient to stand erect, with his arms at his sides, and to bend forward, backward, and to each side. Then, tell him to rotate his upper body. Note any difficulty or pain he has with these movements. Have your patient put on a gown.

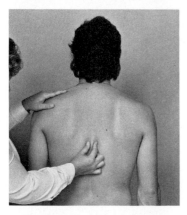

1 If possible, have your patient stand erect, with his arms at his sides. Encourage him to relax. Observe his body build, general posture, and any deformities. Do both of his legs appear to be the same length? Is his pelvis tilted? Is his spine aligned correctly?

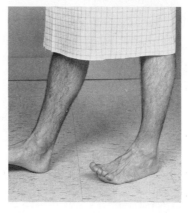

5 To test foot and great toe dorsiflexion, ask your patient to walk across the room on his heels. Note any complaint of pain as well as his posture and balance.

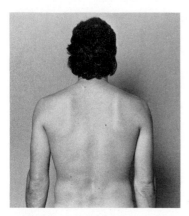

2 With your patient still standing, gently palpate along the spinal column, as shown here. Check for muscle spasms, enlarged nodes, sciatic nerve tenderness, and areas that trigger pain.

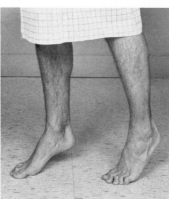

6 Following the same procedure, have Mr. Storz walk on his toes to test calf-muscle function. Note any difficulty he has doing this.

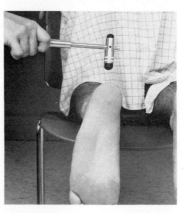

3 Now, compress Mr. Storz's iliac crests, as shown. Note any sacroiliac tenderness.

7 Have Mr. Storz kneel on a chair, with his lower legs extended over the edge of the chair. Use a percussion hammer to check his ankle reflex. Strike the Achilles tendon with the hammer. Then, note how quickly it relaxes after contraction (the muscle should relax in 1 or 2 seconds) as well as any tenderness.

Repeat the test on his left ankle.

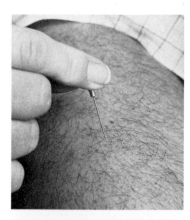

8 Have Mr. Storz remain in the same position while you test his calves and soles for pain sensation. Using a pin, prick his right calf. Ask him to tell you what he feels and when and where he feels it.

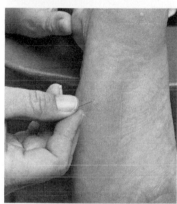

9 Now, following the same procedure, use a pin to prick his sole, as the nurse is doing here. Repeat on his left side.

10 Ask your patient to sit at the edge of an exam table, with his legs dangling. Position yourself facing him. Supporting his right heel with your palm, lift his leg to knee level, as shown here. Return the leg to starting position and repeat on his left leg. Does the movement hurt him? Note it carefully.

11 Now, test your patient's patellar reflex. With your dominant hand, grasp the percussion hammer and strike your patient's patellar tendon, just below the patella. His leg should respond to your action by kicking forward.
Repeat the test on his left knee.

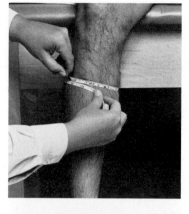

12 Next, measure the widest part of your patient's right calf, as the nurse is doing here. Then, measure the widest part of his left calf. Compare measurements to detect muscle atrophy. Also, measure the widest part of his thighs and note any differences.

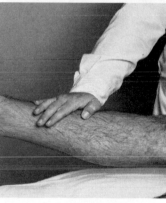

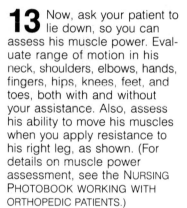

13 Now, ask your patient to lie down, so you can assess his muscle power. Evaluate range of motion in his neck, shoulders, elbows, hands, fingers, hips, knees, feet, and toes, both with and without your assistance. Also, assess his ability to move his muscles when you apply resistance to his right leg, as shown. (For details on muscle power assessment, see the NURSING PHOTOBOOK WORKING WITH ORTHOPEDIC PATIENTS.)

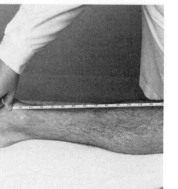

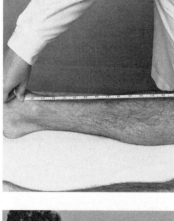

14 Then, measure the length of each leg from the anterior superior iliac spine to the medial malleolus, as the nurse is doing here. Compare measurements, noting any differences.

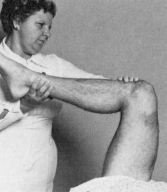

15 Place your palm under Mr. Storz's right heel and bend his knee, guiding his thigh toward his chest, as shown here. Straighten the leg and lower it. Repeat with his left leg. Note any pain or tenderness.

Muscle and bone

Assessing low back pain continued

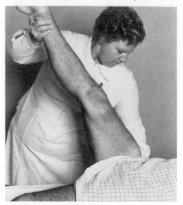

16 Still supporting Mr. Storz's right heel, raise his leg as high as possible. As you do, use your other hand to palpate his spine. Feel for any flat areas that may indicate lumbar lordosis.
Repeat with his left leg.

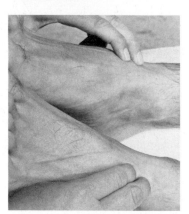

17 Now, check peripheral pulses in his legs bilaterally, as the nurse is doing in this photo.

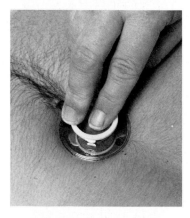

18 Using a stethoscope, auscultate each of your patient's abdominal quadrants. Listen for normal bowel sounds as well as for friction rubs (may indicate a hepatic tumor or splenic infarct), for bruits (may indicate aneurysm or partial arterial obstruction), and for venous hums (may indicate hepatic cirrhosis).

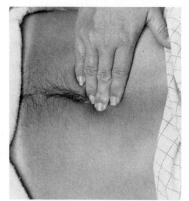

19 If your patient doesn't have any abdominal pain, palpate each abdominal quadrant. Check for tenderness and any masses, which may cause referred back pain.

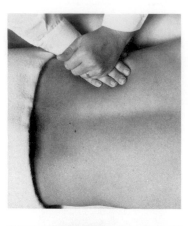

20 Instruct Mr. Storz to lie on his stomach, if possible. Percuss the renal area. To do this, place your right palm on your patient's back, slightly to the right of his costovertebral angle. Hit the back of your right hand with your left fist. Note any tenderness.

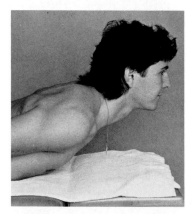

21 Next, palpate your patient's lower back, as the nurse is doing here. Note any local tenderness or muscle spasms.

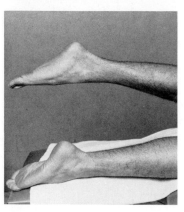

22 Maintaining the same position, have your patient hyperextend his spine. To do this, have him lift his upper body off the table. Tell him to return to starting position. Note any difficulty or pain.

23 Then, have Mr. Storz hyperextend his right leg as high as possible. Instruct him to repeat the exercise with his left leg. Note any difficulty.
You'll also need to perform a rectal and pelvic exam (if your patient's female) and obtain blood and urine specimens for lab tests. If ordered, arrange for lumbar and thoracic X-rays.
Document your findings and observations. If you note any abnormalities, refer the patient, as indicated.

Home care

How to strengthen your back

Dear Patient:

To help reduce your low back pain, you need to build strong and flexible supporting muscles. By exercising for about 30 minutes each day, you can keep your back healthy and fit.

For maximum effectiveness, perform each exercise slowly—don't overdo it. Perform all the exercises the nurse has circled on these sheets in the morning and before dinner. Repeat each exercise five times. *Important:* Don't exercise if you have pain. And if you feel pain while you're exercising, stop immediately and notify your doctor.

Also, be sure to keep in mind the following guidelines as you perform your day-to-day activities.

• When preparing to lift an object, keep your back and upper body straight and flex your knees and hips. Use your palms—not your fingertips—to get a good grip on the object you're lifting. Always hold the object close to your body, and use your leg and hip muscles to stand upright. If the load is too heavy for you to lift by yourself, get help. And remember: To prevent injuries, never lift an object above shoulder level or change direction by twisting your back.

• When standing and walking for long periods, wear comfortable shoes. Remember, too, the importance of maintaining good posture; keep your head erect, shoulders back, back straight, and feet slightly apart. Pull in your abdomen and flex your knees slightly.

• When driving, position the seat so your knees are bent and higher than your hips. Keep both hands on the wheel. Remember that stretching for the pedals and steering wheel increases lower back curve and pain.

• When sitting, select a chair low enough so you can place both your feet on the floor. Hold your head and body erect and keep your hips at a 90° angle to your trunk. Push against the back of the chair. Make sure your weight's resting on your thighs and the widest part of your pelvis.

• When sleeping, select a firm mattress and try lying on your side, with your knees bent.

1 Begin your exercise program by warming up. To proceed, lie on your back, with your knees bent and feet flat on the floor. Keep your arms at your sides. Bend and extend your arms and legs as you alternately tighten and relax your muscles.

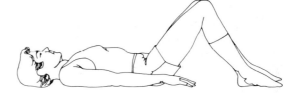

2 To help relax a stiff back, try this exercise. Lie on your back, with your knees bent and feet flat on the floor. Bring your right knee toward your chest. Clasp your hands around your knee and hold for 5 seconds. Return your knee to starting position and repeat with your left knee. Then, repeat the exercise, raising both knees simultaneously. *Note:* Don't lift your legs with your hands.

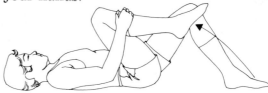

3 This exercise reduces swayback by strengthening your front and back muscles. Maintain the same position—lying on your back with knees bent. Now, tighten your buttock muscles and hold for 5 seconds. Take care to keep your lower spine flat on the floor. Relax your muscles.

Muscle and bone

Home care

How to strengthen your back continued

4 To stretch your hamstrings, lie flat on your back, bend your left knee, and extend your right leg in front of you. Raise your right leg as far as possible and hold for 5 seconds. Lower your right leg and repeat the exercise with your left leg.

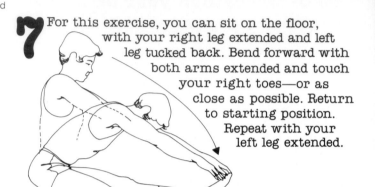

5 To strengthen your abdominal muscles, maintain the same position, with both legs extended in front of you. Clasp your hands under your right knee. Then, as you bring your knee toward your chest, raise your head and touch your nose to your knee. Hold for 5 seconds and return to starting position. Repeat with your left leg.

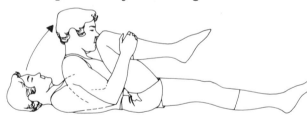

6 To strengthen your abdominal and back muscles, maintain the same position, with your knees bent and feet flat on the floor. As you raise your head and neck to the top of your chest, reach forward with both hands to touch your knees. Hold for 5 seconds and return to starting position.

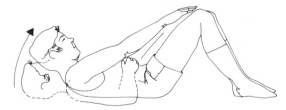

7 For this exercise, you can sit on the floor, with your right leg extended and left leg tucked back. Bend forward with both arms extended and touch your right toes—or as close as possible. Return to starting position. Repeat with your left leg extended.

8 This exercise is more difficult; get your doctor's approval before proceeding.

To begin, lie flat on the floor, with your knees bent, and raise both legs until balanced. Lock your hands behind your head. Slowly move your legs back and forth in a scissorlike motion 10 times, alternating right leg over left leg, then left leg over right leg. Return to starting position and repeat one time.

9 Here's another advanced exercise; get your doctor's approval before proceeding.

Then, lie on your abdomen, with your legs extended. Keeping your legs straight, slowly raise your right leg from the hip and return to starting position. Be sure to keep your pelvis flat against the floor and your leg straight. Repeat the exercise with your left leg.

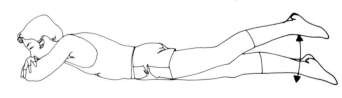

Learning about scoliosis

If you're a school nurse, you see children in an active phase of growth every day. This is why you're in an excellent position to detect early signs of scoliosis, *before* permanent damage can occur. After all, this condition is the most common vertebral column abnormality in adolescents.

As you probably know, scoliosis is a lateral curvature of the spinal column that may be found in the thoracic, lumbar, or thoracolumbar segments of the spine. The curve may be convex to the right, which is more common in thoracic curves, or to the left, which is more common in lumbar curves. Scoliosis is often associated with kyphosis (humpback) and lordosis (swayback). Scoliosis may also cause a rib cage deformity from rotation of the vertebral column around its axis.

Types of scoliosis

Two major forms of scoliosis exist: functional (postural) and structural. *Functional* scoliosis usually results from poor posture or from a discrepancy in leg length because no *fixed* spinal deformity is present. It involves

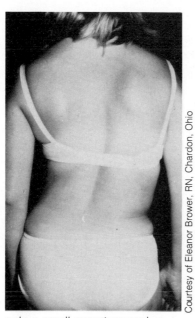

Courtesy of Eleanor Brower, RN, Chardon, Ohio

only a small curvature and corrects itself when the patient bends.

Structural scoliosis, as shown above, results from a vertebral body deformity. This type of scoliosis may be:
• congenital, usually associated with wedge vertebrae, fused ribs or vertebrae, or hemivertebrae
• paralytic or musculoskeletal, developing several months after asymmetric paralysis of trunk muscles caused by cerebral palsy, muscular dystrophy, or polio
• idiopathic, probably hereditary and the most common form of structural scoliosis, accounting for about 75% of scoliosis cases. This form usually appears in a previously straight spine during the child's growing years. Idiopathic scoliosis is subdivided into *infantile,* which affects mostly male infants between birth and age 3, causing left thoracic and right lumbar curves; *juvenile,* which affects boys and girls between ages 4 and 10 equally, causing varying types of curvature; and *adolescent,* which primarily affects girls during the adolescent growth years, beginning around age 10, causing varying types of curvature.

Signs and symptoms

What are the signs and symptoms of scoliosis? Most often, the patient has a major convex curve to the right in the thoracic vertebral area, with compensatory curves to the left in the cervical area above and over the lumbar area below. These compensatory curves develop to maintain body balance and cause or mark the deformity.

Only when the condition's well established may other symptoms develop, such as fatigue, backache, and dyspnea. The family or patient may notice such signs as uneven hemlines or pant legs that appear unequal in length.

Complications

Why is scoliosis assessment so important? If untreated, scoliosis may progress, even *after* skeletal maturity's reached. And progressive scoliosis may cause such complications as compromised cardiopulmonary function, from constriction of the rib cage; neurologic disorders; urinary problems; back pain; degenerative arthritis of the spine; disk disease, sciatica; as well as psychosocial problems stemming from physical deformity. But when scoliosis is detected and treated early, before growth is complete, most mild, progressive curvatures can be arrested without surgery. When surgery's performed at an early stage of the disease, the procedure's usually more successful.

Reviewing scoliosis treatment

Treatment for scoliosis depends on the deformity's severity and the patient's potential for spine growth. Treatment options include close observation, exercise, a brace, surgery, or any combination of these therapies. To ensure effectiveness, treatment should begin early, when the spinal deformity is mild.

For a mild curve

If the patient has a curve of less than 25°, the doctor monitors the deformity by taking spinal X-rays and performing a physical exam every 3 months. He may also recommend exercises, such as situps and pelvic tilts, to strengthen the torso muscles, which keep the curve from progressing. And if the patient's legs are unequal in length, the doctor will suggest that a heel lift be applied to one shoe.

For a moderate curve

If the patient has a curve ranging from 30° to 50°, the doctor may order a brace and exercises to strengthen the patient's spine. The brace halts progression of the condition in about 90% of patients. But it doesn't reverse an existing curve. A brace is most effective when the curve is mild.

If the doctor orders a brace for your patient, he'll probably select a Milwaukee brace, which consists of a leather or plastic girdle that supports an anterior and two posterior metal upright bars connected to a neck ring. It must be worn 23 hours a day until bone growth is complete— about 1 to 4 years, depending on when treatment begins.

The brace can be adjusted as the patient grows. At the end of treatment, he must be weaned gradually from the brace.

Note: The doctor may choose an orthoplast jacket, which serves the same purpose as the Milwaukee brace and is less noticeable under clothing.

For a severe curve

If the patient has a curve of 50° or more, the doctor usually performs surgery (spinal fusion) to correct the deformity. If the curve is 60° or more, surgery is the only method of correcting the deformity. In addition to correcting the curvature, surgery can prevent deteriorating cardiopulmonary function, neurologic dysfunction from distortion of the spinal cord, and severe back pain.

To correct surgically a curvature of more than 60°, the doctor may stabilize the affected vertebral bodies with a Harrington rod. Preoperative preparation may include immobilization in a Risser cast, a localizer cast that immobilizes the trunk in alignment and applies traction longitudinally.

An alternate surgical procedure is the Dwyer instrumentation and spinal fusion. During this operation, the doctor uses a screw to transfix each of the vertebral bodies. Then, he positions grafted bone from a rib or iliac crest segments between the vertebral bodies. Next, a cable is passed through the screw eyes along each of the curve's segments. To facilitate bone fusion, the doctor applies tension to the cable.

Muscle and bone

Performing a scoliosis screening

To detect signs of scoliosis in children, consider setting up a school-sponsored screening program. This way you'll be able to assess a greater number of children. Of course, your assessment will be preliminary. Depending on your working protocol, you'll refer any child with signs of scoliosis to his family doctor or to an orthopedic specialist for further evaluation.

Arrange to screen all children between ages 8 and 15. If necessary, enlist the help of parents, community health nurses, teachers, volunteers, and other trained professionals.

Use an assessment form like the one shown on the opposite page to note your findings. Instruct any co-workers to do the same. Refer to the form frequently during the screening procedure to be sure you cover all assessment points. When you finish a child's screening, review the assessment form. If you've made an entry in the Present block for any item, summarize your findings in the space marked Examiner's observations. *If you detect signs of scoliosis in a child, send a note home with him, explaining your findings and advising the parent or guardian that further evaluation is necessary.*

Before the screening, explain its purpose to the children, teachers, and parents. Tell them the screening helps detect back problems, and assure them the procedure's painless. Answer any questions they may have.

Keep in mind that you'll have to screen the boys and girls separately, so try to schedule the screening during gym class. Instruct the boys to bring gym trunks to wear that day and have them strip to the waist. Tell the girls they can wear underpants and bras (if they wear them) or two-piece swimsuits. Important: *To ensure proper spinal visualization, don't allow the girls to wear one-piece swimsuits or leotards.*

Here's how to proceed.

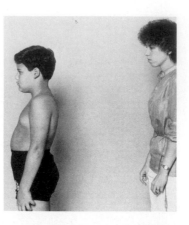

2 Next, ask your patient to turn so his back is facing you. Observe for uneven shoulders, a prominent shoulder blade, uneven hips, and vertebral column deviation to one side. Note your observations on the chart.

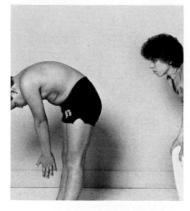

3 Have your patient bend forward, extend his arms toward the floor, and clasp his hands. Look for a bulge or prominence on one side of his back (rib hump). If present, suspect structural scoliosis. Note your observations.

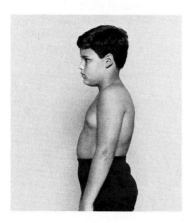

1 First, place a tape strip on the floor where you want the patient to stand. Then, seat yourself about 2' (61 cm) away. Instruct the patient to stand on the tape, with one side facing you. Have him keep his hands at his sides and hold his body erect. As he does, check for postural abnormalities, such as humpback and swayback. Then, have him turn to the other side, so he's facing you. Note all observations on the assessment chart.

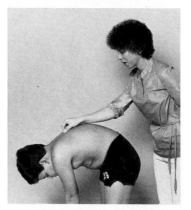

4 Have the patient maintain the same position as you palpate the vertebral processes at the base of his neck. Continue palpating the processes along the length of his spine, as shown here. Check for correct alignment and prominence.

Document your findings on the assessment chart and take action, as indicated.

Using a scoliometer

If, after completing your visual examination, you suspect your patient has a spinal curvature, use a scoliometer (see photo) to determine the angle of his upper body rotation. To do this, ask your patient to clasp his hands and bend forward. This way any rib hump that's present will be as pronounced as possible. Place the scoliometer's axis across the patient's back at the level of maximum deformity. Note the number of degrees. Of course, if your patient's back has two curves, you'll need to obtain two measurements.

If your patient has rotation of 5° or more, refer him for a more detailed evaluation. If the rotation is less than 5°, repeat the screening procedure in 6 months to 1 year.

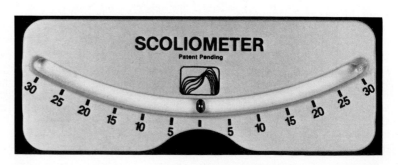

Scoliosis Assessment Chart

Name: _____ Date: _____ Date of follow-up appointment with doctor: _____

Examiner: _____ Appointment kept: Yes _____ No _____

Recommendations: _____

_____

Examiner's observations: _____

_____

1. Head does not line up over crease of buttocks.

☐ Present

☐ Absent

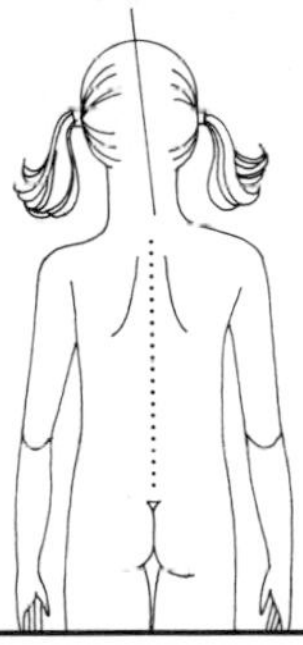

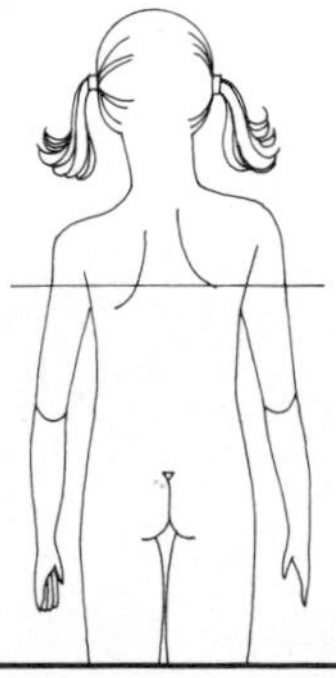

4. Rib cage on one side is prominent.

☐ Present

☐ Absent

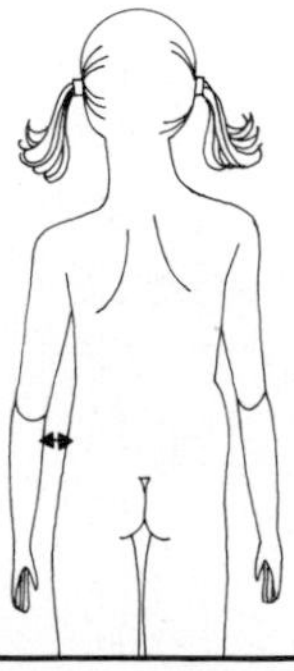

7. One side of waist has deep crease.

☐ Present

☐ Absent

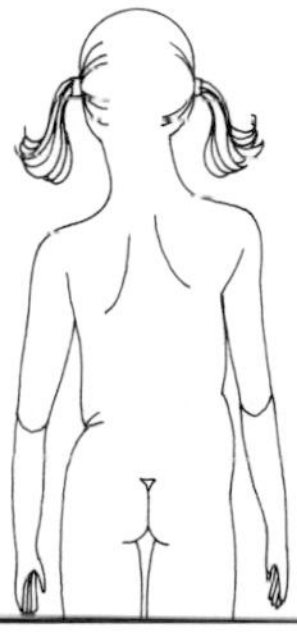

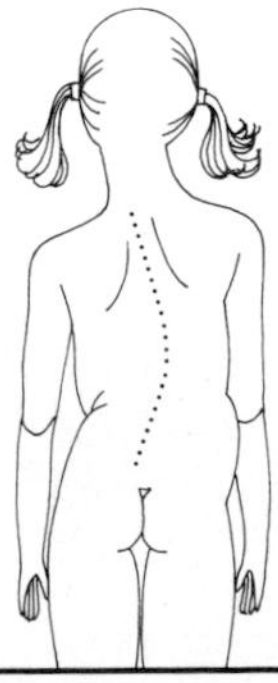

10. Patient tends to lean toward one side.

☐ Present

☐ Absent

2. One shoulder is higher than the other.

☐ Present

☐ Absent

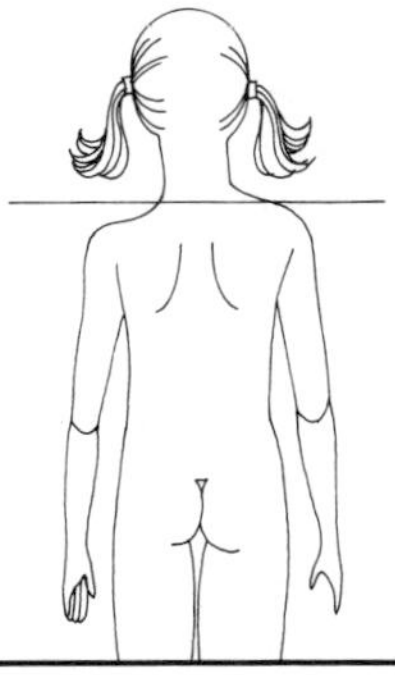

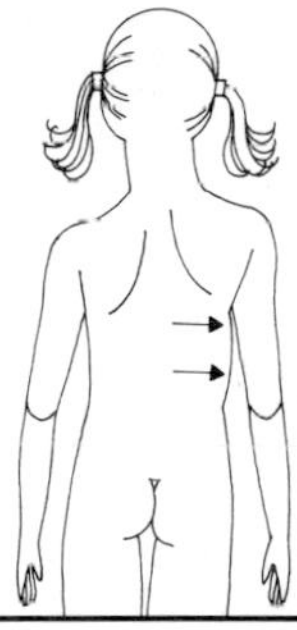

5. Hip on one side is higher or more prominent.

☐ Present

☐ Absent

8. Waist appears fuller on one side.

☐ Present

☐ Absent

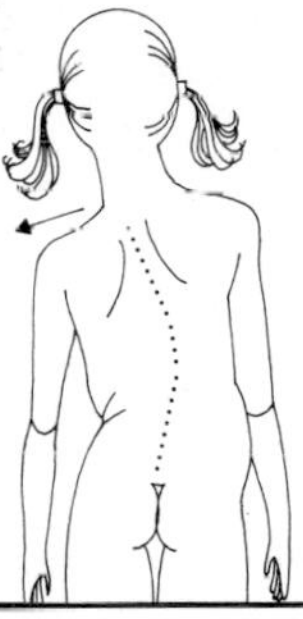

11. One side of back has posterior rib hump.

☐ Present

☐ Absent

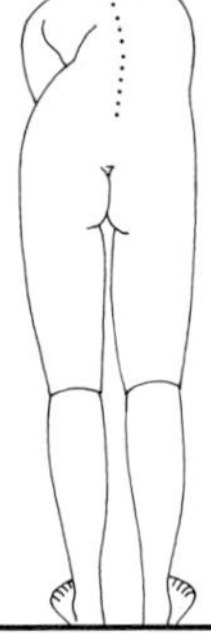

3. Scapula on one side is higher or more prominent.

☐ Present

☐ Absent

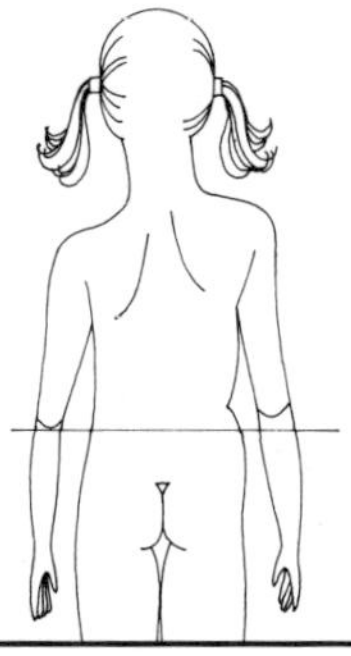

6. When arms are held loosely adducted, distance is unequal between arms and body.

☐ Present

☐ Absent

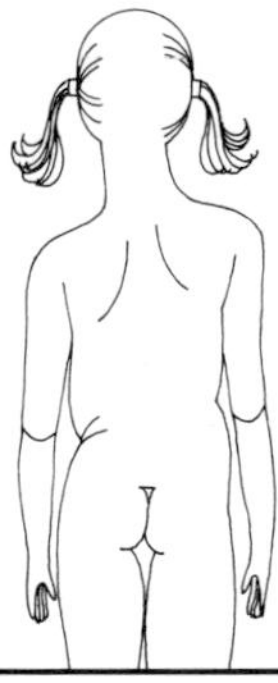

9. Spine appears to curve to one side.

☐ Present

☐ Absent

12. Symmetry of the upper back, and/or lower back is unequal.

☐ Present

☐ Absent

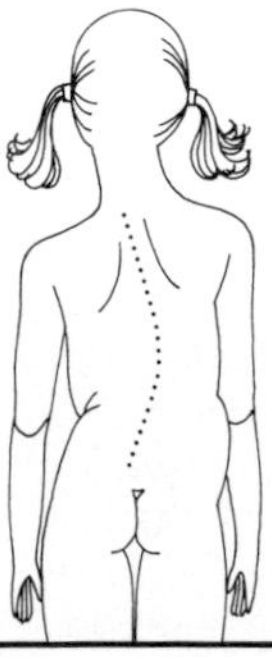

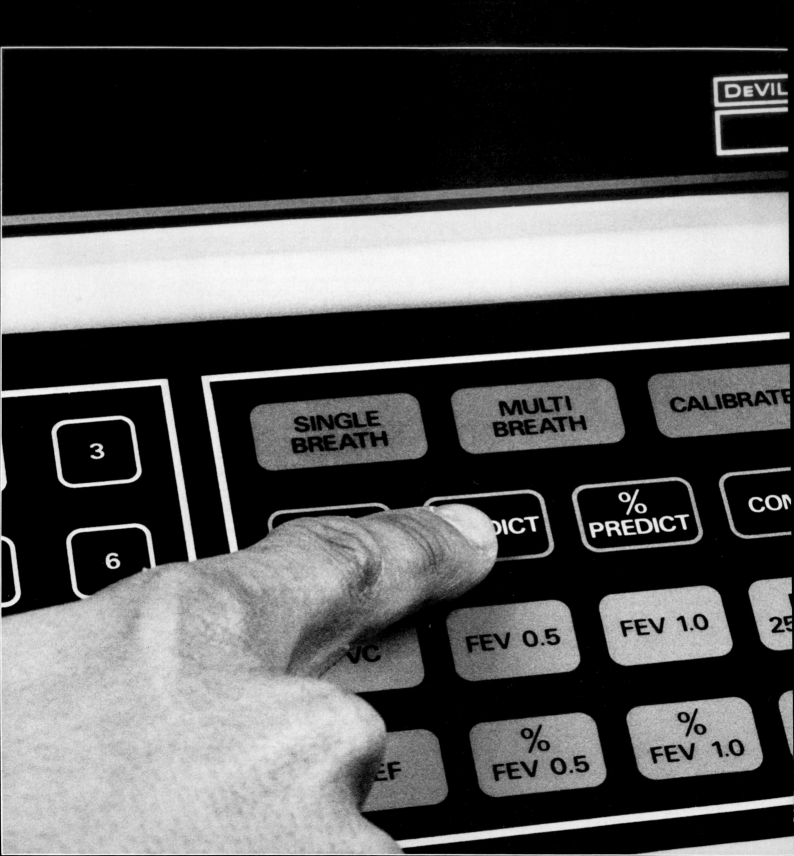

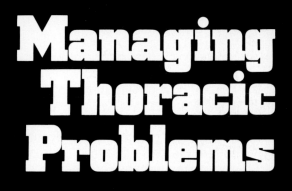

Managing Thoracic Problems

Heart

Lungs

Heart

Detecting and caring for cardiovascular problems can be difficult if you're unfamiliar with the procedures and equipment. How well do you understand stress testing? For example: Do you know how to prepare a patient for this procedure and why it's important?

Can you operate a portable microprocessor electrocardiograph? Do you know what signs and symptoms differentiate a myocardial infarction from angina? Do you know how to teach a patient to take his blood pressure?

On the following pages we answer these questions. So by studying this information, you can assess and care for your patient's heart confidently and knowledgeably.

Cardiovascular warning signs: What they suggest

Many of the cardiovascular warning signs you'll encounter in a patient are detailed here. Study the information carefully. By familiarizing yourself with the signs and symptoms of cardiovascular problems now, you'll be better able to recognize and care for such a patient with these signs and symptoms later.

But first, let's review three common indicators of possible cardiac problems:

• **Peripheral cyanosis**
Check the patient's nail beds and lips for this sign. Consider this sign normal if your patient's anxious or cold. But it may indicate decreased cardiac output, causing vasoconstriction.

• **Central cyanosis**
Check the patient's lips, underside of tongue, tip of the nose, nail beds, and ear helices for this sign. If present, your patient may have a congenital heart defect, especially when blood's shunted from venous to arterial circulation, or prolonged hypoxia.
Important: If your patient's dark-skinned, check the nose, the cheeks, and the mucosa inside the lips. Also look for pale gray facial skin. For details on skin assessment, see pages 65 and 66.

• **Edema**
Check for fluid accumulation in the interstitial tissues (most evident in dependent body parts, such as the feet, legs, and sacrum). If present, your patient may have chronic right-sided heart failure.

Here are additional signs and symptoms that'll alert you to cardiac problems:

Dry, brittle hair
What it suggests: poor nutrition, possibly from cardiac impairment or vascular insufficiency

Diagonal earlobe crease (McCarthy's sign)
What it suggests: coronary artery disease

Subtle up and down head movements in synchronization with heartbeat (Musset's sign)

What it suggests: aortic aneurysm or insufficiency

Yellow plaque (xanthelasma) on eyelids or elbows
What it suggests: chronic elevated serum cholesterol

Gray ring at junction of iris and sclera
What it suggests: elevated serum cholesterol

Pulsation in epigastric aorta
What it suggests: abdominal aortic aneurysm

Absent or sparse body hair
What it suggests: vascular insufficiency (arterial or venous)

Nail clubbing (increased fingertip depth; swollen, spongy nail bases; straight angle between nail and nail base)
What it suggests: cardiac or pulmonary disease from low oxygen saturation of arterial blood

Dry, cool skin
What it suggests: poor nutrition from impaired oxygen delivery to hands and feet

Series of blood pressure readings higher than 140/90
What it suggests: hypertension

Jugular vein distention greater than 3 cm above sternal angle (when patient's head is at a 45° angle)
What it suggests: hypovolemia, right-sided heart failure, pericardial tamponade, or constrictive pericarditis

Hepatojugular reflux (momentary pressure on liver causes sudden jugular vein distention)
What it suggests: right-sided heart failure

Lung rales
What it suggests: left-sided heart failure with pulmonary edema

Taking a cardiovascular history

You're probably aware of the high incidence of heart disease and the seriousness of its complications. Not only does heart disease affect people of all ages, it also occurs in many forms. Heart disease can be congenital or acquired, and it can develop suddenly or insidiously. This is why taking an accurate and complete cardiovascular history is so important. Some questions you may want to ask include:
• Do you have chest pain? How would you characterize the pain? For example, does it burn or produce a squeezing sensation? Where in your chest do you feel the pain? How long does an attack last?
• Have you ever experienced shortness of breath? When?
• Do you tire easily? What activity causes you to feel tired?
• Does your heart pound or beat fast? Does your heart ever skip a beat or seem to jump? Do you ever faint or experience dizziness? When?
• Does your weight fluctuate or have you gained weight recently? How much have you gained?
• Have you experienced any pain or discomfort in your arms or legs? Do you feel pain or cramps in your legs when you walk?
• Have you ever had your blood pressure taken? Can you recall what it was?
• Have you ever been told you have sugar in your urine? Have you ever had a test for blood sugar?
• Did you ever have rheumatic fever or frequent streptococcal infections? Were you ever told you had a heart murmur?
• Have you ever taken diuretic (water or fluid) pills?
• Have you ever been told by your doctor that you have high cholesterol or triglyceride levels?
• Describe what you eat in a typical day.
• Do you drink alcoholic or caffeinic beverages? How much?
• Do you use salt? How much?
• Do you exercise daily? What type of exercise do you do?

Performing a complete blood pressure check

The doctor's ordered weekly blood pressure checks at your clinic for Frank Lott, a 38-year-old accountant with hypertension. To establish a baseline reading, the doctor wants you to take Mr. Lott's blood pressure in both arms while he's sitting, standing, and lying down. Note: When the check is complete, indicate which arm has the higher pressure. In subsequent checks, start with this arm. Do you know how to perform a thorough blood pressure check? If you're unsure, follow these steps:

First, have your patient sit comfortably in a quiet area. Explain the procedure and ask him how he feels. As you talk with him, try to identify any factors that may affect his blood pressure reading, such as recent stress, excessive physical activity, a large meal, or any medications (even over-the-counter drugs) he may be taking. If in response to your questions he says, "I ate dinner about an hour ago," note this on his blood pressure form.

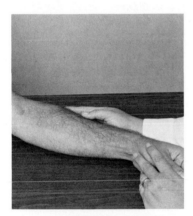

1 Next, tell Mr. Lott to flex his right arm slightly at the elbow and support his forearm at heart level on a smooth surface, such as a table. Then, have your patient roll up his sleeve. Check to be sure the sleeve is not constricting his arm.

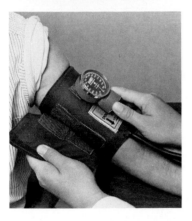

2 Now, wrap the deflated blood pressure cuff around your patient's upper arm so the bottom edge is approximately ¾" (2 cm) above the antecubital space, as shown here. The cuff should be directly over the brachial artery. Check to be sure the inflatable rubber bladder inside the cuff is over the arm's inner aspect—and clear of the rolled sleeve—and that the cuff's secured properly.

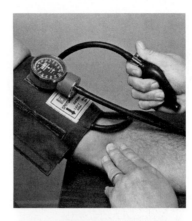

3 Palpate Mr. Lott's brachial artery. As you do, inflate the cuff as quickly as possible. When the pulse you're feeling is gone, pump an extra 20 to 30 mm Hg.

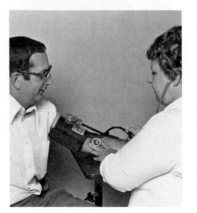

4 Place the stethoscope's diaphragm over Mr. Lott's brachial artery. Now, release the cuff, as the nurse is doing here. At the first return of sound, note the reading. This reading is your patient's systolic pressure.

5 As you continue to release the cuff, listen for a damping or muffling sound. When you hear it, note the reading. This is the diastolic pressure. Then, repeat the procedure on your patient's opposite arm. Document the blood pressure according to the arm used.

Following the same steps, take your patient's blood pressure in both arms while he's lying down and standing. Document your findings.

Ensuring an accurate blood pressure reading

Is your patient's blood pressure reading accurate? It may be falsely elevated if you're:
• using too narrow a cuff. Make sure the cuff bladder is 20% wider than the circumference of the extremity being used for the reading. Keep this in mind when taking a thigh pressure or the blood pressure of an obese person.
• wrapping the cuff too loosely or deflating the cuff too slowly.
• tilting the mercury column away from the vertical.
• viewing the mercury column from more than 3' (91 cm) away.
• holding the mercury column above eye level.
• taking a reading in a patient who is upset, has just eaten or exercised, or has a distended bladder.

Your patient's blood pressure reading may be falsely low if you're:
• using too wide a cuff.
• positioning his arm above heart level.
• holding the mercury column below eye level.
• failing to notice an auscultatory gap; for example, when the sound returns after fading out for 10 to 15 mm Hg. To avoid this, be sure to palpate your patient's radial artery as you pump the cuff.
• unable to hear feeble sounds. If you can't hear any sound, ask your patient to raise his arm before you inflate the cuff again. Doing so usually makes the sounds louder. Have your patient lower his arm, and then deflate the cuff and listen. If you still can't hear anything, document the palpatory systolic pressure.

Heart

Differentiating chest pain

Whenever you assess a patient's chest pain, you'll need to evaluate pain location, radiation, character, onset, and duration as well as associated signs and symptoms, such as nausea, vomiting, dyspnea, and diaphoresis. When combined with other assessment data, this information helps you identify the type of chest pain as well as possible precipitating factors and methods of relief.

Study the chart below to review how to differentiate between various types of chest pain.

Angina pectoris

Description
- Squeezing, vicelike, heavy pressure pain in substernal or retrosternal area (not sharply localized)
- Radiates to back, neck, arms, jaws, upper abdomen, and fingers
- Gradual or sudden onset; pain usually lasts less than 15 minutes and not longer than 30 minutes

Other signs and symptoms
- Dyspnea
- Diaphoresis
- Nausea
- Elevated blood pressure and increased heart rate immediately before or occurring at onset
- Belching
- Apprehension
- Desire to void

Precipitating factors
- Physical exertion, including sexual intercourse
- Cold or hot, humid weather
- Emotional stress
- Eating
- Supine position

Nursing considerations
- Advise the patient to avoid precipitating factors; for example, tell him to eat several small meals a day and not to lie flat on his back.
- Administer nitrates sublingually, as ordered. Remind the patient to take medication before performing activities he knows will precipitate anginal pain.

Esophageal pain

Description
- Burning or dull knotlike pain (simulating angina) in substernal or retrosternal area
- Radiates around chest to shoulders
- Sudden onset; pain usually lasts less than 20 minutes; may occur after meals or when assuming supine position.

Other signs and symptoms
- Nausea
- Regurgitation
- Vomiting

Precipitating factors
- Eating
- May occur spontaneously

Nursing considerations
- Instruct the patient to take antacids, as ordered.
- Tell the patient to avoid lying flat on his back. Suggest he try sitting up for pain relief.
- Advise the patient to eat several small meals daily. Remind him to avoid spicy foods.

Chest wall syndrome

Description
- Localized aching pain or soreness and swelling in costochondral, chondrosternal, or xiphoid sternal joints (pain location simulates angina)
- May begin as dull ache, increasing in intensity over a few days; usually long lasting

Other signs and symptoms
- Edema over pain site
- Local pressure simulates pain
- Pain worsens with deep breathing and movement, causing the patient to display shallow, splinted respirations that may lead to hypoventilation.
- Administration of local anesthetic into affected rib cartilage relieves pain (also a method of relief).

Precipitating factors
- Chest wall movement from exercise, coughing, sneezing, deep breathing
- Chest trauma such as from an automobile accident (patient thrown against steering wheel)

Nursing considerations
- Administer analgesics, as ordered.
- Apply heat to pain site.
- Prepare patient for local anesthetic injection at pain site, as ordered.

Mediastinal emphysema

Description
- Severe pain (simulating myocardial infarction) in substernal, midline, or retrosternal areas; may be associated with spontaneous pneumothorax
- Radiates to jaws, neck, back, shoulder, and one or both arms
- Insidious onset

Other signs and symptoms
- Crunching sound synchronous with heartbeat heard along left sternal border (Hamman's sign)
- Palpable subcutaneous crepitations at base of neck possible
- Dyspnea
- Tactile fremitus
- Tympanic percussion sounds
- X-ray may show air accumulation in mediastinum.

Precipitating factors
- Cigarette smoking
- Deficiency of alpha$_1$-antitrypsin
- Spontaneous pneumothorax

Nursing considerations
- Administer oxygen to treat hypoxia, as ordered.
- Advise the patient to stop smoking and avoid air pollution.
- Administer antibiotics, as ordered, to treat respiratory tract infection; influenza virus vaccine to prevent influenza; and pneumococcal pneumonia vaccine for immunizations.
- Give bronchodilators, such as aminophylline, to reverse bronchospasm and promote mucociliary clearance.

Peptic ulcer disease

Description
- Localized burning pain in epigastric area, with radiation to shoulders
- Sudden onset

Other signs and symptoms
- Heartburn and indigestion
- Severe back pain possible
- Weight loss or gain
- Repeated episodes of massive gastrointestinal bleeding

Precipitating factors
- Empty stomach (more than 2 hours between meals)
- Ingestion of alcoholic or caffeinic beverages, orange juice, or aspirin
- Nocturnal fasting

Nursing considerations
- Instruct the patient to eat several small meals daily. Advise him to avoid spicy foods.
- Administer antacids, as ordered.
- Warn the patient to avoid aspirin-containing drugs, excessive use of caffeinic beverages, stressful situations, and alcoholic beverages.
- Advise the patient to stop smoking, because it stimulates gastric secretions.

Anxiety

Description
- Stabbing pain, tightness or choking sensation, or vague discomfort in left chest area
- Sudden onset; may last less than a minute or for an hour or longer (not brought on by exertion)

Other signs and symptoms
- Dyspnea
- Restlessness, sleeplessness
- Palpitations
- Tachycardia
- Hyperventilation
- Diaphoresis
- Appetite changes
- Repetitive questions
- Skeletal muscle tension (headache; muscle spasm in back, neck, or chest)
- Gastrointestinal disorders (abdominal pain, belching, heartburn, anorexia, nausea, diarrhea, constipation)
- Transient hypertension
- Genitourinary dysfunction (frequent urination, dysuria, impotence, frigidity) possible

Precipitating factors
- Fatigue (sometimes)
- Emotional distress
- Perceived physical threat (inability to meet needs for food, water, necessities of life)
- Perceived psychologic threat (rejection, loss of approval from loved one, unmet emotional needs)

Nursing considerations
- Administer tranquilizers, such as diazepam, chlordiazepoxide, or clorazepate dipotassium, as ordered.
- Instruct the patient to lie down and concentrate on breathing normally.
- Encourage the patient to find alternate ways to deal with anxiety-provoking situations.

Pulmonary origin

(Pleuritis, pulmonary embolism)

Description
- *For pleuritis:* stabbing pain
- *For pulmonary embolism:* angina-like pain
- Sudden onset; may last several days

Other signs and symptoms
- *In pleuritis and pulmonary embolism:* dyspnea
- *In pulmonary embolism:* productive cough possible (sputum may be blood-tinged), low-grade fever, tachycardia, pleural effusion

Precipitating factors
- *In pleuritis:* history of pneumonia, tuberculosis, viruses, systemic lupus erythematosus, rheumatoid arthritis, uremia, Dressler's syndrome, malignancy, pulmonary infarction, and chest trauma
- *In pulmonary embolism:* dislodged thrombi originating in leg veins

Nursing considerations
- Administer antibiotics for infection, as ordered.
- For pulmonary embolism, administer oxygen by mask or nasal cannula, or anticoagulant, as ordered.

Myocardial infarction

Description
- Crushing, heavy, vicelike pain in substernal midline or retrosternal area (approximately 15% of patients are pain-free)
- Radiates to jaws, neck, back, shoulders, and one or both arms (simulates angina)
- Sudden onset; pain usually lasts ½ to 2 hours; residual soreness lasts 1 to 3 days.

Other signs and symptoms
- Dyspnea
- Nausea
- Vomiting
- Diaphoresis
- Sensation of impending doom
- Apprehension
- Weakness
- Gallop heart sound (atrial or ventricular)
- Hypotension
- Marked differences in blood pressures
- Absence of pulses may occur in arms or legs
- Cardiac murmurs
- Bradycardia
- Angina of increasing frequency, severity, or duration

Precipitating factors
- Hypertension
- Smoking
- Positive family history
- Aging
- Stress
- Obesity
- Diabetes
- Elevated triglyceride and cholesterol levels
- May occur at rest or during physical exertion
- Emotional stress
- Sedentary life-style or a Type A personality (aggressive, addiction to work)

Nursing considerations
- Administer morphine or meperidine I.V., as ordered.
- Administer oxygen, as needed.
- Provide complete bed rest to decrease cardiac overload.
- Give atropine I.V., or the doctor may insert a temporary pacemaker to treat heart block
- Administer lidocaine for ventricular arrhythmias and nitroglycerin or isosorbide dinitrate to relieve pain by redistributing blood supply, as ordered. Prepare patient for surgery, if indicated.
- Prepare patient for cardiac catheterization, as ordered.
- Provide emotional support.

Pericarditis

Description
- Mild to severe stabbing pain in substernal area to left of midline
- Radiates to neck, shoulders, back, and arms
- Sudden onset; pain continues for several days

Other signs and symptoms
- Increased pain with movement, inspiration, laughing, coughing
- Precordial friction rub
- Decreased pain with sitting or leaning foward (sitting pulls heart away from diaphragm)
- Fever
- Dyspnea
- Orthopnea
- Tachycardia

Precipitating factors
- Myocardial infarction
- Upper respiratory tract infection
- No relation to physical exertion
- Ingestion of such drugs as hydralazine or procainamide
- Hypersensitivity or autoimmune disease, such as rheumatic fever, systemic lupus erythematosus, and rheumatoid arthritis

Nursing considerations
- To relieve dyspnea and pain, instruct the patient to sit or lean forward.
- Administer oxygen, as needed.
- Administer analgesics, as ordered.
- Bed rest as long as pain and fever persist
- Give nonsteroidal, anti-inflammatory drugs, such as aspirin and indomethacin, to relieve pain and inflammation, as ordered. If these drugs fail to relieve symptoms, administer corticosteroids, as ordered.

Heart

Learning about electrocardiography

Electrocardiography is the most frequently used test to evaluate a patient's cardiac status. This test graphically records electrical current generated by the patient's heart. As you know, this current radiates from the heart in all directions. When the current reaches the skin, it's measured by electrodes connected to an amplifier and strip chart recorder. Let's take a closer look at the standard limb leads: I, II, and III. To run these three leads, you'll place a limb electrode on each of your patient's arms and legs—four electrodes in all. Because the electrode on your patient's right leg acts as the ground, it's inactive.

Now let's look at the augmented limb leads: AVR, AVL, and AVF. In these abbreviations the A means augmented; V means voltage; and R, L, and F mean right arm, left arm, and foot, respectively. These three leads use the same electrode placement as standard limb leads.

But the standard and augmented limb leads are alike in this respect; they both measure electrical potential in the body's frontal plane (see the illustration at right). Simply speaking, they view your patient's heart from the front.

As the illustration shows, the chest leads add still another dimension to the EKG picture. Whereas the standard and augmented limb leads view electrical potential from the body's frontal plane, the chest leads view the electrical potential from a horizontal plane. This added dimension helps pinpoint any damage to the heart's lateral or posterior walls.

The doctor studies the EKG results and compares them with known normals and the patient's previous EKGs to detect changes in wave amplification, duration, intervals, and heart rate. If disturbances in the heart's electrical system exist, the doctor can pinpoint damaged heart muscle (that interrupts or blocks normal electrical activity) by knowing which view each portion of the strip represents.

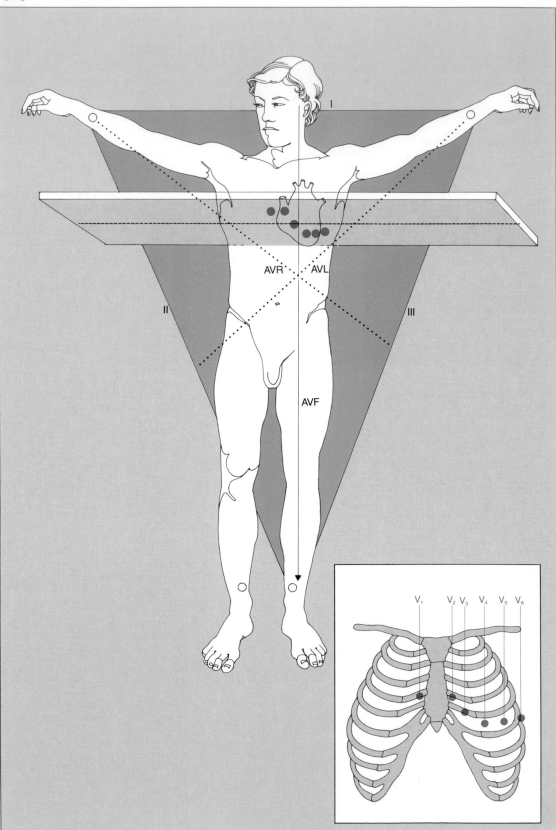

Running a 10-lead EKG

Michael Penn, a 40-year-old production manager, arrives in your office for his annual physical exam. In addition to assessing Mr. Penn's vital signs, you'll want to run a 10-lead EKG. Do you know how to proceed? If you're unsure, follow these steps. Note: In this photostory, the nurse is using the Burdick E200 electrocardiograph. If you're using a different model, check the manufacturer's instructions.

Begin by gathering the equipment you'll need: the EKG machine with 5 or 10 lead wires, four limb-lead sensors, six suction-cup chest sensors, conductive jelly or pads (we're using Lectro-pads® and Liqui-cord®), alcohol pads, 4"x4" gauze pads, and a towel.

Discuss the procedure with your patient even if he's had an EKG. Tell him he can help ensure accurate test results by relaxing during the procedure.

Have him put on a patient gown and pajama bottoms.

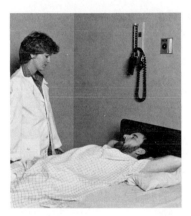

1 Now, ask Mr. Penn to lie flat on his back on the bed. *Note:* If you're using an exam table instead of a bed, be sure it's large enough to support both arms and legs. Place a pillow under his head, and explain what you'll be doing.

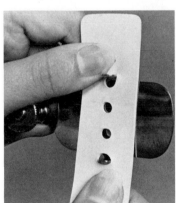

2 Help Mr. Penn take off the patient gown and roll up the legs of the pajamas.
Connect the sensor straps to the ears of the limb sensors, as shown here.

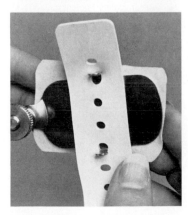

3 Next, place a Lectro-pad (which is presaturated with electrolyte solution) on each sensor. Be sure the pad extends slightly beyond the sensor edge. Allow some electrolyte solution to seep from the pad by stroking the pad lightly, as the nurse is doing here.

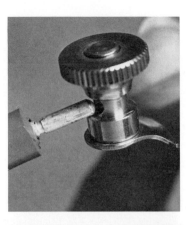

4 Match each limb-lead sensor to the corresponding lead wire. Each lead wire is color coded: white, right arm; black, left arm; green, right leg; red, left leg; and brown, chest.
Connect each limb wire to the appropriate sensor. To do this, plug the lead wire into the sensor's connector. Secure it by turning the sensor screw.

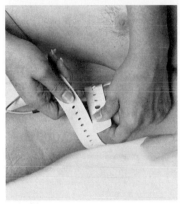

5 Then, apply limb leads to Mr. Penn's arms. Select a smooth, fleshy site; avoid bony or muscular areas. Secure the limb strap so it fits comfortably on the patient's arm. When he relaxes, check to be sure the sensor doesn't press against his body or the bed.
Follow the same procedure to apply a limb lead to his other arm.

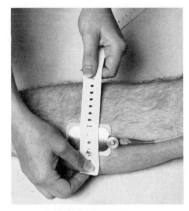

6 Next, choose a smooth, fleshy site on one of Mr. Penn's legs and repeat the procedure. Take care not to position the sensor over the tibia.
Apply the fourth limb lead to his other leg, using the same procedure.

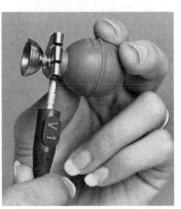

7 Attach the brown lead wires to the corresponding sensors, as the nurse is doing here.

Heart

Running a 10-lead EKG continued

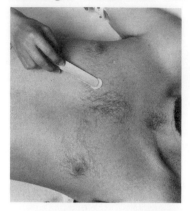

8 Place a dab of conductive jelly at each of the chest sensor sites: V_1, fourth intercostal space to right of sternum; V_2, fourth intercostal space to left of sternum; V_3, halfway between V_2 and V_4; V_4, fifth intercostal space at midclavicular line; V_5, anterior axillary line, halfway between V_4 and V_6; and V_6, midaxillary line, level with V_4. Use a tongue depressor to spread the jelly.

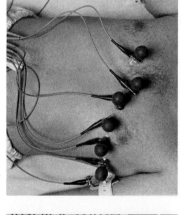

9 Now, pick up the chest sensor and squeeze its rubber bulb between your fingers. Place the sensor on the conductive jelly and release the rubber bulb. The sensor is held in place by suction. To apply the remaining chest sensors, follow the same procedure.

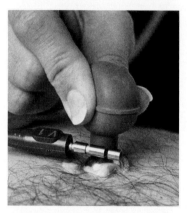

10 Then, check to be sure the leads lie loosely over Mr. Penn's chest. Excess tension on the sensors may result in an inaccurate reading. Also, check that the unit's plugged into a properly grounded wall receptacle. Then, set the front panel controls. The nurse has selected automatic. Place the sequence select switch in the standard (ST'D) position.

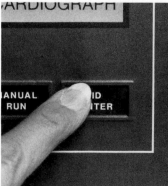

11 To enter patient information, press the ID ENTER switch. The machine shown here allows you to enter up to 10 digits, which appear at the beginning of the patient recording.

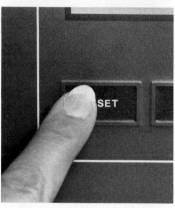

12 Now, depress the AUTO RUN switch. As you do, you'll generate a calibration pulse and, in turn, the 12 leads will record sequentially. You'll see the LED illuminate as each lead's recorded.

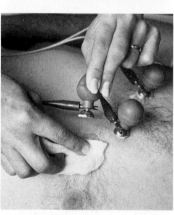

13 When the EKG's complete, press the RESET button to clear the machine for the next patient.

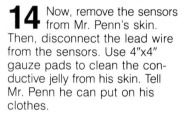

14 Now, remove the sensors from Mr. Penn's skin. Then, disconnect the lead wire from the sensors. Use 4"x4" gauze pads to clean the conductive jelly from his skin. Tell Mr. Penn he can put on his clothes.

15 Next, clean the limb-lead sensors with alcohol pads. To clean the chest sensors, hold them under running water. Dry them with a towel. Then, return them to their package.

Document the entire procedure. Check to be sure each EKG strip includes patient identification, sensitivity, and frequency response information.

Learning about exercise electrocardiography (EKG)

Administering an exercise EKG (stress test) to a patient? Consider the following information before you proceed. As you probably know, this test helps you evaluate your patient's heart action during physical stress. By testing the heart's reaction to increased oxygen demands, you can gather important diagnostic data that can't be obtained from an EKG alone.

When to perform and when to avoid

In most cases, stress testing is performed for these reasons:
• to help diagnose the cause of chest pain
• to determine the functional capacity of the heart after a myocardial infarction or surgery
• to screen for asymptomatic coronary artery disease, especially in men over age 35
• to identify cardiac arrhythmias that develop during physical exercise
• to evaluate the effectiveness of antiarrhythmic or antianginal drug therapy
• to help set limitations for an exercise program.

Contraindications for an exercise EKG include unstable coronary artery disease, uncontrolled hypertension, uncontrolled arrhythmia, severe aortic or mitral stenosis, acute infectious disease, and recent systemic or pulmonary embolism.

Reviewing the basics

You'll remember that the stress test provides standardized conditions for clinically controlled exercise. The results provide valuable information on patients with such conditions as vascular abnormalities, obesity, and diabetes.

The most commonly performed stress test method is walking or running on a motor-driven treadmill, as shown in the photo above. When the patient's positioned on the treadmill, you can increase his workload by changing the treadmill speed and its degree of incline (multistage treadmill test). Be ready to initiate changes at 3-minute intervals either without rest periods (continuous stress testing) or with rest periods (intermittent stress testing). Generally, intermittent stress testing enables your patient to reach a higher stress level, because he can rest between intervals.

One of the treadmill's advantages is that it causes your patient to consume more oxygen and achieve a

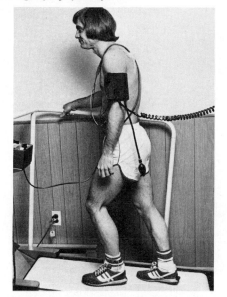

higher heart rate with slightly less hemodynamic stress than the bicycle ergometer. Why? Because walking and running are more familiar to a patient and the exercise strain is more uniformly distributed over a larger muscle mass.

Other stress testing methods include pedaling a bicycle ergometer and climbing stairs or a bench. You can increase the patient's workload on the bicycle ergometer by increasing the wheel resistance. In addition, the bicycle can be used for continuous or intermittent testing. This method, however, usually shows a disproportionate increase in blood pressure and breathing for a specific workload. In many cases, the patient's legs tire before his body.

The least flexible stress tests are step and bench climbing. These methods have no mechanism for controlling the workload level, don't allow for warm-up periods, and require activity too strenuous for some patients and not strenuous enough for others.

During the test

Throughout the stress test you'll monitor your patient's blood pressure, heart rate, and oxygen consumption at 3-minute intervals. His EKG pattern will be continuously monitored. Be prepared to evaluate changes in his general appearance as well as any symptoms that develop.

Keep in mind that if your patient's tolerating the testing procedure satisfactorily, you'll stop the test when he reaches a predesignated heart rate or shows signs of fatigue.

Getting your patient ready for an exercise EKG

If the doctor's ordered an exercise EKG for your patient, one of your responsibilities is to prepare him properly.

Begin by familiarizing your patient with the test procedure. Explain the purpose of the test. Tell him it records his heart's electrical activity and performance under stress. Describe the testing equipment he'll be using—for example, treadmill, bicycle, bench, or stairs—and how it operates.

Explain that during the test he'll work hard and perspire. Tell him to expect to feel tired and slightly breathless. Assure him that he can stop the test if he experiences chest pain or extreme fatigue, but encourage him to exercise as long as possible. If he feels any adverse symptoms, tell him to advise the doctor or attending nurse immediately.

Tell your patient that before the test his complete medical history will be taken, and he'll have a physical exam and a 12-lead EKG. Explain that later the doctor will compare this EKG with the exercise EKG to see how his heart responds to exercise.

Now, review these guidelines with your patient:
• Advise him to wear loose, comfortable clothing for the test. Suggest lightweight shorts or slacks, shirt, socks, and rubber-soled shoes, such as sneakers. If your patient's female, tell her to wear a bra and a short-sleeved blouse that buttons in the front. This way you can measure her blood pressure, apply chest electrodes, and listen to her heart without removing her blouse. Also instruct her not to wear panty hose.
• Explain that several areas on his chest and possibly his back will be cleaned, shaved (if necessary), and abraded to prepare his skin for the electrodes.
• Reassure the patient that he won't feel any electrical current from the electrodes, but the electrode sites may itch slightly.
• Tell your patient that his blood pressure and heart rate will be checked periodically during and after the test.
• Encourage him to report any symptoms during the test.
• Remind him to get a good night's sleep beforehand and to come to the test rested and refreshed. Advise him not to engage in strenuous activity for 12 hours before the test.
• If your patient smokes, tell him to refrain from doing so for 2 hours before the test. Explain that the nicotine elevates his heart rate.
• Instruct your patient not to drink alcohol or caffeinic beverages, such as coffee or cola, for 2 hours before the test.
• Encourage your patient to eat a light meal at least 2 hours before the test.
• Advise your patient to avoid milk and milk products on the day of the test. Explain that this precaution helps prevent nausea during the procedure.

Document all patient teaching and preparations on the appropriate forms.

Heart

Caring for your patient after an exercise EKG

What are your responsibilities in caring for a patient after an exercise EKG? Follow the doctor's instruction for specific orders for each patient's care, but study this list to understand the basics.

• When your patient reaches his targeted heart rate or the doctor stops the test for any reason, the doctor slows the speed of the treadmill. Tell the patient to continue walking for several minutes. Explain that this helps prevent nausea and dizziness.

• Help the patient to a chair, and continue monitoring heart rate and blood pressure for 10 to 15 minutes or until his EKG returns to his baseline.

• Auscultate for S_3 and S_4 heart sounds. In some cases, an S_4 (atrial gallop) develops after exercise, due to increased blood flow volume and turbulence. But an S_3 (ventricular gallop) is more significant than an S_4, indicating transient left ventricular dysfunction.

• Remove all chest electrodes (as shown below) and clean the electrode sites.

• If the patient shows signs of discomfort at the end of the test, tell him to rest until they subside.

• Caution the patient not to drive for at least 1 hour after the test. Suggest he have someone drive him home.

• Instruct the patient to wait at least 1 hour before showering after returning home. Caution him to use warm water rather than hot water; hot water may make him dizzy. Remember, any further vasodilation could produce additional venous pooling and hypotension.

• Instruct the patient to resume his usual diet and to continue taking prescribed medications discontinued before the test.

• Tell your patient to avoid strenuous activity for the rest of the day.

• Encourage your patient to ask questions. Answer them honestly. Provide reassurance and support for your patient. Keep in mind that if he had adverse affects, he may be more anxious about his condition.

• Administer nitroglycerin for chest pain, as ordered.

Document your patient teaching as well as the procedure on the appropriate forms.

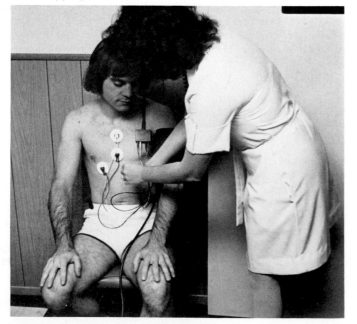

Identifying common cardiovascular disorders

As you probably know, cardiovascular disorders remain the most common cause of death in the United States. And more than one third of these deaths occur suddenly.

As an ambulatory-care nurse, your responsibilities include identifying cardiovascular disorders (both primary and secondary), referring your patient for treatment, teaching him about his disorder, providing emotional support, and monitoring his progress. In many cases, you may be the only health-care professional with whom he has contact, so be alert for possible signs and symptoms of cardiovascular disorders by familiarizing yourself with the information given in the chart below.

But first, review these general guidelines whenever you're caring for a patient with suspected cardiovascular disease:

• Take an accurate patient history.

• Stress the need to control an associated high-risk disease, such as diabetes and hypertension.

• Teach all patients (especially those at high risk) the importance of following a low-cholesterol, low-salt diet and of keeping their weight down, increasing activity, avoiding smoking, getting adequate rest, and minimizing stress.

Coronary artery disease (CAD)
Description
• Decreased coronary blood flow, reducing the amount of oxygen and essential nutrients delivered to myocardial tissue
• More common in men than in women and in Caucasians, the middle-aged, and the elderly
Possible causes
• Atherosclerosis most common cause; less commonly results from dissecting aneurysm, infectious vasculitis, syphilis, and congenital defects
Signs and symptoms
• Burning, squeezing, or crushing pain in substernal or precordial chest that may radiate to left arm, neck, jaws, or shoulder blade
• Anginal episodes following physical exertion, emotional excitement, or temperature changes
• Patient describes pain by clench-ing fist over chest or rubbing left arm.
• Nausea
• Vomiting
• Faintness
• Diaphoresis
• Cool extremities
Nursing intervention
• During anginal episodes, monitor blood pressure and heart rate. Take an EKG before administering nitroglycerin or other nitrates. Note duration of pain, amount of medication required to relieve it, and accompanying symptoms.
• Have nitroglycerin on hand for immediate use. Instruct the patient to notify you immediately whenever he feels chest pain and takes nitroglycerin.
• Prepare the patient for cardiac catheterization by explaining the procedure to him and making sure he knows why it is necessary, understands the risk involved, and realizes that its results may indicate a need for surgery.
• After the catheterization, review the expected course of treatment with the patient and his family. Monitor the catheter site (usually the antecubital fossa or groin) for bleeding. Also check pulses distal to the catheter insertion site. To counter the diuretic effect of the dye used for the test, make sure the patient drinks plenty of fluids. To prevent arrhythmias from muscle irritability, monitor potassium levels closely.
• If the patient is scheduled for surgery, explain the procedure to the patient and his family and answer their questions.
• Emphasize to your patient the importance of taking his medication exactly as prescribed, exercising regularly, and observing any dietary restrictions.
• Stress the need to stop smoking. Refer the patient to a self-help group, if necessary.

Myocardial infarction (MI)
Description
• Decreased blood flow through one of the coronary arteries, leading to myocardial ischemia and tissue necrosis
• Almost half of sudden deaths due to MI occur within 1 hour of the onset of symptoms. Prognosis improves if vigorous treatment begins immediately.
Possible causes
• Predisposing factors to CAD and in turn MI include positive family history; hypertension; smoking; elevated serum triglyceride and cholesterol levels; diabetes mellitus;

obesity or excessive intake of saturated fats, carbohydrates, and/or salt; sedentary life-style; aging; stress or Type A personality. Men are more susceptible than women (incidence is rising in women, especially those who smoke or take oral contraceptives).

Signs and symptoms
• Persistent, crushing, substernal chest pain that may radiate to the left arm, jaws, neck, or shoulder blades; may last for 12 hours. *Important:* Some patients—especially diabetics and the elderly—may be asymptomatic. In other patients, the pain may be mild and mistaken for indigestion.
• In a patient with CAD, angina of increasing frequency, severity, or duration (especially when not precipitated by exertion, ingestion of a heavy meal, or exposure to cold or wind)
• Tachycardia
• Shortness of breath
• Nausea
• Vomiting
• Fatigue
• Sense of impending doom
• Catecholamine responses, such as cool extremities, diaphoresis, anxiety, and restlessness
• Low-grade fever possible several days after MI
• Hypotension or hypertension possible

Nursing intervention
• Plan patient care to allow maximum uninterrupted rest.
• During episodes of chest pain, take EKG; monitor blood pressure, temperature, heart rate, and breath sounds.
• Observe for signs and symptoms of fluid retention, such as rales, cough, tachypnea, and edema. Monitor intake and output. Record daily weight, intake and output, serum enzymes, respirations, and blood pressure.
• Listen for adventitious breath sounds (patients on bed rest frequently have atelectatic rales, which may disappear after coughing) and for S_3 or S_4 gallops.
• To promote compliance with drug regimen and other treatment measures, thoroughly explain the purpose of drugs and dosages and of all procedures. Warn the patient about drug side effects, and advise him to watch for and report signs of toxicity (anorexia, headache, nausea, vomiting, and tinnitus, for example, if the patient is receiving digitalis).
• Review dietary restrictions. If the patient must follow a low-sodium or a low-fat, low-cholesterol diet, provide a list of foods he can eat. It
*Available in both the United States and Canada

may be helpful to have a dietitian discuss the diet with him and his family. Stress what he can have, not what he can't.
• Counsel the patient and partner about resuming sexual activity.
• Advise the patient to report to the doctor any typical or atypical chest pain. Be alert for signs of post-infarction syndrome, such as chest pain, that must be differentiated from recurrent MI, pulmonary infarct, or congestive heart failure.
• If the patient has a Holter monitor in place, explain its purpose and how to use it.
• Stress the need to stop smoking. If necessary, refer the patient to a self-help group.

Congestive heart failure (CHF)
Description
• Myocardial dysfunction, leading to diminished cardiac output, heart pump failure, and abnormal circulatory congestion
• Condition may be acute (a direct result of MI), but it's usually a chronic disorder associated with the retention of water and salt by the kidneys.
• Advances in diagnostic and therapeutic techniques have greatly improved the outlook for patients with CHF, but prognosis still depends on the underlying cause and response to treatment.
• May occur as right, left, or complete heart failure

Possible causes
• Primary heart muscle abnormality (as in infarction), inadequate myocardial perfusion due to CAD, or cardiomyopathy
• Mechanical disturbances in ventricular filling during diastole when there's too little blood for the ventricle to pump
• Systolic hemodynamic disturbances (such as excessive cardiac workload due to volume overloading or pressure overload) that limit the heart's pumping ability

Signs and symptoms
• In *left heart failure:* fatigue, dyspnea (exertional, paroxysmal, nocturnal)
• In *right heart failure:* engorgement of neck veins (when the patient is upright, these neck veins may appear distended, feel rigid, and show exaggerated pulsations), hepatomegaly
• Slight but persistent cold with a dry and productive cough, combined with wheezing, which may be mistaken for an allergic reaction
• Other symptoms include tachypnea, palpitations, dependent edema, unexplained steady weight

gain, nausea, chest tightness, slowed mental response, anorexia, hypotension, diaphoresis, narrow pulse pressure, pallor and oliguria, S_3 gallop rhythm on auscultation, and rales on inspiration; liver may be palpable and slightly tender.
• In later stages, dullness heard over lung bases, hemoptysis and cyanosis, marked hepatomegaly, pitting ankle edema, and in patients confined to bed, sacral edema.

Nursing intervention
• Schedule the patient for an EKG to detect heart strain and ischemia.
• Arrange for the patient to have a chest X-ray to detect heart enlargement, increased pulmonary marking, interstitial edema, and pleural effusion and cardiomegaly.
• Measure the patient for antiembolism stockings, as ordered. Teach him how to apply the stockings.
• Encourage bed rest, as ordered.
• Administer vasodilators, such as prazosin hydrochloride (Minipress*), as ordered.
• Instruct the patient to weigh himself daily at the same time in similar clothing. Tell him to notify you if he gains 1 lb (0.4 kg) or more a day for 3 consecutive days.
• Advise the patient to avoid foods high in sodium content, such as canned or commercially prepared foods, and dairy products to curb fluid overload. Tell him not to add salt to his food.
• Explain to the patient that he must replace the potassium lost through diuretics by taking a potassium supplement and by eating high-potassium foods, such as bananas, apricots, and orange juice.
• Stress the need for frequent checkups.
• Emphasize the importance of taking digitalis exactly as prescribed. Instruct the patient to watch for signs of digitalis toxicity (anorexia, nausea, vomiting, headache, tinnitus, cardiac arrhythmias).
• Teach the patient how to take his own pulse. Have him notify you or the doctor if his pulse rate is unusually irregular or is less than 160 beats per minute; if he experiences dizziness, blurred vision, shortness of breath, a persistent dry cough, palpitations, increased fatigue, paroxysmal nocturnal dyspnea, swollen ankles, decreased urinary output; or if he gains 3 to 5 lb (1.36 to 2.2 kg) in a week.
• Tell the patient to avoid fatigue by pacing activities, simplifying his workload, and obtaining help from others.
• Teach the patient methods of promoting proper respiratory

function, such as getting adequate rest, elevating the head of the bed, limiting exposure to extreme temperature conditions, providing adequate indoor humidity, avoiding persons with respiratory tract infections, and being immunized against influenza.
• Instruct the patient or his family to report signs of unusual fatigue, respiratory status changes, weight gain, or confusion to you or the doctor.

Cerebrovascular accident (CVA)
Description
• Sudden impairment of cerebral blood flow in one or more vessels supplying the brain, which, in turn, interrupts or diminishes the brain's oxygen supply, causing brain tissue damage or necrosis.

Possible causes
• Predisposing factors include history of transient ischemic attacks, atherosclerosis, hypertension, arrhythmia, rheumatic heart disease, EKG changes, diabetes, high serum triglyceride levels, lack of exercise, smoking, and use of oral contraceptives.
• Thrombosis
• Embolism
• Hemorrhage

Signs and symptoms
• *Premonitory:* drowsiness, dizziness, headache, and occasional confusion
• *Generalized:* headache, vomiting, mental impairment, convulsions, coma, nuchal rigidity, fever, and disorientation
• *Focal:* sensory and reflex changes

Nursing intervention
• Instruct the patient and his family to report premonitory signs and symptoms to the doctor immediately.
• Stress the importance of returning for follow-up care.
• If the doctor has prescribed aspirin to inhibit platelet aggregation, tell the patient to be alert for signs of gastrointestinal bleeding, such as vomiting bright red blood. Emphasize that acetaminophen *cannot* be substituted for aspirin.
• Stress the need to control high-risk diseases, such as hypertension and diabetes.
• Provide psychological support. Help the patient set realistic short-term goals and involve his family in his care whenever possible.
• Teach the patient how to manage his activities of daily living. With the aid of an occupational therapist, obtain such appliances as a walker or ramp, as needed. If speech therapy is indicated, encourage the patient to begin as soon as possible.

Heart

Understanding angina pectoris

You're working in a clinic when 45-year-old Jim Falk comes in accompanied by his wife. Mr. Falk tells you that just after completing two sets of tennis with his wife he felt a crushing sensation in his chest. "I feel like someone is standing on my chest," he says, "and this isn't the first time I've felt like this. But the pain usually goes away when I rest for a while."

Based on Mr. Falk's assessment of his pain, you suspect angina pectoris. Although you may care for many patients with angina, never take the condition lightly. If untreated or treated improperly, angina can lead to myocardial infarction (MI) and death. Three major forms of angina exist: *stable* (pain is predictable in frequency and duration and can be relieved with nitroglycerin and rest), *unstable* (pain increases in frequency and duration and is easily induced), and *decubitus* (pain recurs, even at rest).

You'll remember that angina can be triggered by a variety of stimuli; for example, physical exertion, emotional stress, eating a heavy meal, or exposure to temperature extremes. Any of these stimuli (known as the four Es) can increase cardiac output, heart rate, and blood pressure. These, in turn, put stress on the coronary collateral circulation and lead to reduced myocardial oxygenation, ischemia, and pain.

In most cases, anginal pain is relieved by nitroglycerin or beta blockers. If the pain lasts longer than 30 to 60 minutes or is not relieved by medication or rest, suspect MI and notify the doctor immediately. To care for a patient with angina, take these immediate steps:
• Help the patient to a chair or bed. Encourage him to rest. Elevate the head of the bed. Lying in a supine position may aggravate the pain.
• Monitor vital signs closely.
• Perform an electrocardiogram (EKG) immediately.
• Provide emotional support and reassurance to reduce patient and family anxiety.
• Give nitroglycerin or beta-blocking drugs, as ordered, to reduce cardiac workload and oxygen demand. Teach the patient about possible side effects and precautions.
• Document the patient's condition and the location and type of pain. Note the circumstances that evoked the pain.

Because the doctor may want to know more about your patient's heart, he may hospitalize him for further observation and testing; for example, arteriography or an exercise EKG. If so, send a referral form containing your findings and other relevant information to the hospital.

Minimizing the risk factor

Teach the patient and his family how to modify risk factors. Follow these guidelines:
• Explain how the heart is affected by risk factors, such as smoking, high cholesterol and triglyceride levels in the blood, hypertension, uncontrolled diabetes, lack of exercise, obesity, and a family history of atherosclerotic cardiovascular disease. Then, help your patient identify his risk factors. Discuss practical ways to minimize these risks, such as changing exercise or eating habits.
• Emphasize the importance of taking medications as prescribed, even if the patient feels better.
• Explain common emotional responses evoked by angina, such as fear of heart attack or a sudden death in the family.
• Describe how a regular, progressive, physical activity program helps gradually to improve the circulation.
• Teach the patient and his family how to recognize signs and symptoms of a heart attack and to distinguish them from angina.
• Encourage your patient to resume sexual activity as soon as the doctor says it's OK.
• Teach the patient to take his blood pressure.

Teaching your patient about nitroglycerin

If your patient has angina, one of the doctor's first steps will be to initiate drug therapy. Chances are he'll prescribe one or more of nitroglycerin's four forms: sublingual tablets, tablets that are chewed or swallowed whole, or ointment. Explain that nitroglycerin relieves the pain of angina by relaxing the muscles in the arteries and veins, resulting in increased elasticity and greater blood flow—which restores oxygen and nutrients to the heart.

Emphasize to your patient that the success of nitroglycerin therapy depends largely on his cooperation. For example, if the doctor's ordered sublingual medication, the patient must place the tablet under his tongue at the first signs of an attack; the longer he waits, the less effective the tablet will be. Then, give him these general guidelines:
• Take the medication exactly as the doctor prescribes.
• To prevent unpleasant side effects, avoid alcoholic beverages.
• Get out of bed, go up and down stairs, and change positions slowly.
• Lie down at the first sign of dizziness.
• Have the medication on hand at all times.

If your patient's using sublingual tablets:
• Assure freshness by replacing your supply every 3 months.
• Remove the cotton from the container; it absorbs active ingredients in the medication.
• Store the medication in a dark container in a cool place. Don't carry a container of nitroglycerin in your pocket. Your body heat may reduce the drug's effectiveness.
• Expect the medication to cause a headache initially. Take aspirin or acetaminophen to relieve the headache. If you continue to get a headache after taking the medication, notify the doctor; he may adjust the dosage.
• Expect to feel a burning sensation when you place the tablet under your tongue. If the tablet doesn't burn, it's lost its potency. Replace your supply.
• After placing the tablet under your tongue, sit down and rest until the tablet's dissolved. This usually takes several minutes. If you still have pain after the tablet's dissolved, wait 10 to 15 minutes and take another tablet. If you still have pain, repeat the procedure. Suppose after taking three tablets your pain is unrelieved. Call your doctor or go to the hospital emergency department.

If the doctor wants your patient to take nitroglycerin as a preventive treatment, review these considerations:
• If you're taking nitroglycerin tablets that must be swallowed whole or chewed, take them on an empty stomach; for example, 30 minutes before a meal or 1 to 2 hours after a meal.
• If the doctor's prescribed nitroglycerin in ointment form, spread it in a uniformly thin layer in a 2″ (5-cm) circle on a nonhairy area; for example, on your neck. Don't rub it in. Cover the area with plastic wrap to aid absorption and protect your clothing.
• Notify the doctor if you experience continuous headache, nausea, vomiting, fainting, flushing, palpitations, or no pain relief. He may change your dosage.

Learning about hypertension

When we talk about hypertension, we're referring to an intermittent or sustained elevation in diastolic or systolic blood pressure. Generally, patients under age 50 with a blood pressure of $^{140}\!/_{90}$ and those over age 50 with a blood pressure of $^{150}\!/_{95}$ are considered hypertensive. Keep in mind that two major types of hypertension exist: *essential,* which is idiopathic and the most common, and *secondary,* which is due to renal disease or another identifiable cause.

Regardless of the type, hypertension directly results from an increase in cardiac output and arteriolar vasoconstriction. Consequently, a proportionately greater amount of peripheral vascular resistance is necessary to circulate the blood through the body. Hypertension is usually associated with the narrowing of certain blood vessels (vasoconstriction) and may be related to kidney function.

Of course, increased blood pressure may also result from a breakdown or inappropriate response of the following mechanisms:
• Changes in renal arterial pressure that stimulate autoregulation of the blood pressure by the kidneys. This mechanism increases cardiac output.
• Baroreceptors (pressure receptors) in the aortic arch, carotid sinus, and other large central arteries that stimulate the vasomotor center to increase sympathetic stimulation of the heart. This stimulation ultimately increases cardiac output and peripheral vascular resistance.
• Renin-angiotensin system is a neural mechanism that utilizes renin, a renal enzyme, to form angiotensin. Angiotensin directly produces vasoconstriction or indirectly stimulates the adrenal cortex to produce aldosterone. Finally, sodium reabsorption is increased, which, in turn, increases water reabsorption, plasma volume, and cardiac output.

What triggers increased cardiac output—and hypertension? In essential hypertension, this is unknown. Studies show that the condition is more likely to develop between ages 30 and 40 in patients with a family history of hypertension. Other common risk factors include race (more common in blacks), stress, obesity, high dietary intake of saturated fats or sodium, use of tobacco or oral contraceptives, sedentary life-style, and aging.

Secondary hypertension may result from renovascular disease; pheochromocytoma; primary hyperaldosteronism; Cushing's syndrome; dysfunctions of the thyroid, pituitary, or parathyroid glands; and neurologic disorders.

As you probably know, identifying signs and symptoms of hypertension can be difficult. In fact, a high percentage of patients with early-stage hypertension aren't even aware of the problem. Why? Because the condition is usually asymptomatic. Although headache, fatigue, shortness of breath, and dizziness may occur with hypertension, these symptoms are not specific to hypertension. And unfortunately, by the time clinical signs and effects are evident, vascular changes in the heart, brain, or kidneys have usually occurred. But the effects don't stop there. Excessively elevated blood pressure damages the intima of small blood vessels, resulting in fibrin accumulation in the vessels, development of local edema, and possibly intravascular clotting. Symptoms produced by this process depend on the location of the damaged vessels; for example:
• brain: cerebrovascular accident
• retina: blindness
• kidneys: proteinuria, edema, and eventually renal failure.

Hypertension also increases the heart's workload, leading to left ventricular hypertrophy and, eventually, to left ventricular failure, congestive heart failure, and pulmonary edema.

Although the signs and symptoms of hypertension may not be obvious on observation, auscultation may reveal bruits over the abdominal aorta and the carotid, renal, and femoral arteries; ophthalmoscopy may reveal arteriovenous nicking and, in hypertensive encephalopathy, papilledema. Patient history and additional tests—such as urinalysis, intravenous pyelography, serum potassium, BUN and creatinine, EKG, and chest X-ray—may show predisposing factors and help identify an underlying cause, such as renal disease. Prognosis is good if hypertension is detected early and treatment begins before complications develop. Severely elevated blood pressure (hypertensive crisis) may be fatal.

Aiming for control

You'll remember that essential hypertension has no cure. It can be controlled, however, through drugs and modifications in diet and life-style. In most cases, drug therapy begins with a diuretic, which reduces the amount of water and sodium in the body by increasing the amount of urine voided. If this therapy is ineffective, the doctor will probably add a sympathetic nerve blocker or vasodilator to the regimen. Dietary and life-style changes may include weight loss, relaxation techniques, regular exercise, and restriction of sodium and saturated fat intake.

Treatment of secondary hypertension includes correction of the underlying cause and control of hypertensive effects.

Counseling your patient about hypertension

Frank Gray, a 54-year-old engineer, has essential hypertension. You know, of course, that his condition may be controlled with drugs and modification in diet and life-style, but does he follow his treatment plan? If he's like some patients with hypertension, probably not. Why? Because he's not feeling any adverse effects from the condition. Help him adjust his treatment plan by answering his questions.

Patient's question
What is hypertension?
Your answer
Hypertension is high blood pressure. Blood pressure is the force needed to circulate blood through the body's arteries, capillaries, and veins.

Patient's question
How long will hypertension treatment take?
Your answer
Usually the doctor tailors a treatment program to control your hypertension. But finding the right treatment program may take time. Methods he may suggest include weight loss, medication, sodium restriction (sodium is part of salt), or a combination of these. In time, the doctor may adjust your treatment slightly, but expect to follow the same type of treatment program for the rest of your life. You'll also need to have your blood pressure checked regularly.

Patient's question
What causes hypertension?
Your answer
The cause of essential hypertension is unknown. But we do know that it usually occurs between ages 30 and 40. Contributing factors include obesity, high sodium (salt) intake, elevated cholesterol and triglyceride blood levels, and a family history of the condition.

Patient's question
What type of medication will the doctor prescribe?
Your answer
If the doctor prescribes medication, he'll probably order a tablet to reduce the amount of water in your body by increasing the amount of urine voided. In time, he may order additional medications to stimulate your heart or relax your blood vessels.

Heart

Teaching your patient to take his blood pressure

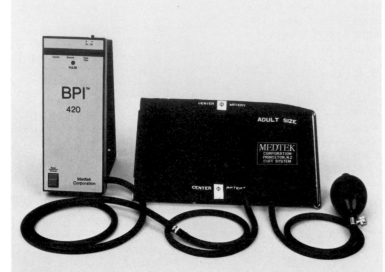

When your patient begins a hypertension treatment program, his doctor may want him to monitor his blood pressure closely. To comply, teach the patient to take his blood pressure. The Medtek BPI™ 420 system, shown here, makes this procedure easy. The system features the BPI 420 unit, the occluding/ sensing cuff, a pressure bulb and AeroMed™ valve, a lockable desk stand/wall bracket, an adapter/charger, and extender tubing connector.

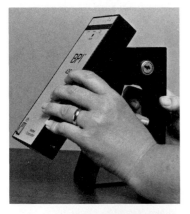

1 Begin by having your patient sit comfortably in a chair. Explain the equipment and procedure to him. Then, instruct him to place the BPI unit in its stand, as the nurse is doing here. Tell him to position the stand so the unit's at his eye level.

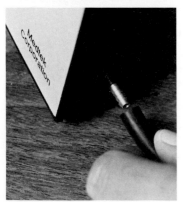

2 Now, show your patient how to attach the tubing to the BPI unit, as shown, and to the unit's extender tubing connector.

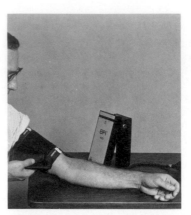

3 Next, tell your patient to rest his arm on a firm surface, such as a table, at heart level. Have him extend his arm and apply the occluding cuff. Check that the cuff's narrow white band is over the brachial artery and that the cuff fits snugly. If the cuff's positioned correctly, the D-ring, or index line, should fall between the two lines indicated on the cuff.

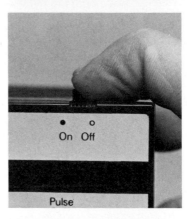

4 When the cuff's in place, have your patient slide the power switch, located on the top of the unit, to ON. As he does, the letters CAL, followed by OCCLUDE, will be displayed on the screen.

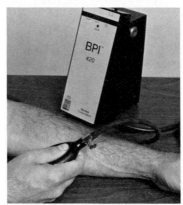

5 To inflate the cuff, have your patient use his opposite hand to pump the pressure bulb rapidly, until the number displayed on the screen is 30 to 40 mm Hg above the patient's expected systolic reading. If the letters LO OCC PRESS are displayed on the screen, tell the patient to pump the pressure bulb once or twice more, until a higher pressure value is shown.

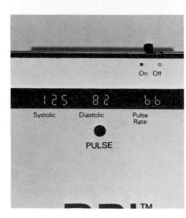

6 Instruct your patient to release the pressure bulb when the cuff is sufficiently occluded. As he does, the cuff automatically deflates at the correct rate. Have him record the pressure values and his pulse rate as they appear on the screen, and the time and date.

Then, show him how to remove the cuff and turn off the unit.

Nurses' guide to antihypertensive drugs

Has the doctor ordered an antihypertensive or diuretic drug for your patient with hypertension? If he has, one of your responsibilities is to teach your patient and his family about the drug.

First, familiarize yourself with the most commonly used drugs by studying the following chart. For more information on antihypertensive and diuretic drugs, see the NURSING82 DRUG HANDBOOK™ or DRUGS in the NURSE'S REFERENCE LIBRARY™ Series. Then, using easy-to-understand terms, explain these important points to your patient and his family:

• What the prescribed drug is called and what it's used for
• What specific side effects it may cause
• What special precautions the patient must observe while taking the drug
• Why initial doses may vary from the maintenance dose
• Why taking the drug exactly as prescribed—even when he's feeling well—is so important.
• Discourage your patient from storing different medications in the same container. Doing so increases the risk of drug errors. Some medications can be mistaken for other drugs; for example, furosemide and digoxin are both white tablets of approximately the same size.

In addition, warn the patient to tell the doctor about any other drugs—including over-the-counter medications—he may use. These drugs may interact with the antihypertensive or diuretic drugs the doctor's prescribed. If the patient develops any side effects (for example, weakness, fatigue, muscle cramps, or blurred vision), tell him to notify the doctor at once. But warn him not to stop the drug abruptly, unless the doctor directs him to do so.

metoprolol tartrate (Lopressor)

Indications and dosage
Hypertension (may be used alone or with other antihypertensives)
Adults: initially, 50 mg b.i.d. P.O. Then dose may be increased to 200 to 400 mg daily in two to three divided doses.
Possible side effects
Fatigue, lethargy, vivid dreams, hallucinations, bradycardia, hypotension, congestive heart failure, peripheral vascular disease, nausea, vomiting, diarrhea, hypoglycemia without tachycardia, rash, and fever
Interactions
• Metoprolol may necessitate insulin and oral hypoglycemic dosage alterations in previously stabilized diabetics.
• Cardiotonic glycosides cause excessive bradycardia and may increase depressant effect on myocardium when given with metoprolol tartrate. Use together cautiously.
*Available in both the United States and Canada

Precautions
• Use cautiously in patients with heart block, congestive heart failure, diabetes, or respiratory disease (including asthma and bronchitis) and in those taking other antihypertensives.
Nursing considerations
• Closely monitor the patient's blood pressure. If severe hypotension develops, administer a vasopressor, as ordered.
• Take apical pulses for 1 minute. Withhold drug and notify doctor if apical pulse rate is less than 60 or more than 120 in an adult, or according to a specific order.
• Instruct the patient to take medication with meals to increase absorption.

prazosin hydrochloride (Minipress*)
Indications and dosage
Mild to moderate hypertension (may be used alone or with a diuretic or other antihypertensive)
Adults: P.O. test dose: 1 mg given before bedtime to prevent first-dose syncope. Initially, 1 mg t.i.d. May increase dose slowly up to 20 mg. *Maintenance dose:* 3 to 20 mg daily in three divided doses. (Some patients require dosages up to 40 mg daily.) *Note:* If the doctor adds another antihypertensive or a diuretic to the patient's regimen, decrease prazosin hydrochloride dosage to 1 to 2 mg t.i.d. and retitrate, as ordered.
Possible side effects
Dizziness, headache, drowsiness, weakness, first-dose syncope, depression, orthostatic hypotension, palpitations, blurred vision, dry mouth, diarrhea, vomiting, abdominal cramps, constipation, nausea, priapism
Interactions
• Propranolol and other beta blockers may cause syncope, with the loss of consciousness. Advise the patient to sit or lie down if he becomes dizzy.
Precautions
• Use cautiously in patients receiving other antihypertensives.
Nursing considerations
• Closely monitor the patient's blood pressure and pulse rate.
• Have the patient sit or lie down during the test dose and for 30 minutes afterward.
• Tell the patient to stand slowly and avoid sudden position changes to prevent dizziness, to limit his alcohol intake, and to restrict strenuous exercise in hot weather.
• Advise the patient that sugarless chewing gum, sour hard candy, or ice chips help relieve mouth dryness.

methyldopa (Aldomet*)
Indications and dosage
Chronic, mild to severe hypertension
Adults: initially, 250 mg P.O. b.i.d. to t.i.d. for the first 48 hours. Increase as needed every 2 days. If other antihypertensives are added to or deleted from therapy, the doctor may adjust dosage.
Maintenance dose: 500 mg to 2 g daily in two to four divided doses. Maximum daily dose is 3 g.

Possible side effects
Hemolytic anemia, reversible granulocytopenia, thrombocytopenia, sedation, headache, asthenia, weakness, dizziness, decreased mental acuity, involuntary choreoathetotic movements, psychic disturbances, depression, bradycardia, orthostatic hypotension, aggravated angina, myocarditis, edema and weight gain, dry mouth, nasal stuffiness, diarrhea, hepatic necrosis, gynecomastia, lactation, skin rash, drug-induced fever, impotence
Interactions
• Norepinephrine, phenothiazines, tricyclic antidepressants, and amphetamines may precipitate hypertension when used with methyldopa.
Precautions
• Use cautiously in patients receiving other antihypertensives or monoamine oxidase inhibitors.
Nursing considerations
• Observe the patient for side effects, particularly unexplained fever. Report side effects to the doctor.
• Monitor the patient's blood pressure and heart rate and rhythm.
• Monitor blood studies (complete blood cell count) before and during therapy.
• If the patient has been on this drug for several months, a positive reaction to direct Coombs' test indicates hemolytic anemia.
• If the patient requires a blood transfusion, be sure he gets direct and indirect Coombs' test to prevent cross matching problems.
• Have the patient weigh himself daily. Tell him to notify the doctor if he gains 1 lb (0.45 kg) or more a day for 3 consecutive days. Salt and water retention may occur but can be relieved with diuretics.
• If the doctor increases the dosage, advise the patient to take initial increased dosage at bedtime to minimize daytime drowsiness.
• Tell the patient that his urine may darken in toilet bowls treated with bleach.
• Tell the patient to stand slowly and avoid sudden position changes to prevent dizziness, to limit his alcohol intake, and to restrict strenuous exercise in hot weather.
• Advise the patient that sugarless chewing gum, sour hard candy, or ice chips help relieve mouth dryness.

nadolol (Corgard*)

Indications and dosage
Hypertension
Adults: initially, 40 mg P.O. once daily. May be increased in 40- to 80-mg increments until optimum response occurs. Usual maintenance dosage ranges from 80 to 320 mg once daily. (Rarely, doses of 640 mg may be necessary.)
Possible side effects
Fatigue, lethargy, vivid dreams, hallucinations, bradycardia, hypotension, congestive heart failure, peripheral vascular disease, nausea, vomiting, diarrhea, hypoglycemia without tachycardia, rash, increased airway resistance, fever
Interactions
• Nadolol may necessitate insulin and hypoglycemic dosage alterations in previously stabilized diabetics.

Heart

Nurses' guide to antihypertensive drugs continued

• Cardiotonic glycosides cause excessive bradycardia and may increase the depressant effect on the myocardium when given with nadolol. Use together cautiously.
• Epinephrine may cause severe vasoconstriction.

Precautions

• Contraindicated in patients with bronchial asthma, sinus bradycardia, greater than first degree conduction heart block, and cardiogenic shock.
• Use cautiously in patients with heart failure, chronic bronchitis, and emphysema.

Nursing considerations

• Teach the patient how to take his pulse, and tell him to take it before taking this drug. If he detects extremes in his pulse rate, advise him to withhold this dose of medication and to call the doctor immediately.
• Monitor your patient's blood pressure frequently. If severe hypotension develops, administer a vasopressor, as ordered.
• Instruct the patient to take this drug at meal-times to increase absorption.
• If your patient's a diabetic, tell him that this drug may mask signs and symptoms of hypogly-cemia. Stress that he should have blood studies performed frequently.

propranolol hydrochloride (Inderal*)

Indications and dosage

Hypertension (usually with thiazide diuretics)
Adults: initially, 80 mg P.O. daily in two to four divided doses. May increase at 3- to 7-day intervals to maximum daily dose of 640 mg. Usual maintenance dose for hypertension: 160 to 480 mg daily.

Possible side effects

Fatigue, lethargy, vivid dreams, hallucinations, bradycardia, hypotension, congestive heart failure, peripheral vascular disease, nausea, vomiting, diarrhea, hypoglycemia without tachy-cardia, rash, increased airway resistance, fever

Interactions

• Propranolol may necessitate insulin and oral hypoglycemic dosage alterations in previously stabilized diabetics.
• Cardiotonic glycosides cause excessive bradycardia and may increase depressant effect on the myocardium when given with propranolol. Use together cautiously.
• Aminophylline may antagonize beta-blocking effects of propranolol. Use together cautiously.
• Isoproterenol and glucagon may antagonize propranolol effect. May be used therapeutically in emergencies.
• Cimetidine may inhibit propranolol's metabolism. Monitor for greater beta-blocking effect.
• Epinephrine may cause severe vasoconstriction when given with propranolol.

Precautions

Contraindicated in patients with diabetes mellitus, asthma, allergic rhinitis, sinus bradycardia, heart block greater than first degree, cardiogenic shock, or right ventricular heart failure secondary to pulmonary hypertension and during adminis-tration of ethyl ether anesthetic.
• Use cautiously in patients with congestive heart failure or respiratory disease and in patients taking other antihypertensives.

*Available in both the United States and Canada

Nursing considerations

• Teach the patient how to take his pulse, and tell him to take it before taking this drug. If he detects extremes in his pulse rate, advise him to withhold this dose of medication and call the doctor immediately.
• Monitor blood pressure frequently.
• If your patient's a diabetic, tell him that this drug masks signs and symptoms of hypoglycemia. Stress that he should have blood studies per-formed frequently.
• If the patient develops severe hypotension, notify the doctor. He may prescribe a vasopressor.
• Instruct the patient to take this drug at meal-times to increase absorption.

furosemide (Lasix*)

Indications and dosage

Acute pulmonary edema
Adults: 40 mg I.V. injected slowly over 1 to 2 minutes; then, 40 mg I.V. in 1 to 1½ hours, if needed.
Edema
Adults: 20 to 80 mg P.O. daily in morning; second dose can be given in 6 to 8 hours, if needed; carefully titrated up to 600 mg daily, if needed; or 20 to 40 mg I.M. or I.V. May increase by 20 mg every 2 hours until optimum response occurs. Give I.V. dose slowly over 1 to 2 minutes.
Hypertensive crisis, acute renal failure
Adults: 100 to 200 mg I.V. slowly over 1 to 2 minutes

Possible side effects

Agranulocytosis, thrombocytopenia, volume depletion and dehydration, orthostatic hypotension, transient deafness with too rapid I.V. injection, abdominal discomfort and pain, hypokalemia, hypochloremic alkalosis, asymptomatic hyperuri-cemia, fluid and electrolyte imbalances (includ-ing dilutional hyponatremia and hypochloremia), hypocalcemia, hypomagnesemia, hyperglycemia and impairment of glucose tolerance, dermatitis

Interactions

• Aminoglycoside antibiotics may potentiate ototoxicity. Use together cautiously.
• Chloral hydrate may cause sweating or flushing with I.V. furosemide.
• Clofibrate potentiates furosemide effects.
• Indomethacin inhibits diuretic response.

Precautions

• Use cautiously in cardiogenic shock compli-cated by pulmonary edema, anuria, hepatic coma, or electrolyte imbalances. Drug is not routinely administered to women of childbearing age, because its safe use during pregnancy has not been established.
• Can lead to profound water and electrolyte depletion.
• May cause an allergic reaction in a patient who is sensitive to sulfonamides.

Nursing considerations

• Monitor the patient's blood pressure.
• Closely monitor the patient's serum electrolyte, blood sugar, and uric acid levels.
• Have the patient weigh himself daily. If he gains 1 lb (0.45 kg) or more a day for 3 consecu-tive days, have him notify the doctor. He may be retaining fluids.
• In elderly patients, be alert for excessive

diuresis, vascular thrombosis, and embolism.
• Instruct the patient to eat plenty of potassium-rich foods, such as citrus fruits, tomatoes, bananas, dates, and apricots.
• Instruct the patient to take oral and I.M. preparations in the morning to prevent nocturia. Have him take the second dose in the early afternoon, if ordered.
• Advise the patient to store tablets in light-resistant container to prevent discoloration (doesn't affect potency).
• Tell the patient to stand slowly to prevent dizziness and to limit alcohol intake and strenuous exercise in hot weather.
• Instruct the patient to notify the doctor imme-diately if he experiences ringing in his ears, severe abdominal pain, sore throat, and fever; these signs and symptoms may indicate a furosemide toxicity.

hydrochlorothiazide (HydroDIURIL*)

Indications and dosage

Hypertension
Adults: 25 to 100 mg P.O. daily or divided dosage. Daily dosage increased or decreased according to blood pressure.
Edema
Adults: initially, 25 to 100 mg P.O. daily or intermittently as maintenance dosage.

Possible side effects

Aplastic anemia, agranulocytosis, leukopenia, thrombocytopenia, fluid volume depletion and dehydration, orthostatic hypotension, anorexia, nausea, pancreatitis, hepatic encephalopathy, hypokalemia, asymptomatic hyperuricemia, hyperglycemia and impairment of glucose toler-ance, fluid and electrolyte imbalances (including dilutional hyponatremia and hypochloremia), metabolic alkalosis, hypercalcemia, gout, derma-titis, photosensitivity, rash, hypersensitivity reactions (such as pneumonitis and vasculitis)

Interactions

• Cholestramine and colestipol decrease intestinal absorption of thiazides. Keep doses separated.
• Diazoxide increases antihypertensive, hyper-glycemic, and hyperuricemic effect of hydrochlo-rothiazide. Use together cautiously.

Precautions

• Contraindicated in patients with anuria or with hypersensitivity to other thiazides or sulfonamide derivatives.
• Use cautiously in patients with severe renal disease, impaired hepatic function, or progressive hepatic disease.

Nursing considerations

• Monitor the patient's intake and output and his serum electrolyte, serum creatine, BUN, and blood uric acid levels.
• Have the patient weigh himself daily. Advise him to notify the doctor if he gains l lb (0.45 kg) or more a day for 3 consecutive days.
• Instruct the patient to eat plenty of potassium-rich foods, such as citrus fruits, tomatoes, bananas, dates, and apricots.
• In elderly patients, monitor for excessive diuresis.
• In patients with hypertension, therapeutic response may be delayed. Monitor blood pressure.
• Tell the patient to take this drug in the morning.

Teaching your patient to use a telephone transmitter

Caring for a patient with a pacemaker? If the doctor wants to check the operation of your patient's pacemaker over the telephone, he may ask you to show her how to use a telephone transmitter. Do you know how to proceed? Follow these steps:
Note: *The equipment shown in this photostory is the Medtronic® model 9407 Teletrace® Telephone EKG transmitter.*

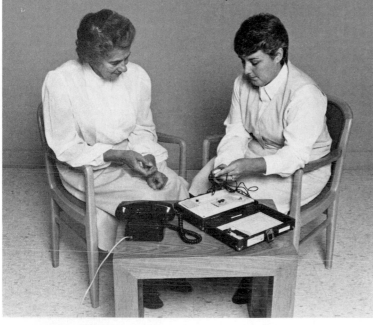

1 First, moisten the inside of your patient's wrist area with water. Then, slip the wrist electrode over her right hand and into position. Check to be sure the electrode plate fits over the moistened area of the wrist, as shown here.
Follow the same procedure on her left wrist.

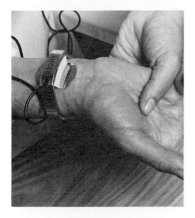

2 Instruct your patient to connect the wrist electrodes to the transmitter. To do this, tell her to insert the white plug into the outlet marked R and the black plug into the outlet marked L.

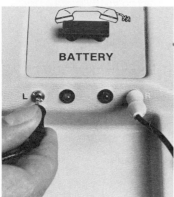

3 Now have your patient dial her doctor's office, as instructed by the doctor. He'll set up a specific date and time for her call.

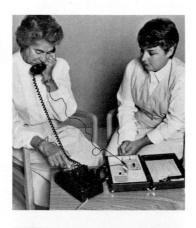

4 When she gets through to the doctor's office, tell your patient that the doctor's nurse will instruct her to place the telephone receiver on the transmitter, as shown here. The mouthpiece should be over the transmitter speaker and the earpiece should rest on the transmitter ON switch. If the unit's properly positioned, tell your patient to expect to hear a high-pitched tone.

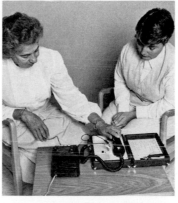

5 When she hears the tone, tell your patient to sit quietly until she no longer hears the tone, usually about 45 seconds.
During this time, the unit in the doctor's office is recording your patient's EKG (see photo).

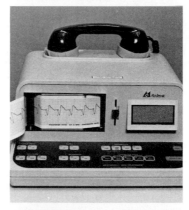

6 Next, have your patient pick up the receiver and follow the nurse's instructions. If the nurse says everything's OK, tell your patient the procedure's complete. Have her hang up the receiver and remove the wrist electrodes.

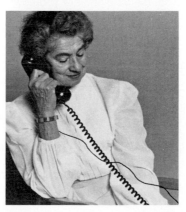

Lungs

Did you know that lung-related disorders are second only to heart disease as the major cause of death in the United States? In addition, acute and chronic lung disorders are common causes of absenteeism and permanent disability.

Because many patients with lung problems are cared for in an ambulatory setting, you'll need to detect change in lung function quickly and accurately. To help provide the care your patient needs, read the following pages closely. You'll find information on:
• what pertinent questions to ask your patient during your assessment.
• how some occupations may cause chronic lung diseases.
• how to use a spirometer to measure your patient's lung function.
• what your patient can do if he's short of breath.

Obtaining a patient profile

Before physically assessing your patient's lung function, part of your health evaluation and screening is to obtain a profile of his condition, including his history. By doing so, you'll gather clues that may help you identify and treat your patient's problem.

As part of your patient's profile, consider asking him the following questions:
• Do you frequently feel the need to clear your throat?
• Do you ever cough? If so, describe what it sounds and feels like. How frequently do you cough? Is the cough more severe at a particular time of day? Does anything make the cough worse? Better? Have you recently been exposed to anyone with a similar cough? Was this person's cough caused by a cold or flu?
• Is there any sputum when you cough? If so, how much? Is it thick? What color is it? Does it contain any blood? Does it have an odor? Is the amount of sputum increasing? When, during the day, do you cough up the most sputum?
• Do you ever feel short of breath? When does it occur? Does it occur when your body's in a particular position? Does any type of activity seem to trigger the shortness of breath? How many pillows do you use while sleeping?
• When you're short of breath, do you also cough, sweat, or have chest pain?
• Do you make a whistling sound when you breathe? Or, a harsh, high-pitched sound?
• Do your nostrils flare when you breathe?
• Does your breathing seem rapid or shallow?
• Do you smoke (cigarettes, pipes, or cigars)? How much do you smoke? How long have you smoked?
• Do you feel any pain in your chest? Describe what it feels like. How often does the pain occur? How long does it last? Does it occur only when you inhale or cough? Is the pain accompanied by coughing, sneezing, or shortness of breath?
• Do you or members of your family have a history of any of the following: Fever or chills? Sweating at night? Tuberculosis? Emphysema? Asthma? Bronchitis? Upper respiratory tract infections? Recurring pneumonia? Congenital or trauma-related chest deformities? High blood pressure, heart attack, or congestive heart failure?
• What medications are you now taking? Do you take any prescription or over-the-counter drugs for cough control, expectoration, or nasal congestion?
• Describe your typical daily diet.
• What type of work do you do? What types have you done in the past? What kinds of hobbies do you have? Have you ever been exposed to any chemicals, toxic fumes, dust, or asbestos while on the job?
• Do you travel frequently? Have you traveled in the past? Where did you go?
• Have you ever been immunized against tuberculosis, pneumonia, influenza, or whooping cough?
• Do you have any allergies to medications, foods, pets, dust, or pollens? Have you ever been treated for any allergies?

Nurses' guide to acute respiratory disorders

You'll probably encounter patients with acute respiratory disorders more than patients with any other type of condition. Acute respiratory disorders are one of the major causes of absenteeism in schools and industry. Because acute respiratory disorders are so common, you need to know how to identify and care for a patient with one.

To refresh your memory of various types of acute respiratory disorders and your role in caring for these patients, read the following chart.

Acute bacterial sinusitis
Inflammation of the paranasal sinus mucosa; recurrence may lead to chronic condition
Cause
• Bacterial (pneumococci)
• Viral (*Hemophilus influenzae*)
• Allergy
Signs and symptoms
• Nasal congestion, followed by gradual buildup of pressure in the affected sinus
• Possibly purulent nasal discharge
• Low-grade fever
• Sore throat
• Malaise
• Pain and swelling over the affected sinus
Nursing intervention
• Stress to your patient the importance of taking the antibiotic medication ordered by the doctor.
• Advise your patient to take an oral antihistamine-decongestant combined with aspirin or acetaminophen.
• Teach your patient how to use nasal decongestant spray correctly.
• Encourage fluid intake to mobilize secretions and promote drainage.
• Tell your patient to watch for and report any of the following signs and symptoms of complications: vomiting, chills, fever, edema of forehead or eyelids, blurred or double vision, or personality changes.

Croup
Severe inflammation and obstruction of the upper airway; may be mistaken for and usually follows upper respiratory tract infection; more common in children. Three types exist: acute laryngotracheobronchitis, laryngitis, and acute spasmodic laryngitis. Laryngotracheobronchitis is the most common type of croup.
Causes
• Viral (parainfluenza, influenza, and measles viruses)
• Bacterial (pertussis and diphtheria)
Signs and symptoms
• Inspiratory stridor
• Hoarse or muffled sounds
• Sharp, barklike cough
• Inflammatory edema and possibly spasm, which may obstruct airway and compromise ventilation
For laryngotracheobronchitis:
• Fever
• Edema of the bronchi and bronchioles
• Expiratory rhonchi

- Scattered rales

For laryngitis:
- Sore throat and cough, possibly progressing to marked hoarseness

For acute spasmodic laryngitis:
- Mild to moderate hoarseness and nasal discharge, followed by cough and noisy inspiration
- Labored breathing with retractions, rapid pulse, clammy skin
- Suprasternal and intercostal retractions, dyspnea, diminished breath sounds, restlessness

Nursing intervention
- Promote bed rest.
- Administer aspirin or acetaminophen in recommended dosages.
- Obtain throat specimen for culture to help identify infecting organism (if bacteria's the cause).
- Urge use of cool-mist humidifier during sleep.
- Instruct parents to monitor cough and breath sounds, hoarseness, cyanosis, respiratory rate and character, restlessness, and fever.
- To relieve a croup spell, tell parents to carry child into the bathroom, shut the door, and turn on the hot water.
- To help control coughing, encourage parents to position two or three pillows under the child's head.
- To relieve the child's sore throat, have parents provide water-based ices, such as fruit sherbet and Popsicles. Tell parents to avoid giving milk-based fluids if child is expectorating thick mucus or has difficulty swallowing.
- Warn parents that ear infection and pneumonia are complications of croup that may appear within 5 days after recovery. Tell them to watch for and report the following signs and symptoms immediately: earache, productive cough, high fever, or increased shortness of breath.

Bronchitis
Inflammation of the tracheobronchial tree; more common in adults, especially those with chronic lung disease
Cause
- Usually viral; secondary bacterial infections are common

Signs and symptoms
- Cough; may or may not be productive
- Coarse rhonchi or wheezes on lung auscultation
- Nasal discharge
- Fever
- Malaise

Nursing intervention
- Promote bed rest.
- Administer aspirin or acetaminophen in recommended dosages.
- Urge patient to take all the antibiotic medicine prescribed by the doctor, if appropriate.
- Recommend use of cool-mist vaporizer to help loosen secretions.
- Tell patient to use cough medicine with an expectorant to remove secretions.

Influenza
Acute, highly contagious respiratory tract infection; occurs sporadically or in epidemics, especially during winter
Cause
- Viral

Signs and symptoms
- Fever
- Malaise
- Myalgia
- Headache
- Sore throat
- Sudden onset of chills
- Cough

Nursing intervention
- Promote bed rest.
- Suggest increased fluid intake.
- Administer aspirin or acetaminophen in recommended dosages.
- Administer cough medicine with an expectorant to enhance expectoration of secretions.
- If signs and symptoms persist, instruct patient to return to the doctor for further evaluation. He may develop secondary complications, such as pneumonia.

Nasopharyngitis
Infection causing mucosal edema and vasodilation
Cause
- Viral (usually rhinovirus)

Signs and symptoms
- Possibly fever, especially in infants and young children
- Dry, irritated nose and throat, possibly accompanied by sneezing and coughing
- Irritability and restlessness
- Chills
- Muscle soreness
- Vomiting or diarrhea possible in infants and young children

Nursing intervention
- Promote bed rest.
- Administer aspirin or acetaminophen in recommended dosages.
- If ordered, obtain a throat specimen for culture to test for streptococcal infection.
- Encourage increased fluid intake.
- Teach patient how to use nose drops to relieve nasal congestion.
- Also tell patient to use antihistamine-decongestant tablets to relieve nasal congestion.

Pharyngitis
Acute or chronic inflammation of the pharynx; may precede nasopharyngitis; usually lasts 3 to 10 days; most common throat disorder; often occurs in adults who live or work in dusty or dry environments, habitually use tobacco or alcohol, or suffer from chronic sinusitis, persistent coughs, or allergies
Causes
- Viral
- Bacterial (usually streptococcus)

Signs and symptoms
- Sore throat
- Difficulty swallowing
- Sensation of lump in throat
- Constant urge to swallow
- On physical exam, posterior wall of pharynx appears red and edematous; mucous membranes studded with white or yellow follicles
- Exudate, usually confined to lymphoid areas
- May be accompanied by mild fever, headache, and muscle and joint pain (especially if bacteria's the cause)

Nursing intervention
- Obtain throat specimen for culture to identify causative organism.
- Promote bed rest.
- Administer aspirin or acetaminophen in recommended dosages.
- Teach patient with chronic pharyngitis how to minimize throat irritation; for example, using a humidifier while sleeping.
- Tell your patient to gargle with warm salt water to relieve sore throat pain.
- Administer throat lozenges containing a mild anesthetic.
- Encourage increased fluid intake.
- Administer penicillin, as ordered (if bacteria's the cause).
- Refer patient to a self-help group to stop smoking.

Tonsillitis
Inflammation of the tonsils; may be acute or chronic; acute form usually lasts 4 to 6 days and commonly affects children between ages 5 and 10.
Causes
- Bacterial (usually beta-hemolytic streptococcus)
- Viral

Signs and symptoms
For acute tonsillitis:
- Mild to severe sore throat
- Loss of appetite (in young child)
- Dysphagia
- Fever
- Chills
- Swelling and tenderness of lymph glands in submandibular area
- Muscle and joint pain
- Malaise
- Headache
- Possibly earache
- Generalized inflammation of pharyngeal wall
- Possibly edematous and inflamed uvula
- Swollen tonsils with white or yellow exudate

For chronic tonsillitis:
- Recurrent sore throat
- Purulent drainage in tonsillar crypts
- Frequent attacks of acute tonsillitis
- Peritonsillar abscess

Nursing intervention
- Administer aspirin or acetaminophen in recommended dosages.
- Administer antibiotics, as ordered (if bacteria's the cause).
- Obtain throat specimen for culture to determine infecting organism and appropriate antibiotic therapy (if bacteria's the cause).
- Use differential diagnosis to rule out infectious mononucleosis and diphtheria.
- Suggest gargling to soothe the throat, unless it exacerbates the pain
- Make sure the patient and parents understand the importance of completing prescribed course of antibiotic therapy.
- Encourage increased fluid intake.
- Promote bed rest.
- Suggest that parents give child ice cream or flavored drinks and ices.
- If tonsil removal is necessary, explain the procedure.

Lungs

Learning about influenza immunization

Of course, one of your primary responsibilities as an ambulatory-care nurse is preventing disease when possible. And for influenza—an acute, highly contagious respiratory tract disease—immunization is the most effective method of prevention.

You're probably aware that influenza is spread rapidly and easily throughout the community and can lead to serious complications, such as pneumonia. The elderly and those with chronic illnesses (such as cardiac, pulmonary, renal, or neurologic metabolic diseases) are particularly susceptible.

If your patient has influenza, the first signs and symptoms will appear 24 to 72 hours after he contracts the disease. These signs and symptoms include:
* sudden onset of fever
* chills
* headache
* muscle ache
* general malaise
* coughing
* sore throat.

The viruses that cause influenza constantly change, preventing the buildup of natural immunities. Therefore, you'll have to know which strain of virus is prevalent at the time so you can give your patient the appropriate vaccine. Vaccine content is based on the previous year's virus and is usually 75% effective.

In addition, because of the large number of influenza viruses and their constantly changing nature, you won't routinely immunize all your patients for influenza. Annual immunizations at the start of the flu season are usually given to the elderly, those persons with chronic or debilitating diseases, and those providing services essential to the community (for example, police officers, fire fighters, and hospital personnel).

Note: Mass immunizations are ordered only when an epidemic's declared.

The influenza vaccine provides about 3 to 12 months of protection. Some persons may still develop the disease after immunization, but it'll probably be less severe.

Before administering the vaccine, be sure to explain to your patient such possible side effects as discomfort at the vaccination site, fever, and malaise. Remember, because the vaccine's made from chicken embryos, avoid administering it to patients who are allergic to chicken, chicken feathers, or eggs.

You'll inject the influenza vaccine into your patient's subcutaneous skin or muscle layers, depending on the type of vaccine you're using. For large-scale immunizations, you may use an immunization gun. (For details on using the immunization gun, also called a jet injection apparatus, see the photostory that follows.)

Using a jet injection apparatus for immunizations

Suppose you're a community health nurse and have to administer a measles vaccine to several hundred schoolchildren. To do so, use a jet injection apparatus. The highly pressurized air in this device forces the vaccine through the patient's pores, into the subcutaneous skin layer. For large-scale immunizations, the device is faster and more efficient than a needle and syringe.

Before you begin, enlist the help of two or three co-workers. Be sure to obtain a signed consent form from each child's parent or guardian. Then, have your co-workers check that the patient's shirt sleeve is rolled up, and briefly explain to each patient that he may feel slight discomfort as the vaccine's injected, but assure him the injection won't hurt. Important: Keep 1:1,000 epinephrine handy in case of anaphylactic shock.

Note: *Don't use the jet injection apparatus unless you've received the proper training and certification.*

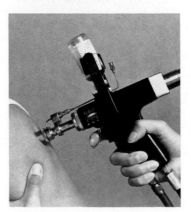

1 To prepare the apparatus, hold a bottle of the prescribed vaccine in your left hand. Then, pick up the apparatus with your right hand, invert it, and insert the needle in the bottle's rubber top. Make sure the bottle is firmly in place. Don't allow anything to touch the needle, because you may contaminate the vaccine.

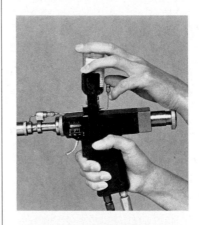

2 Place your foot on the hydraulic pump's foot pedal. Press and release the pedal to activate the apparatus. Remember, you'll have to do so for every injection.

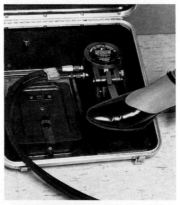

3 To locate the injection site, measure about one handbreadth down from the top of your patient's shoulder. Have a co-worker clean the skin with an alcohol swab. Support the patient's arm as you position the apparatus' tip firmly against the patient's skin. Then, pull back on the trigger to inject the vaccine.

Finally, have your co-worker massage the site with a clean alcohol swab.

Learning about chronic lung diseases

As you probably know, a chronic lung disease results from the persistent obstruction of airflow entering or leaving the lungs. As the air passages narrow, gas exchange is compromised.

But are you aware that chronic lung disorders affect millions of persons and that the incidence of these disorders is rising? Today, more than ever, you need to know and understand all you can about chronic lung disorders. Because a patient with a chronic lung disorder usually isn't hospitalized, you'll have to help him cope by teaching him about the disease and how he can manage it.

Here are some general guidelines for you to follow when caring for such a patient:
• Make sure your patient understands the importance of taking his medication as prescribed.
• Alert your patient to factors that may make his condition worse. These include stress or anxiety; pollution; excess work, eating, or exercise; and fatigue or lack of sleep.
• Help your patient find ways to avoid or deal with stress or anxiety.
• Show the patient how to breathe through pursed lips to help increase his lung capacity. Also demonstrate relaxed breathing techniques.
• Demonstrate chest physiotherapy and postural drainage techniques to your patient and his family members. This way they can perform these techniques at home.
• Develop an exercise program for your patient, keeping in mind his limited capability. Help the patient and family adjust his life-style to accommodate the limitations caused by the disorder.
• Teach the patient and family how to recognize early signs and symptoms of an upper respiratory tract infection; for example, sore throat and fever. Warn your patient to avoid contact with people who currently have respiratory tract infections.
• Emphasize the importance of

*Available in both the United States and Canada

good mouth care to your patient to help reduce the risk of further infection.
• Encourage your patient to express his feelings about his condition. Because his degree of activity may be limited, he may become angry or depressed.
• Assist your patient in developing a high-calorie diet to maintain his weight. Tell him to eat small, frequent meals that are high in protein and to supplement them with nutritional snacks.
• If your patient's receiving oxygen therapy, tell him and his family to administer it in low concentrations.

Now, read the following chart to become more familiar with the various types of chronic obstructive lung disorders.

Asthma

Increased bronchial reactivity to stimuli, producing episodic bronchospasm and airway obstruction

Causes
• *Extrinsic asthma:* exposure to specific allergens, such as ragweed, animal dander, tree and grass pollens, foods, or such drugs as aspirin
• *Intrinsic asthma:* respiratory tract infections; smoke, cold air, atmospheric pollutants; exercise, resulting in hypocapnia; overuse of medications, such as narcotics and sedatives, resulting in hypoventilation and bronchoconstriction; emotionally stressful situations, such as fear or excitement, which cause hyperventilation and hypocapnia

Signs and symptoms
• History of intermittent attacks of dyspnea and wheezing
• Audible wheezing
• Chest tightness (patient feels like he can't breathe)
• Productive cough with thick mucus
• Prolonged expiration
• Intercostal and supraclavicular retraction on inspiration
• Nostril flaring
• Use of accessory muscles during breathing
• Increased chest circumference
• Tachypnea
• Tachycardia
• Perspiration
• Flushing
• Possibly signs and symptoms of

eczema or allergic rhinitis
• Absent or diminished breath sounds during severe obstruction
• Chest X-ray reveals hyperinflated lungs with trapped air during attack; normal chest X-ray when in remission
• Pulmonary function tests during an attack show decreased forced expiratory volumes, which improve after use of bronchodilator; increased residual volume and, occasionally, total lung capacity may be normal between attacks.

Nursing intervention
• Administer aerosol containing beta-adrenergic agents or oral beta-adrenergic agents and oral methylxanthines.
• Prepare patient to undergo skin test to try to determine specific allergens causing the condition. If specific allergens are identified, teach patient how to avoid them.
• Show patient how to use antihistamines, decongestants, and oral or aerosol bronchodilators, if appropriate.
• Explain how stress and anxiety affect asthma, and teach patient ways to avoid them.
• Warn patient of asthma's association with exercise (particularly running) and cold air. Tell him to avoid both, if possible.
• If patient requires emergency treatment, administer oxygen, corticosteroids, and bronchodilators, such as intravenous aminophylline, and inhaled agents, such as isoproterenol, following approved protocol.

Emphysema

Abnormal, irreversible enlargement of air spaces distal to terminal bronchioles, from destruction of alveolar walls; results in decreased elastic recoil properties of lungs

Cause
• Unknown but believed to be related to deficiency of alpha$_1$-antitrypsin; this deficiency allows release of proteolytic enzymes, which destroy lung tissue; loss of lung-supporting structure results in decreased elastic recoil and airway collapse on expiration; destruction of alveolar walls decreases surface area available for gas exchange; factors that may be involved include cigarette smoking, respiratory tract infections, air pollution, and allergens.

Signs and symptoms
• Insidious onset
• Dyspnea
• Chronic cough

• Anorexia
• Weight loss
• Chronic malaise
• Increased chest circumference (barrel-chest appearance)
• Use of accessory muscles during breathing
• Prolonged expiratory period with grunting
• Pursed-lip breathing
• Tachypnea
• Peripheral cyanosis
• Digital clubbing
• In advanced disease: flattened diaphragm, reduced vascular markings at lung periphery, overaeration of lungs, vertical heart, enlarged anteroposterior chest circumference, and large retrosternal air space may be visible on chest X-ray.
• Pulmonary function tests show increased volume, total lung capacity, and compliance; decreased vital capacity, diffusing capacity, and expiratory volume.

Nursing intervention
• Teach your patient to use bronchodilators to reverse bronchospasm and promote mucociliary clearance.
• Stress to your patient the importance of taking antibiotics as ordered, to prevent a respiratory tract infection; a flu vaccine to prevent influenza; and Pneumovax* to prevent pneumococcal pneumonia.
• Promote fluid intake to help loosen secretions.
• Teach patient and his family how to perform postural drainage and chest physiotherapy at home, if ordered.
• Urge patient to stop smoking. If necessary, refer him to a self-help group. Also, have the patient try to avoid contact with air pollutants.

Cancer

Usually develops within the wall or epithelium of the bronchial tree; various types include squamous cell (epidermoid), oat cell (small cell), adenocarcinoma, and anaplastic (large cell). Lung cancer is the most common form of cancer death.

Cause
• Most likely, the inhalation of carcinogenic pollutants; direct relationship between increased incidence of cancer and cigarette smoking; increased susceptibility for persons working in industries using carcinogenic substances or with family history of cancer

Signs and symptoms
• Usually do not appear until

Lungs

Learning about chronic lung diseases continued

disease's later stages; depends on the type of cancer and how far it's spread.
• Initially, productive cough, possibly containing mucopurulent or blood-tinged sputum
In squamous cell or oat cell:
• Hemoptysis
• Wheezing
• Dyspnea
• Smoker's cough
• Chest pain later in disease
In adenocarcinoma and anaplastic carcinoma:
• Weight loss, anorexia
• Weakness; fatigue
• Lesion visible on chest X-ray

Nursing intervention
• Since surgery, radiation, and chemotherapy are the most common treatments, your care involves identifying people at risk, early detection of disease, teaching the patient about the procedures and helping prepare him for them, and providing emotional support during treatment.
• Explain the possible side effects of radiation or chemotherapy treatments.
• If patient smokes, urge him to quit. Refer him to a self-help group, if necessary.
• Recommend that all heavy smokers over age 40 have chest X-rays and sputum cytologies annually. Tell your patient to contact his doctor if he detects any change in the character of his cough.

Chronic bronchitis
Excessive mucus production in the tracheobronchial tree with productive cough for at least 3 months a year for 2 successive years; severity related to amount and duration of smoking; may worsen during respiratory tract infection; rarely develops into significant airway obstruction.

Cause
• Hypertrophy and hyperplasia of the mucus-secreting glands of the trachea, bronchi, and bronchioles, resulting in damage to cilia lining the lungs; cilia's function of clearing the lungs is impaired, and mucous plugs form, becoming a culture media for bacterial infections.

Signs and symptoms
• Insidious onset
• Productive cough
• Dyspnea on exertion
• Abundant sputum production; may be gray, white, or yellow
• Weight gain from edema

• Cyanosis
• Tachypnea
• Wheezing
• No use of accessory muscles noted during respirations
• Prolonged expirations
• Rales and wheezing on auscultation
• Neck vein distention
• Nasopharyngitis associated with increased sputum and worsening dyspnea may take longer to resolve.
• Hyperinflation and increased bronchovascular markings may be visible on X-ray.
• Pulmonary function tests show increased residual volume, decreased vital capacity and forced expiratory volumes, normal static compliance and diffusing capacity.

Nursing intervention
• Remind patient of the importance of complying with antibiotic therapy prescribed by the doctor.
• Urge patient to quit smoking. Refer him to a self-help group for assistance.
• Tell patient to avoid air pollutants.
• Encourage fluid intake to promote secretions.
• Teach patient and his family how to perform chest physiotherapy and postural drainage.
• Instruct patient and family on the proper use of nebulizers and oxygen therapy.

Diffuse interstitial pulmonary fibrosis
Progressive thickening and scarring of interalveolar septa, with steadily progressive dyspnea; may result in death from lack of oxygen or heart failure.

Cause
• Inhalation of dust, industrial irritants, allergens, irritant gases, or chemicals

Signs and symptoms
• Chest pain
• Dyspnea on exertion
• Dry, irritating cough, progressing to productive hemoptysis
• Wheezing
• Tachypnea
• Cyanosis on exertion
• If chemicals are the cause: burning of eyes, nose, throat, and trachea; possibly nausea and vomiting

Nursing intervention
• Tell patient to control dyspnea by limiting his activity.
• After taking patient's history and determining the cause, warn him to avoid contact with cause.

Lung diseases: Some occupational causes
Occupational lung disease develops when the patient breathes air containing a damaging substance. The disease usually develops gradually over months or years. But some lung hazards, such as phosgene gas, can cause instantaneous lung damage.

A patient may dismiss or ignore early signs of lung disease because they're relatively minor. These signs may include lingering colds; an increasing need to cough up mucus; occasional complicating infections, such as bronchitis or pneumonia; and slight breathlessness on exertion. If the hazard's allowed to persist and the patient's condition worsens, life-threatening complications may develop.

Occupational lung hazards come in various forms. They include:
• dusts; for example, coal dust, dust from the processing of plant products (cereal grains), or chemical dusts (pesticides, dye). These may cause bronchitis, asthma, and cancer.
• fumes and smoke from metal welding, burning wood, and cigar, cigarette, and pipe smoking. These may cause lung inflammation, bronchitis, metal fume fever, and lung cancer.
• gases and vapors; for example, from a chemical reaction in industry or from welding, smelting, or furnace work. These can cause hypersensitivity reactions.
• mists or sprays from paints, lacquers, hair spray, pesticides, cleaning products, acids, and solvents. These may irritate or damage the lungs.
• radiation; for example, from working with substances or devices that emit radiation, such as X-rays, in industry or in medicine. This increases the risk of cancer.

Types of occupational lung disease
Several types of occupational lung disease exist, varying according to the substance involved and the concentration at which it's inhaled. Some common diseases include:
• silicosis: a pneumoconiosis caused by the inhalation of silica dust; this usually affects workers in the ceramics and building materials industries
• asbestosis: inhalation of asbestos fibers, which may lead to fibrosis and cancer; primarily affects workers in the construction and fireproofing industries and those involved in the mining and milling of asbestos
• berylliosis: inhalation of dust, fumes, or mists containing beryllium, a metal used in the metallurgy, machine tools, and nuclear power industries; related to rising incidence of lung, liver, and gallbladder cancers
• pneumoconiosis of coal workers: known as black lung; afflicts coal miners who continually inhale coal dust
• byssinosis: inhalation of fibers, such as cotton, flax, or hemp, primarily by textile industry workers.

Your role
The role of an ambulatory-care nurse in assessing a patient with suspected chronic lung disease involves more than an examination. In addition, you should:
• take an accurate history, including a description of the patient's job, materials he works with, and how long he's been working with them.
• perform various pulmonary function tests.
• evaluate working conditions for lung hazards.
• educate workers about possible lung hazards and show them ways to avoid these hazards by using protective equipment, such as a respirator.
• work with management and workers to alleviate hazards.
• provide follow-up physical examinations to determine the effectiveness of preventive measures.

Learning about respirators

One way of reducing the risk of work-related lung disorders is to have the workers wear respirators. Keep in mind, though, that other methods of controlling lung hazards include changing the operational procedure that's causing the hazard and constructing a ventilation system to remove the hazardous material.

The respirator should be worn only when no other protection's available or as a temporary measure while other hazard-control equipment's being installed or repaired.

The two basic types of respirators are:
• An air-filtering device consists of a mask that fits over the nose and mouth, cleaning the air as the worker breathes. Because unfiltered air may seep in around the mask's edges, the worker shouldn't use the mask around a dangerous hazard. In addition, filters are designed to handle only one specific type of hazard.
• Supplied-air respirators come in two styles: those that supply air as the worker needs it and those that continuously pump air into the mask to maintain a pressure that's higher than the surrounding air. The latter style, called a positive-pressure system, is the only one that can be used in an immediately hazardous situation, because the increased pressure keeps out the hazardous air.

What's your role? If you're an occupational health nurse, you'll need to help each worker determine which type of respirator is best for him and teach him how to use it.
• Show him how to clean the respirator after each use to ensure effectiveness. Stress that the respirator *must* be cleaned after each use.
• Emphasize the importance of wearing the respirator. He may find it uncomfortable and decide not to wear it.

Supplied-air respirator

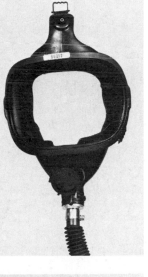

Air-filtering respirator

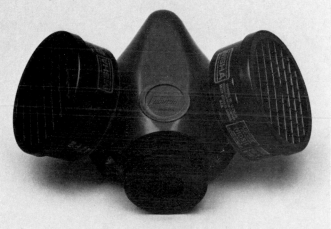

Learning about pulmonary function tests

If you suspect your patient has some type of pulmonary dysfunction, confirm your suspicion by performing a series of pulmonary function tests. You'll also use these tests for screening persons working in high-risk environments. These tests help measure your patient's lung volume and capacity—the elasticity of his lungs and his ability to move air in and out of them.

By studying the results of pulmonary function tests, you can determine if your patient has a chronic lung disease and identify the type of disease. You can also use the results to assess the effectiveness of specific therapeutic measures.

Of course, you'll use a spirometer to measure pulmonary function. Types of spirometer vary from simple mechanical devices to sophisticated electronic equipment. But they all work on the same principle: They measure your patient's lung function as he breathes into a tube connected to the machine.

Values
Average values for pulmonary function tests are predicted based on a patient's age, weight, height, and sex. These average values are then compared with actual measurements, which are recorded as a percentage of the average value. If your patient's test results are less than 80% of the predicted value, consider them abnormal. Refer him to a doctor.

These are the measurements you'll receive on the pulmonary function tests:
• *Tidal volume:* amount of air inhaled or exhaled during normal breathing
• *Expiratory reserve volume:* amount of air that can be exhaled after normal expiration
• *Minute volume:* total amount of air your patient breathes per minute
• *Inspiratory reserve volume:* amount of air inspired over the above-normal inspiration
• *Residual volume:* amount of air remaining in the lungs after forced expiration
• *Vital capacity:* total volume of air that your patient exhales after maximum inspiration
• *Inspiratory capacity:* amount of air your patient inhales after normal expiration
• *Functional residual capacity:* amount of air remaining in the lungs after normal expiration
• *Total lung capacity:* total volume of the lungs when maximally inflated
• *Forced vital capacity:* dynamic measurement of amount of air exhaled after maximum inspiration
• *Forced expiratory volume:* volume of air expired in the first, second, or third second of the forced vital capacity test
• *Maximal voluntary ventilation* (maximum breathing capacity): greatest volume of air breathed per specific unit of time.

Of all the tests listed above, tidal volume, expiratory reserve volume, vital capacity, inspiratory capacity, forced vital capacity, forced expiratory volume, and maximal voluntary ventilation are direct spirographic measurements. The others are indirect measurements that you'll calculate individually for your patient.

Your role
If you're administering pulmonary function tests, follow these guidelines:
• Explain the procedure and equipment to your patient.
• Advise him that the test's accuracy depends on his cooperation.
• Instruct your patient not to eat a heavy meal before the test and not to smoke for 4 to 6 hours before it.
• Make sure your patient hasn't taken any medication—for example, an analgesic or bronchodilator—that may depress respirations before the test.

Lungs

Performing a pulmonary function test

Forty-two-year-old Betty Donlevy works at a glass manufacturing plant. To determine whether the dust Ms. Donlevy inhales on the job is affecting her lungs, you'll use a spirometer to measure her lung capacity and volume. In this photostory, we'll use the DeVilbiss® Surveyor I spirometer, which contains a microcomputer that measures and analyzes test results as your patient breathes into a tube connected to the machine. Then, the results are displayed on a screen above the keyboard.

You can perform two types of test with the DeVilbiss I spirometer: single-breath and multibreath tests. Before beginning, explain the procedure for both tests to Ms. Donlevy. Important: If you're administering the single-breath test to an elderly person or one with a suspected heart disorder, allow him to rest between tests. But before administering the multibreath test, be sure such a patient checks with his doctor.

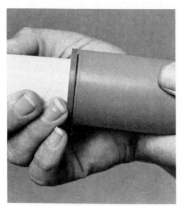

1 Turn on the spirometer and allow it to warm up for about 10 minutes. Then, firmly attach the breathing hose to the spirometer and insert a disposable mouthpiece about halfway into the breathing hose, as shown.

Now, follow the manufacturer's instructions to program the computer with patient information, date, and time.

Have your patient hold the breathing hose and mouthpiece in one hand.

2 To start the single-breath test, press the button marked SINGLE BREATH on the keyboard. Keeping your finger on the button, instruct your patient to take a deep breath and hold it while placing her lips around the mouthpiece. Then, lift your finger off the button, and tell her to exhale forcefully for as long as possible. The spirometer will automatically measure the results.

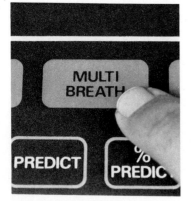

3 To perform the multibreath test, press the MULTIBREATH button on the keyboard. Release the button and tell Ms. Donlevy to breathe rapidly and deeply.

After the test is complete, follow the manufacturer's instructions to obtain a printed summary of the test results.

Discard the mouthpiece and document the procedure.

Learning about chest X-rays

As you know, a chest X-ray allows you to visualize what's taking place inside your patient's chest and lungs. And X-ray films will help you and the doctor identify relationships between bone and tissue and surrounding structures. X-rays penetrate your patient's chest, and then react on a photographic plate. Because normal lung tissue is radiolucent, such abnormalities as fluids, tumors, infiltrates, and foreign bodies appear as densities on the film. The illustrations below distinguish between normal and diseased lungs.

As a diagnostic tool, the chest X-ray is most valuable when compared with previous X-rays of the patient or when studied along with other tests; for example, a sputum culture. *Note:* Because of radiation risks, chest X-rays are no longer routinely ordered.

Depending on your working protocol, a chest X-ray may be taken to assess your patient's pulmonary status and to detect pulmonary disorders. For example, suppose you suspect your patient has pneumonia. You may use chest X-rays as part of a screening procedure for tuberculosis. Or, you may use a chest X-ray to help confirm your suspicion. Finally, if you're an occupational health nurse, a chest X-ray may help you determine whether if dust inhaled on the job is affecting his lungs.

If you're taking a chest X-ray of your patient, keep these guidelines in mind:
• Before you begin, have your patient remove all clothing above the waist and any jewelry that may obstruct the view of the area.
• Explain that he'll receive only a small amount of radiation during the procedure. Assure him that the procedure is safe.
• Tell your patient to take a deep breath and hold it momentarily while you take the X-ray. This helps separate pulmonary structures and provides a clearer view on the film.
• To avoid radiation exposure, leave the room or immediate area while taking the X-rays. If you must stay in the area (for example, to position the patient correctly), wear a lead apron or protective clothing and a monitor.

Remember: Chest X-rays are usually contraindicated for patients in the first trimester of pregnancy; if they're absolutely necessary, place a lead apron over your patient's abdomen to shield the fetus.

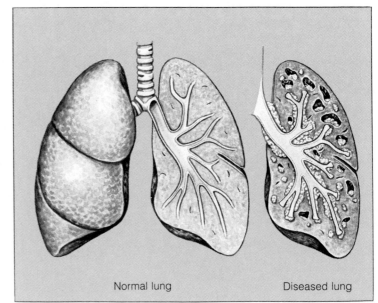

Normal lung   Diseased lung

Positioning your patient for a chest X-ray

Sheila Adams, a 24-year-old law student, arrives at the clinic where you work complaining of chest pain, fever, productive cough, and shortness of breath. After you take Ms. Adams' history and perform a physical examination, you suspect she has pneumonia. In this situation, help confirm your suspicions by taking a chest X-ray, according to your working protocol. As you know, a chest X-ray is an important tool in diagnosing a lung disorder.

Begin by explaining the procedure and its purpose to Ms. Adams. Describe the equipment she'll see in the X-ray area. Then, ask her to remove her clothing above the waist and put on the patient gown you've provided. Also ask her to remove any jewelry from around her neck. Take care to protect her privacy, and provide emotional support throughout the procedure.

Note: Ask Ms. Adams if she's pregnant. If she is, a chest X-ray may be contraindicated.

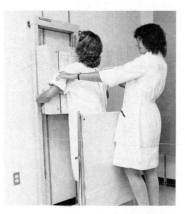

1 Ask Ms. Adams to face the X-ray machine and place her hands on either side of the machine, as shown. Assist her as necessary. This position, the posteroanterior (PA) view, shows more lung area than other views because of the lower diaphragm position.

Note: Remind Ms. Adams to hold her breath and remain very still as you take the X-ray.

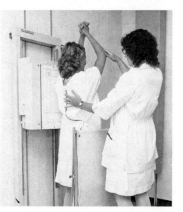

2 Now, ask Ms. Adams to turn to her right, so her *left* side's facing the X-ray machine. Tell her to raise her arms above her head and clasp her hands. This position's called the left lateral (LL) view and provides a better picture than the right lateral (RL) view because the heart's left of midline and not as magnified.

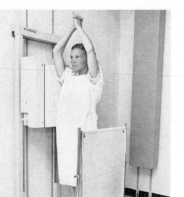

3 Finally, instruct Ms. Adams to turn around so her right side's facing the X-ray machine. Again, have her raise her arms above her head. This position provides an RL view of her lungs. Lateral views may show abnormalities that aren't visible on a PA view.

Document the procedure and any patient teaching.

Learning about tuberculosis

Although the incidence of tuberculosis has declined greatly in developing countries, the disease is by no means eradicated.

Because a patient with tuberculosis is no longer confined to a sanitorium—and usually isn't even admitted to a hospital—you may be responsible for his follow-up care. You can help such a patient deal with this disease by teaching him about it and stressing the importance of following treatments. You're also responsible for detecting new cases of tuberculosis through accurate assessment and screening programs.

As you probably know, tuberculosis is an acute or chronic bacterial infection that usually affects the lungs. Mycobacteria may exist in other parts of the body, however, such as the kidneys and lymph nodes.

Tuberculosis-causing bacteria (*Mycobacterium tuberculosis* or other strains of mycobacterium) are spread by droplets emitted when an infected person speaks, coughs, or sneezes. Another person may inhale droplets containing the bacteria, which usually become implanted in the lungs. A primary infection may result, but often it's so minor that the body's defense system controls it by walling it up in a tiny nodule (tubercle). The signs and symptoms of the primary infection are similar to other respiratory tract infections: fatigue, weakness, anorexia, weight loss, night sweating, and low-grade fever. Normally, no serious illness results, and the tuberculosis remains hidden.

After years of dormancy, the tubercle bacilli may become reactivated, especially when the patient's defense system is lowered. Those who are susceptible include the elderly; patients with pneumonia, diabetes, cancer, or alcoholism; and those patients receiving cortisone or similar drugs.

After the bacilli are reactivated, they produce tissue necrosis, accompanied by fibrosis in any organ they attack. Liquid necrosis may cause a cavity in the organ, such as a lung, and spread the disease to other organs, such as the joints, lymph nodes, peritoneum, genitourinary tract, and bowels.

After reactivation, the patient may exhibit the following signs and symptoms: fatigue, anorexia, weight loss, fever, occasional hemoptysis, chest pain, and a prolonged productive cough.

Assessing the patient

To determine whether your patient's been exposed to tuberculosis, perform a skin test. Two types of skin test exist: a single-injection test (the Mantoux), which is more accurate, and multi-puncture tests (Tine or Mono-vacc), which are slightly less accurate but easier to administer to large groups. Both types involve an intradermal injection of tuberculin antigen. If the patient has active or dormant tuberculosis, he'll have induration of 10 mm or more in diameter around the injection site within 48 to 72 hours after the injection. Remind your patient to return in about 72 hours so you can assess the test results.

The skin test, however, can't detect whether the disease is active. To confirm the presence of active bacilli, you'll have to use other assessment methods, such as physical examination (crepitant rales, bronchial breath sounds, wheezes, and whispered pectoriloquy on auscultation, dullness over the affected area on percussion), chest X-ray (nodular lesions, patchy infiltrates especially in the upper lobes, cavity formation, scar tissue, and calcium deposits), and sputum stains and cultures (heat-sensitive, nonmotile, aerobic, acid-fast bacilli).

Treatment of tuberculosis

The doctor will probably order several oral medications, such as isoniazid, ethambutol, and rifampin. After the first few weeks of treatment, the signs and symptoms of tuberculosis should disappear. Emphasize the importance of complying with long-term treatment and follow-up examinations.

Lungs

Teaching your patient about tuberculosis treatment

As you probably know, drug therapy—along with rest—is the principle way to treat tuberculosis. Of course, how effective the treatment is depends on your patient. Be sure to tell your patient about the importance of taking his medication on time—exactly as prescribed. Suggest that after he takes his pills, he check off the date on the calendar. Recommend that he keep the pills in a place where he'll be sure to see them; for example, on the kitchen table. But tell him to make sure the pills are out of the reach of children. Explain that skipping a dosage will give the tuberculosis bacteria a chance to grow stronger, making them harder to kill. Remind your patient that he must continue taking the medication for the amount of time prescribed by the doctor. And finally, instruct your patient to cover his nose and mouth when he coughs or sneezes.

If you're caring for a patient with tuberculosis, you should know the medications commonly used in tuberculosis treatment. Read the following information to familiarize yourself with several of these medications.

Isoniazid (INH)

Because this drug is considered a primary treatment against active, growing tubercle bacilli, it is the most frequently prescribed drug in tuberculosis treatment. Be alert for these possible side effects: agranulocytosis, aplastic anemia, peripheral neuropathy, nausea, vomiting, epigastric distress, hepatitis, hyperglycemia, and possibly hypersensitivity reaction.

Keep in mind that isoniazid's contraindicated in patients with liver or kidney disease, arthritis, epilepsy, convulsions, or joint stiffening; it's also contraindicated if your patient's pregnant or an alcoholic.

Tell a patient taking isoniazid to notify his doctor immediately if he notices any of these signs and symptoms, which may indicate liver impairment: loss of appetite, fever, nausea, weakness, sore muscles, dark urine, or yellowing of the skin or eyeballs. Also, tell him to take the medication at least 1 hour before taking aluminum-containing antacids or laxatives.

Ethambutol hydrochloride

This drug's used as adjunctive treatment in pulmonary tuberculosis. It's usually not prescribed for children younger than age 13.

Remember that ethambutol hydrochloride is contraindicated in patients with optic neuritis and should be used cautiously in patients with impaired renal function, cataracts, recurring eye inflammations, gout, and diabetic retinopathy.

If your patient's taking this drug, be alert for any of these possible side effects: headache, dizziness, possibly mental confusion, optic neuritis, anorexia, nausea, vomiting, elevated uric acid level, and dermatitis or pruritus.

Rifampin

This drug's used in the primary treatment of pulmonary tuberculosis. As you know, rifampin must be used cautiously in patients with hepatic disease. If your patient's taking this drug, be alert for these side effects: drowsiness, headache, dizziness, mental confusion, thrombocytopenia, transient leukopenia, hemolytic anemia, visual disturbances, epigastric distress, anorexia, serious hepatotoxicity, as well as transient abnormalities in liver function studies.

Inform your patient that rifampin causes drowsiness and that he should avoid activities requiring alertness and good psychomotor coordination, such as driving. Also, warn him that this drug may color his urine, feces, saliva, perspiration, and tears red-orange.

Note: For more information on these drugs, see DRUGS in the NURSE'S REFERENCE LIBRARY™ Series.

Teaching effective coughing

Sam Washburn, a 42-year-old carpenter, has emphysema. As a result of the disease, Mr. Washburn's lungs easily become clogged with secretions. If these secretions remain in his lungs, they may breed infection, leading to such complications as pneumonia.

To help Mr. Washburn remove the secretions from his lungs and thereby prevent complications, teach him how to cough effectively. But remember, Mr. Washburn may be afraid to cough because doing so causes him to become short of breath. Assure him that the procedure's safe and will help clear his lungs when performed correctly. Do you know how to proceed? If you're unsure, follow these steps. Note: *Tailor this procedure to your patient, based on his disease, age, and general physical condition.*

First, tell Mr. Washburn to sit in a chair with his feet firmly on the floor.

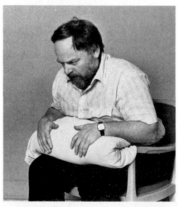

1 Now, instruct Mr. Washburn to relax his shoulders and roll them forward slightly. Give him a pillow to hold on his lap or have him fold his arms across the pillow. Tell him to inhale slowly through his nose and push his abdomen against the pillow.

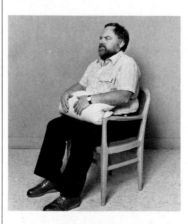

2 Next, tell him to drop his head, sink his chest, and slowly bend forward. Have him exhale, with his lips slightly parted or pursed. Then, tell him to sit up and inhale slowly by sniffing. This technique increases air volume in the lung area and propels mucus out of the passageways.

Have Mr. Washburn repeat this procedure three or four times.

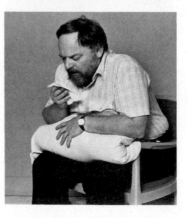

3 When Mr. Washburn's ready to cough, tell him to take a deep breath. Now, tell him to bend forward and cough twice. Expect the first cough to be soft and the second progressively more forceful. Offer tissues so he can remove the sputum from his mouth. Document your findings.

Home care

Learning breathing techniques

Dear Patient:

You have a lung disease that impairs your normal breathing. To help you feel better and be more active, the doctor wants you to strengthen your abdominal muscles. This way they can help your diaphragm with some of the work of breathing. To strengthen your abdominal muscles, perform the exercises shown here. The doctor will tell you which ones he wants you to do and how much time to spend on each one. Try to do these exercises two to four times every day; for example, when you wake up in the morning, before meals, in the late afternoon or evening, and just before you go to bed.

Note: If the doctor's ordered medication for your lung congestion, be sure to use it before performing these exercises.

Whenever you perform the exercises, wear loose clothing. Also, blow your nose to be sure your nasal passages are clear. Take your time as you perform the exercises. Rest whenever you feel tired.

1 ☐ To perform this exercise, sit in a chair or on the edge of your bed, with your feet flat on the floor. Allow your neck and shoulders to droop. Place your hands over your lower ribs and upper abdomen, as shown. Then, purse your lips as you would to whistle. Blow air out through your lips slowly and evenly. Press firmly on your ribs and abdomen as you do. Then, release the pressure slightly and start to inhale. Now, gently cough and try to produce mucus.

2 ☐ For this exercise, lie flat on the floor, not on the bed. Keeping your feet flat on the floor, bend your knees and pull up your thighs toward your chest as far as possible. Rest one hand across the middle of your chest and the other hand on your abdomen. Place the thumb of the hand on your abdomen just below your navel.

Keep your mouth closed and inhale deeply through your nose. Let your abdomen come out as far as possible, but try to keep your chest still. Then, exhale slowly through pursed lips, and press your abdomen firmly inward and upward at the same time. Again, try to keep your chest still.

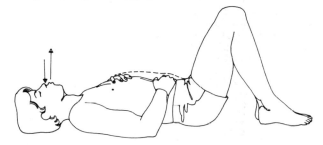

3 ☐ Begin this exercise by lying flat on the floor, in the same position as the previous exercise. Place your arms around your legs, as shown. As you do, breathe in through your nose and let your abdomen rise as much as possible. Then, as you pull your legs toward your chest, as far as possible, exhale through pursed lips. Be sure to lift your feet off the floor.

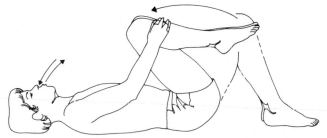

Lungs

Teaching a patient to perform her own IPPB

Lynn Davidson, a 36-year-old plumber, was recently treated at the local hospital's emergency department for an asthma attack. As part of her treatment, the doctor has ordered her to use an intermittent positive pressure breathing (IPPB) machine at home. You'll have to show Ms. Davidson how to use the machine correctly.

In this photostory, we'll use the Bennett pressure breathing therapy unit, which compresses, regulates, and delivers room air to the patient. The unit also delivers medication and can be connected to an oxygen source (if oxygen's ordered by the doctor). Remind Ms. Davidson to use the machine as directed to get quick relief from an asthma attack. Stress the importance of continuing to take her oral medication, as ordered.

Note: If you're teaching your patient to use another type of IPPB machine, follow the manufacturer's instructions.

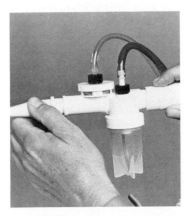

1 Tell Ms. Davidson to begin by plugging the machine's power cord into a nearby electrical outlet. Next, have her connect the main tube to the unit, the blue tube to the unit's nebulizer outlet, and the clear tube to the expiration valve outlet. Finally, tell her to place the mouthpiece on the manifold.

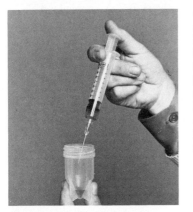

2 Because the doctor's ordered medication for Ms. Davidson's IPPB treatments, tell her to remove the nebulizer vial from the manifold, place the medication into the vial, and reconnect it to the manifold. Remind Ms. Davidson that she can use distilled water to add humidity to the air when no medication's prescribed.

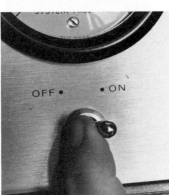

3 Instruct Ms. Davidson to sit in a straight-back chair, close to the front of the unit. Advise her to check the tube to make sure it isn't kinked. Then, tell her to push the unit's power button to the ON position.

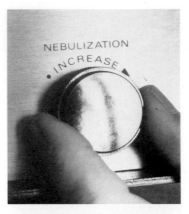

4 Tell Ms. Davidson to open the nebulizer control until a very light fog's produced, to make sure it's working correctly.

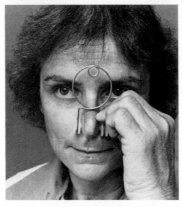

5 Have your patient pinch her nostrils closed with the noseclip to prevent air from leaking from her nose. This ensures that she'll receive maximum benefits from the therapy.

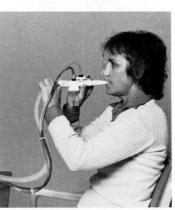

6 Have Ms. Davidson turn the pressure control to a low setting. Then, have her fit the mouthpiece into her mouth. Instruct your patient to make a tight seal with her lips around the mouthpiece and to inhale very slowly. As she does, the air from the machine will fill her lungs. When the machine stops providing air, encourage her to hold her breath for a few seconds to allow the medication to settle. Tell her to exhale slowly.

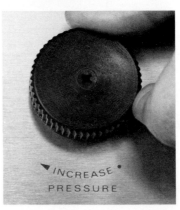

7 Ask your patient to adjust the pressure control knob until the gauge reaches the pressure prescribed by the doctor. Instruct Ms. Davidson to inhale deeply enough to keep the gauge needle at the prescribed level for as long as possible.

Have your patient continue the treatment until all the medication's gone. When she's finished, tell her to cough to remove secretions.

Understanding blunt chest trauma

While sitting on the sidelines of a high school baseball game, you see a student swing the bat and accidentally let go of it. The bat strikes 15-year-old Marie Russo in the chest, and she immediately crumples to the ground in pain. What should you do?

The above situation is just one example of how blunt chest trauma can happen. Keep in mind that this type of injury can occur in many different settings, in a variety of ways. And since you may be the first health-care professional on the scene of such an injury, you need to know how to recognize blunt chest trauma and what life-threatening complications can result.

If you're caring for a patient with blunt chest trauma, follow these guidelines to perform an emergency assessment:
- Make sure your patient's airway is open.
- Check your patient's vital signs and determine his level of consciousness.
- Observe for signs and symptoms of cardiac tamponade.
- Listen to heart and lung sounds carefully.
- Assess the adequacy of your patient's ventilation. Compare the length of his inspirations with his expirations. Determine the depth of his respirations and whether he's using his accessory muscles to breathe.
- Observe the position of your patient's trachea.
- Inspect your patient for jugular vein distention and paradoxical chest motion.
- Check for subcutaneous emphysema (crepitation).
- Assess the integrity of your patient's rib structure.
- Obtain a history of the injury. If your patient can speak, ask him how the injury occurred and how long ago it occurred. Ask him where he has pain and if he's having trouble breathing.
- Refer the patient to the local hospital. If the injury's minor, refer him to his doctor.

Remember: If the injury was inflicted by a weapon, contact the appropriate authorities.

Now, familiarize yourself with these common types of blunt chest trauma:

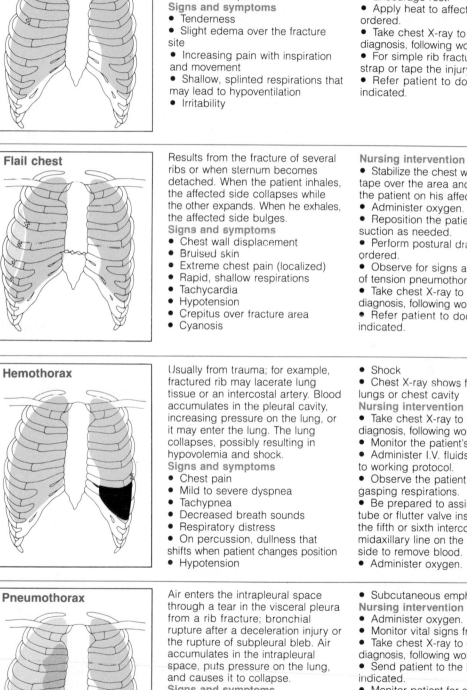

Rib fracture

Usually occurs at the point at which maximum force is applied. The rib may also be fractured posteriorly at its weakest point.

Signs and symptoms
- Tenderness
- Slight edema over the fracture site
- Increasing pain with inspiration and movement
- Shallow, splinted respirations that may lead to hypoventilation
- Irritability

Nursing intervention
- Administer mild analgesic in recommended dosages.
- Encourage rest.
- Apply heat to affected area, if ordered.
- Take chest X-ray to confirm diagnosis, following working protocol.
- For simple rib fractures, don't strap or tape the injury.
- Refer patient to doctor, as indicated.

Flail chest

Results from the fracture of several ribs or when sternum becomes detached. When the patient inhales, the affected side collapses while the other expands. When he exhales, the affected side bulges.

Signs and symptoms
- Chest wall displacement
- Bruised skin
- Extreme chest pain (localized)
- Rapid, shallow respirations
- Tachycardia
- Hypotension
- Crepitus over fracture area
- Cyanosis

Nursing intervention
- Stabilize the chest wall by applying tape over the area and positioning the patient on his affected side.
- Administer oxygen.
- Reposition the patient frequently; suction as needed.
- Perform postural drainage, if ordered.
- Observe for signs and symptoms of tension pneumothorax.
- Take chest X-ray to confirm diagnosis, following working protocol.
- Refer patient to doctor, as indicated.

Hemothorax

Usually from trauma; for example, fractured rib may lacerate lung tissue or an intercostal artery. Blood accumulates in the pleural cavity, increasing pressure on the lung, or it may enter the lung. The lung collapses, possibly resulting in hypovolemia and shock.

Signs and symptoms
- Chest pain
- Mild to severe dyspnea
- Tachypnea
- Decreased breath sounds
- Respiratory distress
- On percussion, dullness that shifts when patient changes position
- Hypotension
- Shock
- Chest X-ray shows fluid level in lungs or chest cavity

Nursing intervention
- Take chest X-ray to confirm diagnosis, following working protocol.
- Monitor the patient's vital signs.
- Administer I.V. fluids, according to working protocol.
- Observe the patient for pallor and gasping respirations.
- Be prepared to assist with chest tube or flutter valve insertion at the fifth or sixth intercostal space at midaxillary line on the affected side to remove blood.
- Administer oxygen.

Pneumothorax

Air enters the intrapleural space through a tear in the visceral pleura from a rib fracture; bronchial rupture after a deceleration injury or the rupture of subpleural bleb. Air accumulates in the intrapleural space, puts pressure on the lung, and causes it to collapse.

Signs and symptoms
- Sudden pleuritic chest pain
- Coughing
- Tachypnea
- Restlessness and anxiety
- Dyspnea
- Faint or absent breath sounds on affected side
- Decreased fremitus
- Subcutaneous emphysema

Nursing intervention
- Administer oxygen.
- Monitor vital signs frequently.
- Take chest X-ray to confirm diagnosis, following working protocol.
- Send patient to the hospital, as indicated.
- Monitor patient for signs and symptoms of tension pneumothorax, such as tachycardia, progressive dyspnea, increased tympany on involved side, and tracheal shift. If suspected, assist the doctor with insertion of a spinal or 14G to 16G needle to decompress chest.

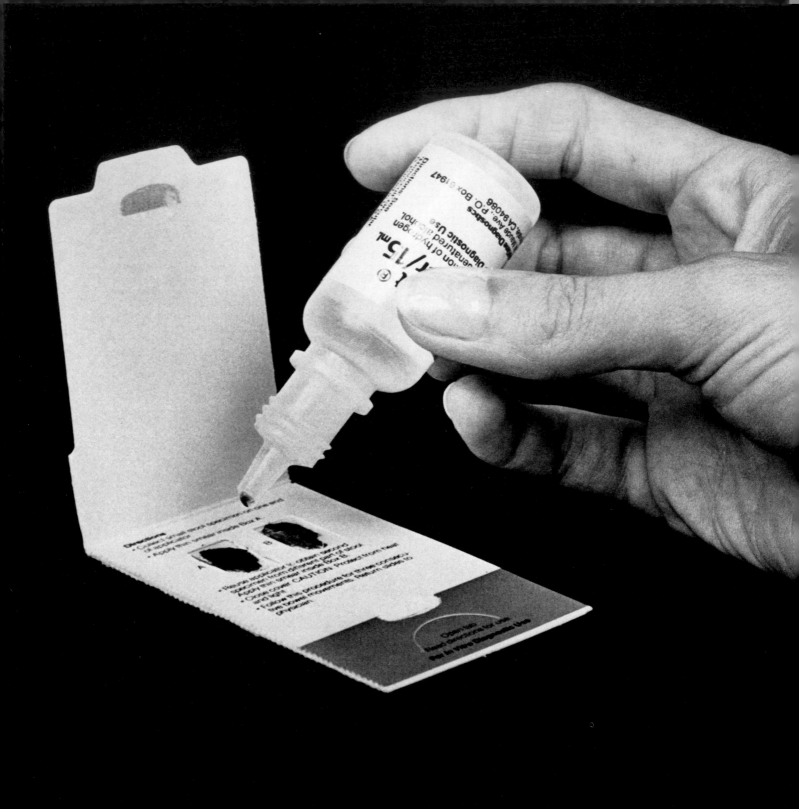

Managing Abdominal/Pelvic Problems

GI system

GU system

GI system

The patient coming to you with a gastrointestinal (GI) problem may have such nonspecific signs and symptoms as nausea, vomiting, diarrhea, and constipation.

Of course, successful management of GI problems depends on accurate history taking and assessment. In the box at right, we give you the guidelines you need for taking an accurate history. You'll also find tips on performing a GI assessment.

Then, we discuss common types of abdominal disorders and show you an easy step-by-step method for assessing abdominal pain. In addition, we tell you how to detect GI bleeding in a patient and familiarize you with possible causes of a patient's diarrhea.

Do you know how to teach a patient to collect a stool specimen or perform a Hemoccult test? In the following pages, we'll provide you with the facts to share with your patient.

Finally, we tell you how to differentiate types of hemorrhoids and suggest ways to help relieve your patient's discomfort.

Read these pages carefully.

Taking a GI history

Let's suppose a week-long bout of diarrhea brings 36-year-old Milton Urbansky into the clinic where you work. Besides determining what's causing his diarrhea, consider the possibility of dehydration and electrolyte imbalance.

For a patient like Mr. Urbansky, the doctor may order an upper and lower gastrointestinal (GI) X-ray series in addition to a thorough oral, abdominal, and rectal examination. Keep in mind that signs of GI problems, such as diarrhea, vomiting, and constipation, may have a variety of causes, ranging from viral infection and food poisoning to diverticulitis and colorectal cancer. This is why you first need to obtain an up-to-date and accurate GI history. By gathering information about your patient's medical and emotional history, diet, life-style, and present condition, you can begin to rule out some possible causes of his problem.

Here are some questions you may want to ask:
• Do you wear dentures? How long have you been wearing them? How do they fit? Do you use dental adhesive?
• Describe the condition of your teeth. When was your last dental exam? What did the doctor find? Did you have any pain, cavities, or infections? Do changes in temperature affect your teeth?
• Do you experience any difficulty or pain when chewing or swallowing food? Point to where you feel the pain or discomfort. Does it occur when you eat solid foods or when you drink liquids?
• Do your gums bleed? Do you have sores on your gums or tongue?
• Do you ever have abdominal pain, cramping, or distention? Do you have hemorrhoids?
• Have you ever had indigestion, heartburn, or gas? Does it occur after you eat certain foods?
• Have you ever vomited blood? Is your vomitus ever dark brown or black? Does it have an unusual odor?
• How often do you have a bowel movement? Are you constipated? Do you take laxatives? How frequently?
• Do you ever experience diarrhea? What color is it? What did you eat before the diarrhea's onset? Do periods of diarrhea alternate with periods of constipation?
• How would you describe the size and character of your bowel movements?
• Describe what you've had to eat and drink in the past 24 hours. Do you have any allergies? What are they? Have you recently lost weight? How much?
• Are you currently taking any medications? What are you taking and how often?
• Have you ever been X-rayed for an ulcer? When? Have you ever been treated for one? When? Do you still have pain from your ulcer?
• Has your colon ever been X-rayed?
• Have you ever had a colonoscopy or proctoscopy?
• Do you have a colostomy or an ileostomy? How long have you had it? Why was it done?
• Have you ever seen a doctor for abdominal or intestinal problems? For what reason?
• What do you feel is your major problem?
• Does anyone in your immediate family have a gastrointestinal problem? How is it being treated?
• Do you smoke? How much and how often?
• Do you drink alcoholic beverages or beverages with caffeine? How much and how often?

Assessing the GI system: Some tips

What's the first step in caring for a patient with a gastrointestinal (GI) disorder? Compiling an up-to-date patient history, of course. Then, you'll want to apply the information from the history to perform a thorough patient assessment. Not only must you collect as much data as possible in a limited time, but you must also act on the data you've collected. As you can see, your patient assessment skills will help you identify and manage your patient's problem. So before you perform another patient assessment, take a moment to review these tips:
• Begin your physical assessment with an overall visual inspection.
• Auscultate your patient's abdomen before you palpate or percuss it. Palpation and percussion may change the frequency of peristaltic sound.
• Observe the patient's position. For example, a patient with acute appendicitis may draw his right leg up to his chest to reduce the pain.
• Determine the location of your patient's pain, and palpate this area last.
• Carefully note when the pain began. This may help you differentiate food poisoning from other GI disorders, such as acute pancreatitis.
• Place the stethoscope's diaphragm directly on each abdominal quadrant. Dragging the diaphragm across tender muscle causes guarding.
• To assess high-frequency sounds, position the entire diaphragm on the patient's skin.
• To improve diaphragm contact and reduce extraneous noise, apply water-soluble jelly to your patient's skin before you auscultate.
• Never exert pressure on the stethoscope's bell. Doing so may cause the patient's skin to act as a diaphragm, making it difficult to hear low-frequency sounds.
• Suspect peritonitis if your patient's abdomen is boardlike and extremely tender.

Nurses' guide to abdominal disorders

Chances are you care for a lot of patients suffering from various degrees of abdominal pain. And, as you know, signs and symptoms associated with abdominal pain can be disturbingly similar—nausea, vomiting, and diarrhea. This is why taking an accurate patient history, recognizing early signs and symptoms, and knowing what additional signs and symptoms to look for are so important. Clearly, any type of abdominal disorder—whether peptic ulcer, ulcerative colitis, or gallbladder disease—may threaten your patient's health and even his life. Learn how to differentiate signs and symptoms of these disorders and how best to care for your patient by studying this chart.

Gastroenteritis
(intestinal flu, traveler's diarrhea, viral enteritis, food poisoning)
A self-limiting disorder that occurs in patients of all ages but may be life-threatening in children and in elderly or debilitated patients

Possible causes
• Food poisoning from *Staphylococcus aureus* and *Clostridium botulinum;* ingestion of toxins, such as certain plants and toadstools, and of heavy metals
• Bacteria, such as *Salmonella, Shigella, Escherichia coli,* and *Clostridium perfringens*
• Amoebae, such as *Entamoeba histolytica*
• Parasites, such as *Ascaris, Enterobius,* and *Trichinella spiralis*
• Viruses (may be responsible for traveler's diarrhea), such as adenovirus, echovirus, and coxsackievirus
• Drug reactions; for example, from antibiotics
• Enzyme deficiencies
• Food allergens

Signs and symptoms
• Vary, depending on causative agent, patient's condition, length of time in the body, and on the level of gastrointestinal tract involvement, but usually include anorexia, nausea, vomiting, fever, malaise, abdominal discomfort ranging from cramping to pain, and diarrhea (with or without blood and mucus)

Nursing considerations
• Obtain stool specimen for culture to identify causative organism.
• Encourage bed rest.
• Administer medication, as ordered.
• Tell patient to coordinate medication dosages with meals; for example, take antiemetics 30 to 60 minutes before meal.
• If patient can eat, encourage him to have broth, ginger ale, and lemonade, as tolerated. Warn him to avoid milk and milk products, which may provoke recurrence of symptoms.
• Instruct patient how to record intake and output. Have him notify you if he notices any of these signs of dehydration: dry skin, fever, sunken eyes.
• Notify the doctor if patient has signs of dehydration or if vomiting or diarrhea persists. The doctor may hospitalize the patient to provide I.V. fluid replacement.
• To ease anal irritation, tell patient to take warm baths and apply witch hazel compresses to the anal area.
• Teach good hygiene to prevent recurrence.
• Instruct patient to cook foods thoroughly, especially pork; to refrigerate perishable foods, such as milk, mayonnaise, potato salad, and cream-filled pastry; to always wash hands with soap and warm water before handling food, especially after using the bathroom; to clean utensils thoroughly; to avoid dairy products, untreated drinking water, and raw fruit or vegetables when visiting a foreign country; and to exterminate flies and roaches in the home.
• If food poisoning is probable, contact public health authorities so they can interview patients and food handlers and take samples of suspected contaminated food or water.

Diverticular disease
(diverticulitis)
Diverticula, which appear as bulging pouches on the gastrointestinal wall, push the mucosal lining through the surrounding muscle. The most common site for diverticula is in the sigmoid colon, but they may develop anywhere from the proximal end of the pharynx to the anus. Keep in mind that diverticular disease has two clinical forms: diverticulosis (diverticula are present but do not cause symptoms) and diverticulitis (diverticula are inflamed and may cause a potentially fatal bowel obstruction, perforation, infection, or hemorrhage). Diverticular disease is most common in men over age 40.

Possible causes
• High intraluminal pressure on areas of weakness in the gastrointestinal wall where blood vessels enter
• Contributing factors include a diet lacking natural bulk and fiber.

Signs and symptoms
• *In diverticulosis:* usually no symptoms, but recurrent lower left quadrant pain, possibly accompanied by alternating constipation and diarrhea that's relieved by defecation or passage of flatus
• In elderly patients, possibly hemorrhage of diverticulum in the right colon. Bleeding is usually mild to moderate and easily controlled but may be massive and life-threatening.
• *In mild diverticulitis:* moderate lower left abdominal pain, mild nausea, gas, irregular bowel habits, low-grade fever, leukocytosis
• *In severe diverticulitis:* rupture of diverticula, producing abscesses or peritonitis and causing abdominal rigidity; lower left quadrant pain. Peritonitis follows release of fecal matter from the rupture site and causes sepsis and shock. Rupture of the diverticulum near a blood vessel may cause microscopic or massive hemorrhage, depending on the ruptured vessel's size.
• *In chronic diverticulitis:* narrowing of bowel's lumen from fibrosis and adhesions, leading to bowel obstruction; constipation; ribbonlike stools; intermittent diarrhea; abdominal distention. As obstruction progresses, abdominal distention causes abdominal rigidity, diminishing or absent bowel sounds, nausea, vomiting, and abdominal pain.

Nursing considerations
• *In mild diverticulosis without signs and symptoms of perforation:* Explain what diverticula are and how they form, and teach patient the importance of dietary roughage and the harmful effects of constipation and straining when defecating. Encourage him to increase intake of foods high in digestible fiber, such as fresh fruits and vegetables, whole-grain bread, and wheat or bran cereals. Warn that a high-fiber diet may temporarily cause flatulence and discomfort. Advise the patient to relieve constipation with stool softeners or bulk-forming cathartics. Caution against taking bulk-forming cathartics without plenty of water; if swallowed dry, they may absorb enough moisture in the mouth and throat to swell and obstruct the esophagus or trachea.
• *In mild diverticulitis:* Administer medications, as ordered, explain diagnostic tests and preparations for such tests, and teach patient how to evaluate bowel movements and maintain accurate records of pulse rate, respirations, and intake and output.
• Prepare patient for surgery to resect diverticula, as ordered.
• Stress importance of follow-up care.

Peptic ulcers
Circumscribed lesions in the gastric mucosal membrane that can develop in the lower esophagus, stomach, pylorus, duodenum, and jejunum from constant contact with gastric juice (especially hydrochloric acid and pepsin). About 80% of all peptic ulcers are duodenal, which affect the proximal part of the small intestine and occur most often in men between ages 20 and 50.

Possible causes
• Unknown, but decreased mucosal resistance, inadequate mucosal blood flow, and inadequate mucus production have been associated with development of peptic ulcers.

Signs and symptoms
• *For a gastric ulcer:* heartburn and indigestion at onset of pain; after a large meal, pain in left epigastrium and feeling of fullness and distention; weight loss; repeated episodes of massive gastrointestinal bleeding.
• *For a duodenal ulcer:* heartburn, well-localized midepigastric pain (relieved by food), weight gain, sensation of hot water bubbling in the back of the throat. Attacks usually occur about 2 hours after meals, when the stomach is empty, and after consumption of orange juice, coffee, alcohol, or aspirin.
• Both types may be asymptomatic or may cause severe back pain. Complications include bowel perforation, hemorrhage, and pyloric obstruction.

Nursing considerations
• *For gastric ulcer:* Encourage patient to get plenty of rest, and give sedatives and tranquilizers, such as chlordiazepoxide and phenobarbital, as ordered.
• Administer medications, as ordered. Be alert for cimetidine and anticholinergic side effects, such as dizziness, rash, mild diarrhea, muscle pain, and leukopenia and gynecomastia, dry mouth, blurred vision, headache, constipation, and urinary retention.
• Instruct patient to take anticholinergic 30 minutes before meals to ensure maximum effectiveness.
• Tell patient to take antacids 1 hour after

GI system

Nurses' guide to abdominal disorders continued

meals. Instruct patient with a history of cardiac disease or on a sodium-restricted diet to take only low-sodium antacids. Warn that antacids may cause changes in bowel habits; for example, diarrhea with magnesium-containing antacids, constipation with aluminum-containing antacids.
• Warn the patient to avoid aspirin-containing drugs as well as reserpine, indomethacin, and phenylbutazone, because they irritate the gastric mucosa. For the same reason, warn against excessive use of coffee, stressful situations, and alcoholic beverages during exacerbations. Advise patient to stop smoking, because smoking stimulates gastric secretions.

Ulcerative colitis

Inflammatory, often chronic disease affecting the mucosa and submucosa of the colon. It usually begins in the rectum and sigmoid colon and often extends upward into the entire colon; it rarely affects the small intestine except for the terminal ileum. The disease produces congestion, edema, and ulcerations that eventually develop into abscesses. Severity ranges from a mild localized disorder to a fulminant disease that may cause a perforated colon, progressing to potentially fatal peritonitis and toxemia. Ulcerative colitis occurs primarily in young adults, especially women; it is also more prevalent in higher socioeconomic groups.

Possible causes
• Unknown, but predisposing factors include family history of the disease; bacterial infection; allergic reaction to food, milk, or other substances that release inflammatory histamine in the bowel; overproduction of enzymes that break down the mucous membranes; emotional stress; autoimmune reactions, such as arthritis, hemolytic anemia, erythema nodosum, and uveitis.

Signs and symptoms
• Recurrent bloody diarrhea, which usually contains pus and mucus, interspersed with asymptomatic remissions
• Spastic rectum and anus
• Abdominal pain
• Irritability
• Weight loss
• Anorexia
• Nausea
• Vomiting
• Complications may include anemia from iron deficiency, coagulation defects from vitamin K deficiency, erythema nodosum on the face and arms, pyoderma gangrenosum on the legs and ankles, uveitis, pericholangitis, sclerosing cholangitis, cirrhosis, possibly cholangiocarcinoma, arthritis, ankylosing spondylitis, loss of muscle mass, hemorrhoids, strictures, pseudopolyps, anal fissures, abscesses, stenosis, and perforated colon.

Nursing considerations
• Prepare patient for sigmoidoscopy, colonoscopy, or barium enema, as indicated.
• Ask patient to record what he eats and drinks as well as the frequency, color, and amount of his stools.
• Instruct patient to observe for signs and symptoms of dehydration (dry skin, fever, sunken eyes), hypokalemia (muscle weakness, numbness), and hypernatremia (fast pulse rate, flushed

skin, fever, and dry tongue).
• Tell patient to thoroughly clean the area around the rectum after each bowel movement.
• Administer medications, as ordered. Watch patient for side effects of prolonged corticosteroid therapy, such as moonface, hirsutism, edema, gastric irritation. Be aware that such therapy may mask infection.
• Prepare patient for hyperalimentation, as needed.
• Monitor patient for signs of such complications as perforated colon or peritonitis (fever, severe abdominal pain, abdominal rigidity and tenderness, cool and clammy skin) and toxic megacolon (abdominal distention, decreased bowel sounds).
• Prepare patient for surgery, if necessary.
• Encourage patient to verbalize his feelings. Provide emotional support and a quiet environment.

Pancreatitis

Inflammation of the pancreas that occurs in acute and chronic forms. In men, this disease is commonly associated with alcoholism, trauma, and peptic ulcers; in women, with biliary tract disease. Prognosis is good when pancreatitis results from biliary tract disease but poor when it's caused by alcoholism.

Possible causes
• Biliary tract disease
• Alcoholism
• Pancreatic carcinoma
• Trauma, such as blunt, penetrating, or surgical
• Drugs, such as glucocorticoids, sulfonamides, chlorothiazide, and azathioprine
• May be complication of peptic ulcers (especially duodenal), mumps, hypothermia
• Rarely, stenosis or obstruction of the sphincter of Oddi; hyperlipemia; metabolic endocrine disorders, such as hyperparathyroidism; vasculitis or vascular disease; viral infections; mycoplasmal pneumonia; and pregnancy

Signs and symptoms
• Steady epigastric pain close to the umbilicus, radiating between the 10th thoracic and 6th lumbar vertebrae; unrelieved by vomiting
• In severe attack, extreme pain, persistent vomiting, abdominal rigidity, diminished bowel activity, rales at lung bases, left pleural effusion, extreme malaise, restlessness, mottled skin, tachycardia, low-grade fever, and cold, sweaty extremities
• Complications may include paralytic ileus, diabetes mellitus, massive hemorrhage, and total destruction of the pancreas, resulting in diabetic acidosis, shock, or coma

Nursing considerations
• Administer antibiotics, as ordered. Watch for adverse reactions to antibiotics, such as nephrotoxicity with gentamicin, pseudomembranous enterocolitis with clindamycin, and blood dyscrasias with chloramphenicol.
• Administer analgesics, as needed, to relieve pain and anxiety. Remember that anticholinergics reduce salivary and sweat gland secretions. Warn the patient that he may experience dry mouth and facial flushing.
• Instruct patient to have blood studies performed, as ordered. Observe for signs and symptoms of hyperglycemia.

Gallbladder disease
(cholelithiasis, choledocholithiasis, cholangitis, cholecystitis, cholesterolosis, biliary cirrhosis, gallstone ileus)
Inflammation of the gallbladder and/or biliary tract that's commonly associated with deposition of calculi; usually requires surgery and may be life-threatening.

Possible causes
• *For cholelithiasis* (gallstones): stones or calculi in the gallbladder from changes in bile components; may be associated with sluggishness in gallbladder from pregnancy, oral contraceptives, diabetes mellitus, celiac disease, cirrhosis of the liver, and pancreatitis
• *For choledocholithiasis* (stones in the bile duct): stones pass from the gallbladder, lodge in the hepatic and common bile ducts, and obstruct the flow of bile into the duodenum
• *For cholangitis* (bile duct infection): may be associated with choledocholithiasis and may follow percutaneous transhepatic cholangiography. Predisposing factors include bacterial or metabolic alteration of bile acids. Widespread inflammation causes common bile duct fibrosis or stenosis.
• *For cholecystitis* (acute or chronic inflammation of the gallbladder): usually associated with a gallstone impacted in the cystic duct
• *For cholesterolosis* (cholesterol polyps or deposits of cholesterol crystals in the gallbladder's submucosa): may result from bile secretions containing high concentrations of cholesterol and insufficient bile salts
• *For biliary cirrhosis* (ascending infection of the biliary system): primary cause unknown
• *For gallstone ileus:* gallstone lodged at terminal ileus

Signs and symptoms
• *For acute cholelithiasis, choledocholithiasis, acute cholecystitis, and cholesterolosis:* acute abdominal pain in the upper right quadrant, which may radiate to the back between the shoulders or to the front of the chest after a meal rich in fats or in the middle of the night; recurring fat intolerance; biliary colic; belching that leaves a sour taste in the mouth; flatulence; indigestion; diaphoresis; nausea; vomiting; and chills; with choledocholithiasis, low-grade fever, jaundice, and clay-colored stools.
• *For cholangitis:* rise in eosinophils, jaundice, abdominal pain, high fever, and chills
• *For biliary cirrhosis:* jaundice, related itching, weakness, fatigue, slight weight loss, and abdominal pain
• *For gallstone ileus:* nausea, vomiting, abdominal distention, and absence of bowel sounds, if bowel is completely obstructed

Nursing considerations
• Provide emotional support and reassurance.
• Prepare patient for X-ray and hospitalization, as indicated.
• Prepare patient for diagnostic testing and surgery, as indicated.
• Stress importance of follow-up evaluations after surgery.
• Encourage patient to maintain a fat-free diet and avoid foods that trigger attacks.
• For cholangitis, administer antibiotics, as ordered. Also, encourage patient to drink plenty of fluids.

How to assess abdominal pain

Suppose you're caring for a patient with a constant ache in her midepigastric area, nausea, indigestion, and, occasionally, diarrhea. After you take her history, perform an abdominal assessment to help relate her symptoms to specific organs in her abdomen. Here's how:

Before assessing for abdominal pain, have your patient empty her bladder and put on a patient gown. Then, have her lie on an exam table.

Expose your patient's abdomen from the xiphoid process to the symphysis pubis. Drape the other areas to keep her warm and protect her privacy.

Always examine the painful area last. Examine the lower quadrants first and then the upper quadrants, from the perimeter inward. This way any pain you elicit from the trouble area doesn't tighten the rest of your patient's abdominal muscles.

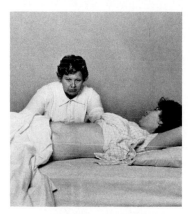

1 First, inspect your patient's abdomen for possible asymmetry, which may indicate an intraabdominal mass. Check for visible lumps, masses, and pulsations and for any redness, swelling, or herniation of the umbilicus. Also look for a bluish umbilicus (Cullen's sign), which may indicate intraabdominal hemorrhage, and for visible peristaltic movements.

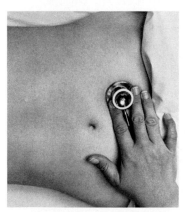

2 To auscultate your patient's abdomen, place the stethoscope's diaphragm lightly on her lower left quadrant and listen for intermittent rumbling and gurgling, which are normal bowel sounds. If everything's OK, you should hear 5 to 34 of these sounds per minute.

If you don't hear any sounds, auscultate each quadrant.

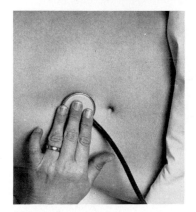

3 Use the stethoscope's bell to auscultate for vascular sounds, such as bruits, venous hums, and friction rubs. Move the bell at 2″ to 3″ (5- to 7.6-cm) intervals as you auscultate each area.

Friction rubs over the liver and spleen may indicate a hepatic tumor or splenic infarct; bruits in the abdomen may indicate an aneurysm or partial arterial obstruction.

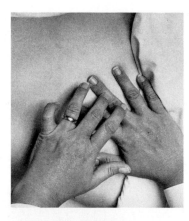

4 Moving clockwise, percuss all your patient's abdominal quadrants. As you do, mentally note where the percussion sounds change from tympanic to dull. This information helps you identify the location of her abdominal organs and possible abdominal masses.

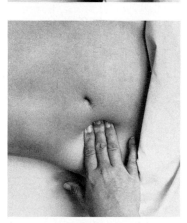

5 Now, again moving clockwise, lightly palpate your patient's abdomen by quadrants. Note her skin temperature and any unusual pigmentation. Also check for tenderness and possible large masses.

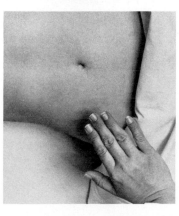

6 Deeply palpate your patient's abdomen in each quadrant, following the same order. Note organ location and abdominal masses, bulging, or swelling. If you detect a mass, document its location, size, shape, consistency, tenderness, and mobility. Also note any pulsations you may feel.

7 If you detect a painful area in your patient's abdomen, check for rebound tenderness. To do this, slowly press your fingertips into the tender area, and then quickly release them. If your patient complains of sharp pain, suspect rebound tenderness, which may indicate peritoneal inflammation. Document all your findings on the appropriate forms.

GI system

Caring for a patient with GI bleeding

Late Wednesday afternoon, 28-year-old Susan Parks comes into your clinic feeling cold, sweaty, and faint. She tells you she vomited bright red blood nearly an hour ago and confesses that she's scared. You know, of course, that vomiting bright red blood almost always indicates upper gastrointestinal (GI) bleeding. But how much do you know about this life-threatening symptom? Let's take a closer look at GI bleeding.

As you probably know, GI bleeding may be red and obvious—as in the case of Ms. Parks—or it may be brown and obscure. Brown blood, which produces *coffee-ground* vomitus, results from upper GI blood mixing with gastric acid. But regardless of color, vomited blood almost always indicates bleeding somewhere above the ligament of Treitz. *Remember:* Be sure to rule out other possible causes of bloody vomitus, such as blood swallowed from a nosebleed or contained in sputum.

Blood from an upper GI hemorrhage may pass through the intestine. When more than 300 ml pass through the intestine rapidly, the patient's stools may contain red blood. But when 50 to 300 ml of blood pass through the intestines slowly, the patient may pass black, tarry stools (melena). Other possible causes of black stools include rapidly eliminated bile or ingestion of beets, greens, or berries.

If your patient's stool is bloody, she may also have a lower intestinal bleed. If the stool is blood-streaked or has clots on its surface, suspect bleeding from the distal colon. Stool with dark red blood throughout indicates bleeding above the level of the distal colon.

Causes of GI bleeding vary as much as the bleeding sites. The illustration above shows some possible bleeding sites. The most common causes include esophageal varices; gastroesophageal lesions (A); gastritis (B); cancer of the stomach or colon (C); gastric ulcer (D); peptic ulcer (E); diverticulitis (F); Meckel's diverticulum; ulcerative colitis; polyps; and hemorrhoids.

Specific signs and symptoms of GI bleeding depend on the bleeding site, rate and amount of blood loss, and existence of associated conditions. If your patient has bleeding, look for these signs and symptoms: weakness, fatigue, anorexia, irritability, palpitations, faintness, headache, and insomnia. Anemia will probably be present if your patient has chronic bleeding. Shock or renal failure are a risk in a patient with massive bleeding.

As you can see, GI bleeding is a sign of an underlying problem. But before you work toward detecting this problem, attempt to stabilize your patient's condition.

Notify the doctor and follow these steps:
● Reassure the patient as much as possible, and provide emotional support.

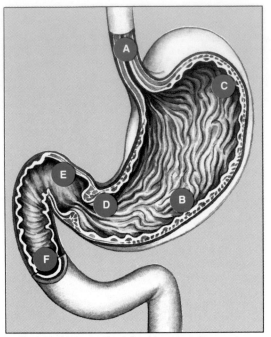

● Assess your patient for signs and symptoms of shock: cool, clammy skin; hyperventilation; weakness; chills; restlessness; confusion; decreased blood pressure; and rapid, thready pulse.

If any of these signs are present, insert an I.V. line, according to your working protocol.
● Determine how much blood your patient has vomited. Transport her to a hospital as soon as possible, and prepare her for blood transfusions.
● Check pulse rate and blood pressure every 15 minutes.
● Provide oxygen, as needed, to improve tissue perfusion.
● If your patient is still vomiting blood, insert a nasogastric tube, so iced gastric lavage can be performed to control bleeding.
● Monitor urinary output and insert a catheter, according to your working protocol.

When your patient's condition has stabilized, begin looking for the underlying cause of the bleeding. To do this, you must rely on physical clues, patient history, and physical examination.

To determine the bleeding site, the doctor will probably order aspiration of gastric contents. Be prepared to assist, as ordered.

In addition, if the doctor suspects an upper GI bleed, he may order such diagnostic tests as fiber-optic endoscopy, an upper GI series, and abdominal angiography. If he suspects a lower GI bleed, he may order sigmoidoscopy, barium enema, and arteriography. Prepare your patient as indicated, and reassure her as much as possible.

Document all your findings and any procedures in your notes.

Diarrhea: Identifying causes

Diarrhea is an increase in stool frequency, fluidity, and/or volume as compared with the normal bowel pattern. It may be spurred by bacteria, viruses, parasites, medication, diseases, and surgery. Acute diarrhea can be life-threatening in elderly or debilitated patients. Chronic diarrhea may lead to malabsorption, anemia, and an increased susceptibility to other diseases.

Recognizing underlying causes
Because diarrhea is only a sign, identifying the underlying cause is important. Associated signs and symptoms vary, depending on the cause, duration, and severity of the diarrhea; the area of the bowel affected; and the patient's general condition. Begin your assessment by taking your patient's history. Be sure to note the time, place, and circumstances of onset, the duration, and the severity of the diarrhea.

Then, inquire about the frequency and timing of his bowel movement; any evidence of fatty, greasy, or oily stools with a foul odor; and associated changes in weight or appetite. Learn when the diarrhea occurs and if it's associated with cramping or abdominal pain, fever, chills, nausea, weakness, a change in dietary habits, or traveling. Also check to see if the patient experiences any rectal or anal pain when he has a bowel movement. If he does, suspect inflammation, a hemorrhoid, an anal fissure, or a tumor. *Important:* If the patient is alternating between constipation and diarrhea, suspect partial bowel obstruction.

Obtain a stool specimen. Then, carefully note the color, consistency, and appearance of stool for clues to other conditions. Also, check your patient for signs of dehydration. If present, refer the patient to his doctor for further evaluation.

Home care

Collecting a bowel movement specimen

Dear Patient:

Carefully follow these instructions for collecting a bowel movement specimen at home. Doing so will help you avoid contaminating the specimen, which would interfere with the test results and necessitate retesting.

First, make sure you have a clean, dry bedpan (to collect the bowel movement specimen), a tongue depressor or small piece of cardboard, and a waterproof container with a tight-fitting lid (which the nurse or lab technician will give you). If you don't have a bedpan, use a large glass jar that you've cleaned and boiled.

When you feel the urge to move your bowels, urinate into the toilet as you usually would. Then, close the toilet's lid and position the bedpan or glass jar on the lid, as shown.

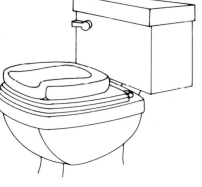

Position yourself on the bedpan and move your bowels. When you're finished, don't urinate or place toilet tissue in the bedpan. Doing so contaminates the stool. Clean your genital area with toilet tissue, using one top-to-bottom motion, and get dressed.

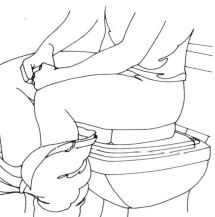

Remove the lid from the container and place it flat side down. Make sure you don't touch the inside of the lid or container.

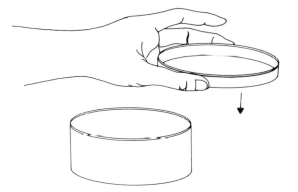

Using the tongue depressor, transfer some of the bowel movement into the container, being careful not to overfill it. Avoid touching the outside of the container with the tongue depressor. Place the filled container on the sink and discard the tongue depressor.

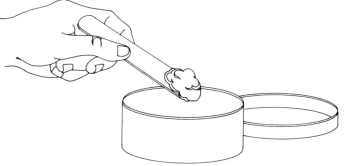

Put the lid on the container and wash your hands thoroughly. Then, depending on the instructions you were given, return the specimen container to the nurse, the lab, or the doctor's office within 30 minutes. If this is impossible, place the container in a paper bag and store it in the refrigerator—away from food—until you can deliver it to the proper person or place.

GI system

Your role in stool specimen collection

If your patient has abdominal pain or diarrhea, one of the doctor's first steps may be to ask the patient to collect a stool specimen. He has good reason for this. Stool specimen analysis is almost always necessary to diagnose infectious disease, gastrointestinal (GI) bleeding, and other GI tract disorders. By analyzing a patient's stool, the doctor can study the digestive efficiency and integrity of the patient's stomach and intestines.

Reviewing the basics

Before reviewing what you can do to help your patient obtain a quality stool specimen for the Hemoccult test, let's consider GI physiology.

As you probably know, food and fluid intake, medications, exercise, and rate of digestion affect normal defecation patterns. These patterns may vary from two or three bowel movements daily to two or three weekly.

Remember, too, that stool consists of 75% water and 25% solids, such as cellulose and other indigestible fiber, bacteria, unabsorbed minerals, fat and fat derivatives, desquamated epithelial cells, mucus, and small amounts of digestive enzymes and secretions. Stool is usually light to dark brown, soft, and slightly acidic. Color depends on the patient's diet, drugs, absorption efficiency, and bilirubin concentration. Stool pH depends on dietary influences. For example, a high-carbohydrate intake results in acidic pH; a high-protein intake results in alkaline pH. Stool odor is determined by indole and skatole, which are end products of protein catabolism by bacterial action in the large intestine.

Stool is usually about 1" (2.5 cm) in diameter and has the tubular shape of the colon. Depending on the colon's condition, stool shape may be larger or smaller. Stool color may, in turn, reflect the condition of the abdominal structure. For example, if the colon is partially obstructed or loses its elasticity, the passage of stool may traumatize the colon and cause bleeding; blood in the stool may also result from hemorrhoids. Black, tarry stool can result from bleeding high in the intestinal tract. Large, bulky, foul-smelling stool that floats on water may indicate malabsorption of fat or the presence of a large quantity of air or other gases in the stool. Stool containing mucus may indicate colitis or a tumor. The presence of pus, detected in microscopic analysis, can result from rectal abscess or ulcerative colitis.

Stool testing

Stool evaluation begins with gross examination and documentation of color, consistency, odor, and other characteristics and concludes with microscopic or bacterial analysis. The Hemoccult test helps detect occult blood in the stool. The doctor usually orders this test when he suspects your patient may have GI bleeding. You'll remember that small amounts of blood—for example, 2 to 2.5 ml a day—normally appear in the stool. The Hemoccult test is designed to detect quantities larger than this.

To prepare a patient for the Hemoccult test, explain that the test helps detect abnormal GI bleeding. Tell your patient not to collect the specimen during a menstrual period or while suffering from bleeding hemorrhoids. Advise him this test requires collection of three stool specimens.

How to perform a Hemoccult test

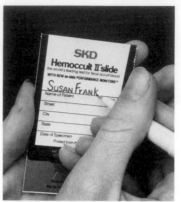

1 You've taught your patient how to collect a stool specimen. But suppose you want to check her stool for occult blood. Teach her how to apply a specimen to the Hemoccult II® slide, following these guidelines:

First, have your patient fill in the information blanks on each slide.

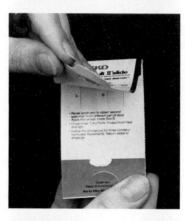

2 Then, tell her to take a small amount of stool from the specimen container, using an applicator stick. Instruct her to open the first slides.

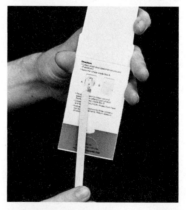

3 Have her smear the stool inside box A.

Then, tell her to reuse the stick and take a specimen from a different part of the stool. Ask her to apply this specimen inside box B.

Instruct your patient to close the flap and store the slide away from heat and light. Have her repeat this procedure for her next two bowel movements. Tell her to return the slides to you.

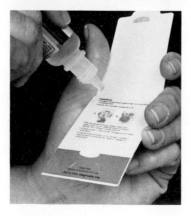

4 When you receive the slides, open the flaps. Apply two drops of Hemoccult developer to each smear. Wait 30 to 60 seconds, and then read the results. If you see a trace of blue on or at the edge of either smear, consider the slide *positive* for occult blood. Document the results and refer the patient to the doctor, if necessary.

Learning about hemorrhoids

When veins in the anal canal dilate, hemorrhoids result. These veins, situated in the hemorrhoidal plexus, may appear as swellings and may cause bleeding and pain.

Basically, two types of hemorrhoid may develop: internal and external. *Internal hemorrhoids* (shown at right) are covered with mucosa and bulge into the rectal lumen. These hemorrhoids are usually painless and easily seen. They may prolapse when a patient strains and disappear when he relaxes.

As shown in the bottom illustration, *external hemorrhoids* are covered with skin and protrude from the rectum. They appear as tan or gray, soft swellings; are usually painless; and rarely bleed.

Thrombosed hemorrhoids, however, are a different matter. These hemorrhoids result from a blood clot that has formed inside the hemorrhoid. Because the clot stretches the anal skin, these hemorrhoids—which look like small, blue-purple lumps—can be painful. They may develop suddenly and, in many cases, require surgical removal.

Identifying causes

Wondering what causes hemorrhoids? Usually, hemorrhoids result from a diet low in fiber and high in refined foods. This type of diet makes normal bowel elimination difficult. As a result, waste matter collects in the sigmoid colon and forms a stool of abnormal density. The longer the stool remains in the colon, the more water the body draws from it. In time, the stool becomes hard and compact. This, in turn, makes the stool harder to pass, causing constipation, which results in the patient straining on the toilet. Clearly, straining increases pressure on veins in the anal canal. Ongoing pressure, then, causes the veins to dilate

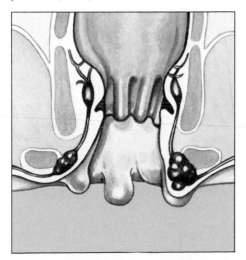

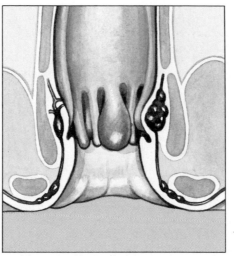

and become hemorrhoids.

Other factors causing hemorrhoids to develop include occupations that require prolonged sitting or standing; prolonged diarrhea, coughing, sneezing, or vomiting; hepatic disease; alcoholism; anorectal infection; loss of muscle tone from aging; pregnancy; rectal surgery or episiotomy; and anal intercourse.

Recognizing signs and symptoms

Because signs and symptoms of hemorrhoids may be subtle, you'll need to count on your assessment skills to recognize them. Initially, hemorrhoids develop in two or three clusters around the wall of the anal canal. At this point, they may be painless and cause only occasional bright red blood on the stool or on toilet paper used to wipe the anal area. Bleeding results from injury to the mucosa covering the hemorrhoids during defecation and is considered the classic sign of hemorrhoids. Other signs include mucus discharge and ongoing pain.

Assessment

If you suspect your patient has hemorrhoids, your first step is to perform a visual inspection of the external anal area. Look for swollen, gray, or tan areas. Depending on your working protocol, follow your visual inspection with a digital rectal examination. *Important:* If your patient has thrombosed hemorrhoids, perform only an external inspection. To perform a rectal examination, insert a well-lubricated, gloved finger into the patient's anal canal. Note any lumps or swollen areas. When you withdraw your finger, check for blood on it. If present, your patient may have an internal hemorrhoid. Perform anoscopy to confirm your suspicions. Be sure to document your findings, and refer your patient to the doctor, as necessary.

Caring for a patient with hemorrhoids

How do you care for a patient with hemorrhoids? This depends on the type and severity of the hemorrhoids and the patient's overall condition. As you know, you'll be responsible for teaching your patient methods to ease pain, combat swelling, and regulate his bowel habits. Explain to him that these methods may mean readjusting his life-style, but they may also make more involved treatment, such as surgery, unnecessary.

Changing eating habits

Begin by encouraging your patient to establish a bowel pattern and eat a well-balanced diet. Stress the importance of closely monitoring his intake of alcohol and highly refined foods, such as cold cuts, canned vegetables, and frozen dinners.

Then, teach your patient specific precautions to take, using the following points as guidelines. Emphasize that these precautions must be ongoing.
• Use stool softeners and laxatives only when necessary. Explain that overuse of laxatives can lead to constipation.
• Use enemas only as ordered by the doctor.
• Empty your bowels as soon as the urge is felt.
• Sit on the toilet only as long as necessary. Don't read while on the toilet or sit on the toilet for prolonged periods. Doing so increases pressure on the veins in the anal canal.
• Apply temporary relief measures, such as lotions, creams, or suppositories, to the hemorrhoidal area as indicated by the doctor.
• Wipe the anal area, with soft, white, preferably moistened toilet paper. The fixative used in colored paper can irritate your skin. Avoid wiping the area with washcloths or using harsh soaps.

To help reduce external thrombosed hemorrhoids, suggest the patient get plenty of rest and apply ice to the area. To do this, tell him to put a few ice cubes in a plastic bag and apply the bag to the hemorrhoidal area for a few minutes at a time over several hours. In most cases, the pain subsides in a few days and the clot disappears within a few weeks.

To help relieve pain, especially after bowel movements, tell your patient to sit in 3" to 4" (7.6 to 10 cm) of warm—not hot—water.

But remember, if these methods do not relieve your patient's symptoms, prepare him for surgery, as indicated. As you know, hemorrhoidal bleeding may lead to anemia and can mask more serious conditions. Instruct your patient to return to the doctor if signs and symptoms recur.

GU system

You know the importance of accurately assessing your patient's genitourinary tract and reproductive system. By recognizing abnormalities in your patient's renal function or reproductive system, you can help prevent serious complications. On the following pages, you'll find important information related to:
● taking your patient's history.
● assessing urine color changes.
● recognizing testicular problems.
  Read these pages carefully.

Taking a patient history

Diseases of the genitourinary tract and reproductive system can have far-reaching implications for your patient. For example, a urinary tract disorder can produce a wide range of signs and symptoms. And a reproductive system disorder not only affects your patient physically but may cause emotional and psychological problems as well.

Obviously, assessment of a patient with a genitourinary tract or a reproductive system problem can be difficult. But you can meet this challenge by starting with an accurate patient history. Consider asking your patient these questions:
● Have you noticed a change in the amount of your urine? When did you first notice the change? Does it happen only if you drink a lot of fluids?
● How frequently do you usually urinate? How many times a day have you been urinating? Has your urine stream changed in size? After you've urinated, do you feel as if some urine remains in your bladder? Do you frequently feel the urge to urinate but only produce a small amount? Do you ever have trouble starting the flow? Do you frequently wake up during the night to urinate? Do you have trouble controlling the urge to urinate?
● What color is your urine? Have you noticed any change in the color recently? How long has it been this color?
● Do you ever experience pain or a burning sensation when you urinate? How often does this occur? Does your abdomen ever swell?
● Have you ever had kidney or bladder stones? When did you have them and how were they treated?
● Have you ever had a urinary tract or genital infection or a sexually transmitted disease?
● Have you ever been treated for diabetes, tuberculosis, multiple sclerosis, hypertension, hepatitis, or frequent streptococcal infections?
● Do you have any allergies?
● Are you taking any medications? What are you taking and why?
● Have you ever had surgery for a urinary tract disorder? What was the problem and how was it treated? How long ago was surgery performed?
● Do you have trouble sleeping at night? Are you ever awakened by leg or thigh cramps? Do you feel like sleeping during the day?
● Is your sexual life satisfying? Is there anything about it you'd like to change?
● Do you ever feel short of breath, particularly when lying down? Do you ever wake up in the middle of the night feeling breathless?
● Do you ever have a metallic taste in your mouth?
● Do you frequently feel tired or lethargic?
● Are you experiencing recurring headaches?
● What type of work do you do?
● Do you feel under stress at work or at home?

When assessing a male patient, consider asking these questions:
● Have you noticed any discharge on your penis? What color and consistency is it?
● (For the uncircumcised patient) Do you have trouble retracting your foreskin? After it's retracted, can you return it to its normal position?
● Do your testes ever feel painful or look swollen?
● Have you recently suffered injury to your genitals?
● Have you noticed any mass or lump in your genital area? When did you first notice it? Is the mass or lump painful? Does it disappear when you lie on your back?
● Do you have nocturnal or morning erections? Do you have trouble sustaining an erection? Can you achieve an erection by fantasizing or masturbating?
● Have you ever suffered injury to your back or spinal cord?

When assessing a female patient, consider asking these questions:
● Have you noticed any lumps or masses in your breasts? Have you noticed any lumps around your vagina? When did you first notice the lump? Has it changed since you first noticed it? Can you feel the lump without touching it? Does the lump feel hard or soft and tender? Is it painful?
● Have you noticed any unusual discharge from your vagina? When did you first notice it? What does it look like? Does it have an odor? How much discharge is there? Has your sexual partner had abnormal discharge recently?
● When was your last menstrual period? When was the menstrual period before your last one? How frequently do you get your period? How long do they usually last?
● When were your last Pap test and pelvic examination performed?
● Do you ever have pain or cramping with your periods? Does the pain develop suddenly or gradually? How long does it last? Can you describe it? Do you ever experience pain during sexual intercourse or at any other time?
● Do you have heavy flow with your periods? Has the flow increased gradually or suddenly? Have you noticed any blood clots in the flow? During your period, how many tampons or sanitary napkins do you use per day?
● Have you noticed any spotting between periods? Does the bleeding occur only after intercourse or the use of intravaginal objects? Are you taking any medications containing estrogen?
● Have you missed any periods recently? Did you experience an acute illness during the month before the missed period?
● Have you recently experienced emotional stress or have you suddenly begun to exercise strenuously?
● Do you douche? How often do you douche? What type of douching solution do you use?
● Does your vagina itch? When is the itching worse?
● Have you ever tried to become pregnant, without success? Have you ever been treated for fertility problems?
● Do you practice birth control? What method do you use? How long have you used this method? Is it satisfactory?
● Have you ever been pregnant? How many times? Describe each pregnancy.

Assessing kidney tenderness

Alvin Leahy, a 24-year-old television cameraman, has come with a urinary problem to the clinic where you work. He tells you he has to urinate frequently and admits that he often experiences back pain and burning when he does. From his comments, you suspect he has a kidney infection. Of course, you'll take a patient history and perform a detailed assessment to help confirm your suspicion. As part of your physical examination and assessment, you'll perform direct or indirect percussion to his kidneys to check for pain or tenderness. Here's how to proceed.

Begin by explaining the procedure to Mr. Leahy. Be sure to answer any questions he may have. Then, ask him to remove his clothing above the waist and sit on the examining table. Wash your hands.

Note: *Make sure you also check Mr. Leahy's abdomen and genital area for pain or swelling.*

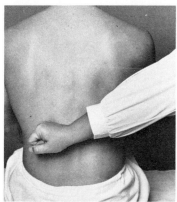

1 Before you begin percussion, determine the location of your patient's kidneys. To do this, locate his 12th rib and his costovertebral angle. The kidneys are located slightly to the right and left of this area, as shown in the illustration.

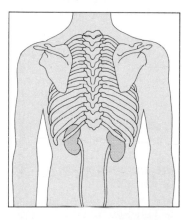

2 Perform direct percussion by making a fist with your right hand and striking his back directly to the right of his costovertebral angle. As you strike the area, observe Mr. Leahy's reaction. Ask him if this causes him any pain. Repeat the procedure slightly to the left of his costovertebral angle.

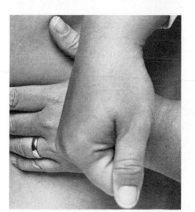

3 To perform indirect percussion, place your left palm on Mr. Leahy's back, to the right of his costovertebral angle. Then, make a fist with your right hand and strike your left hand with it. Repeat the procedure slightly to the left of his costovertebral angle. If Mr. Leahy experiences pain during the procedure, refer him to a doctor. Then, document everything in your notes.

Assessing urine color

Besides assessing the amount and consistency of your patient's urine, assess the color, which can provide you with clues to his condition. Normal urine color ranges from straw-colored to amber. But several possible urine color changes may or may not involve damage to the urinary system. They can result from diet, drugs, metabolic disorders, infections, or inflammation. Knowing what these changes mean will help you assess your patient.

Here are color changes you may encounter and their possible causes:

• *Colorless (diluted):* excessive fluid intake (especially alcohol), chronic renal disease, diabetes insipidus, emotional disturbance

• *Dark yellow (concentrated):* low fluid intake, acute febrile disease, dehydration, vomiting, diarrhea, such drugs as chlorpromazine hydrochloride and sulfonamides

• *Yellow-orange:* such drugs as furosemide and sulfasalazine

• *Yellow to amber, with pink sediment:* hyperuricemia, gout

• *Orange-red to orange-brown:* urobilinuria and such drugs as phenazopyridine hydrochloride and rifampin

• *Red or red-brown:* porphyria, hemoglobin, erythrocytes, hemorrhage, ingestion of beets, such drugs as pyrvinium pamoate

• *Tea-colored:* obstructive jaundice

• *Green-brown:* bile duct obstruction, phenol poisoning

• *Dark brown or black:* acute glomerulonephritis, chorea, typhus, bile

• *Blue or blue-green:* medication containing methylene blue dye, such drugs as triamterene

• *Green:* foods containing carotene, *Pseudomonas* infection, such drugs as amitriptyline hydrochloride

Hematuria—blood in the urine—is probably the most common urine color change you'll see. In most cases,

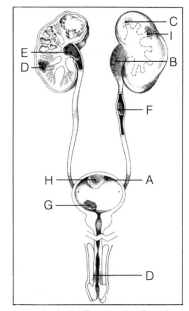

hematuria indicates genitourinary tract bleeding.

As shown above, possible causes of hematuria include infection, such as cystitis (A); obstruction, such as hydronephrosis (B); inflammation, such as acute pyelonephritis (C); trauma (D); calculi in the kidney (E), ureter (F), or bladder (G); cancer (H); acute or chronic glomerulonephritis; renal hypertension; lupus nephritis; renal vein thrombosis; subacute bacterial endocarditis; hemorrhagic disorders; allergic purpuras; and renal tuberculosis (I).

If your patient has hematuria, use the urination stage at which hematuria occurs to aid your diagnosis. For example, when blood appears early in urination and then disappears, suspect a urethral disorder, such as urethritis or cystitis. If hematuria occurs throughout urination, the source of the problem is usually above the bladder neck, where blood has mixed with the urine. This may also indicate the presence of active bleeding. Hematuria throughout urination may be from sickle cell anemia, calculi, infection, cancer, trauma, filtration and reabsorption disorders, or collection and excretion disorders.

GU system

Home care

How to examine your testicles

1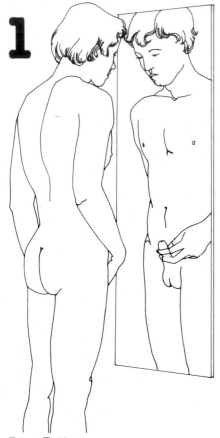

2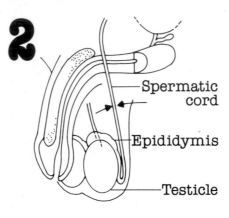

Spermatic cord

Epididymis

Testicle

Next, you'll feel your testicles for lumps and masses. First, locate the cordlike structure at the back of your testicles. This is called the epididymis. Your spermatic cord extends upward from the epididymis.

3

Gently squeeze the spermatic cord above your right testicle between the thumb and first two fingers of your right hand. Then, using the thumb and first two fingers of your left hand, examine the spermatic cord above your left testicle. Check for lumps and masses by squeezing along the entire length of the cords.

Dear Patient:
To help detect abnormalities early, you should examine your testicles once a month. Eventually, you'll become familiar with them and will be able to recognize anything abnormal.

Here's how to examine your testicles: Remove your clothes and stand in front of a mirror. With one hand, lift your penis and check your scrotum (the sac containing your testicles) for any change in shape or size and for red, distended veins. Expect the scrotum's left side to hang slightly lower than the right.

4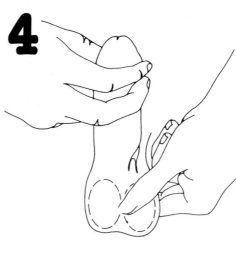

To examine your right testicle, place your right thumb on the front of the testicle and your index and middle fingers behind it. Gently press your thumb and fingers together. They should meet. Make sure you check your entire testicle. Then, use your left hand to examine your left testicle in the same manner. Your testicles should feel smooth, rubbery, and slightly tender, and you should be able to move them.

If you notice any lumps, masses, or changes, notify your doctor.

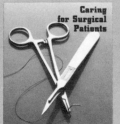
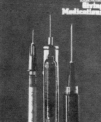
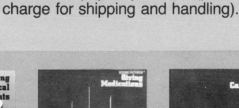
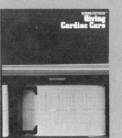
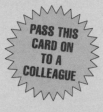
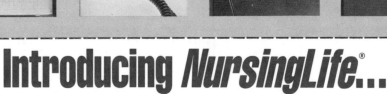

Get acquainted with the incomparable NURSING PHOTOBOOK series and learn important new procedures, step by step.

Hundreds of crystal-clear photographs, diagrams, sketches, and tables give you "how to" instructions quickly. The concise, clearly written text amplifies each highly detailed photostory.

The NURSING PHOTOBOOK series is a remarkable breakthrough in nursing education that can change your career. You actually watch experts at work. You'll learn how to ● administer drugs safely ● effectively teach your patient about his disorder and its treatment ● minimize trauma ● understand doctors' diagnoses ● increase patient comfort ● control pain ● and much more.

Each handsomely bound PHOTOBOOK offers you 160 illustrated, fact-filled pages ● brilliant, high-contrast photographs ● convenient 9"x10½" size ● durable hardcover binding ● carefully chosen bibliography ● complete index.

See for yourself how much you get out of this exciting series and how much your nursing will improve. Return the postage-paid card today.

© 1984 Springhouse Corporation

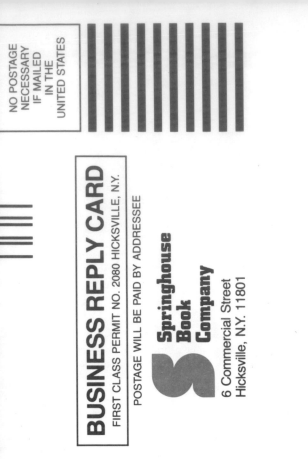

You can examine each NURSING PHOTOBOOK at your leisure...for 10 days *absolutely free.*

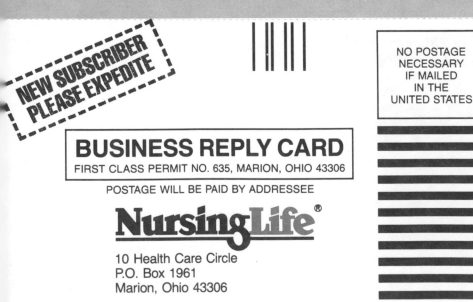

At last! A journal that helps you with "the other side" of nursing. The things they didn't (and couldn't) teach you in nursing school.

NursingLife tells you how to be a better nurse... how to find greater fulfillment in your career... how to grow on the job.

It's all about the skills today's nurses need to round out their professional lives.

Become a subscriber to this exciting new professional journal. Just tear off and mail this card today. There's no need to send money now. This is a no-obligation, free trial offer!

If order card is missing, send your order to:

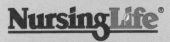

Nursing Life ®

10 Health Care Circle
Marion, Ohio 43306

Nurses' guide to testicular problems

Testicular problems you're most likely to encounter as an ambulatory-care nurse are detailed in the chart below. When undetected and untreated, these problems can lead to serious complications, such as ureteral obstruction and sterility.

Keep in mind that your patient may be hesitant to talk about such a problem. This is why you must be well acquainted with possible signs and symptoms and know how to intervene.

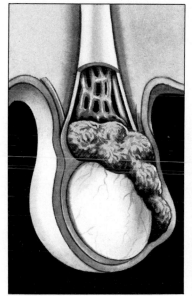

Epididymitis
Infection of the epididymis, the testis' cordlike excretory duct; one of the most common male reproductive tract infections; usually affects adults; may spread to the testes, causing orchitis. Bilateral epididymitis may cause sterility.
Causes
• Bacterial (streptococci, staphylococci, or *Escherichia coli*), secondary to urinary tract infection or prostatitis
• Trauma
• Sexually transmitted disease
• Chlamydial infection
Signs and symptoms
• Pain
• Extreme tenderness
• Swollen groin and scrotum, from enlarged lymph nodes in the spermatic cord
• Possibly scrotal warmth
• Fever
• Malaise
• Waddletype walk
• Possibly acute hydrocele
Nursing intervention
• During acute stage, encourage bed rest. Tell patient to keep scrotum elevated by placing a rolled-up towel beneath it.
• Recommend use of ice bag to reduce swelling and relieve pain.
• Administer analgesics and broad-spectrum antibiotics in recommended dosages.
• Emphasize the importance of completing prescribed antibiotic therapy, even after symptoms subside.
• After pain and swelling subside, recommend use of athletic supporter when walking.
• Promote fluid intake.
• Observe patient closely for abscess formation (localized, red, hot, tender area) or spread of infection to testes.
• If sterility results, suggest supportive counseling.

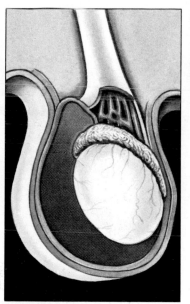

Hydrocele
Abnormal accumulation of fluid within the scrotum around the testis
Cause
• Inadequate reabsorption or overproduction of hydrocele fluid from trauma, infection, or lymphatic or venous obstruction
Signs and symptoms
• Scrotum enlargement
• Usually painless until fluid accumulates, causing pressure
• Smooth, fluctuant mass on examination; mass is undistinguishable on transillumination with flashlight.
• Testis doesn't retract when patient coughs.
Nursing intervention
• Refer patient to doctor for evaluation and treatment.
• Aspiration gives temporary relief but increases risk of secondary infection.
• Assess patient for complications of aspiration, such as infection or hemorrhage into the scrotal tissues.
• If problem persists, prepare patient for surgery, as indicated.

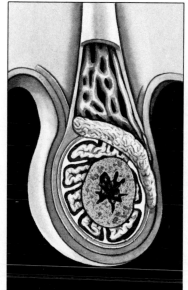

Testicular cancer
Malignant tumor of testis; usually originates in gonadal cells but may spread through the lymphatic system to other areas of the body; most common in Caucasian men between ages 15 and 40
Cause
• Unknown but believed to be associated with cryptorchidism, infection, endocrine disorders, and a family history
Signs and symptoms
• Firm, smooth mass that may be painless
• Mass will appear as opaque shadow on transillumination exam.
• Sensation of heaviness
• Possibly associated breast enlargement and nipple tenderness
• In late stages, may metastasize and lead to ureteral obstruction, abdominal mass, cough, hemoptysis, shortness of breath, weight loss, fatigue, pallor, and lethargy
Nursing intervention
• Provide encouragement and support. Treatment usually involves radiation, chemotherapy, and surgery.
• Explain possible side effects of radiation and chemotherapy. Give antiemetics, as needed, to prevent severe nausea and vomiting. Suggest small, frequent meals to maintain weight.
• Promote fluid intake.

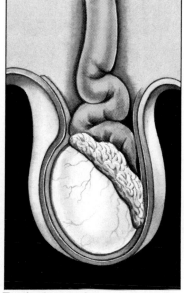

Testicular torsion
Abnormal twisting of the spermatic cord caused by rotation of the testis or mesorchium (a fold in the area between the testis and epididymis); results in strangulation of the testis and, if untreated, eventual infarction; most common between ages 12 and 18
Causes
• *In adolescents* (intravaginal): abnormality of the tunica vaginalis (serous membrane covering the front and sides of the testis and epididymis), resulting in abnormal position of the testis, or narrowing of the mesentary support
• *In neonates* (extravaginal): loose attachment of the tunica vaginalis to the scrotal lining, causing spermatic cord rotation above the testis
Signs and symptoms
• Severe pain in the affected testis or iliac fossa
• Nausea
• Vomiting
• Tachycardia
• Diaphoresis
• Pallor
• Tense, tender swelling in the scrotum or inguinal canal
• Hyperemia of the overlying skin
• Sound of pulsating blood flow absent from affected testis
Nursing intervention
• Refer patient to doctor for treatment (usually surgical repair) immediately.
• Administer analgesics in recommended dosages to relieve pain after surgery. Also recommend use of ice bag to reduce swelling and relieve pain.
• Tell patient to return periodically for examinations.

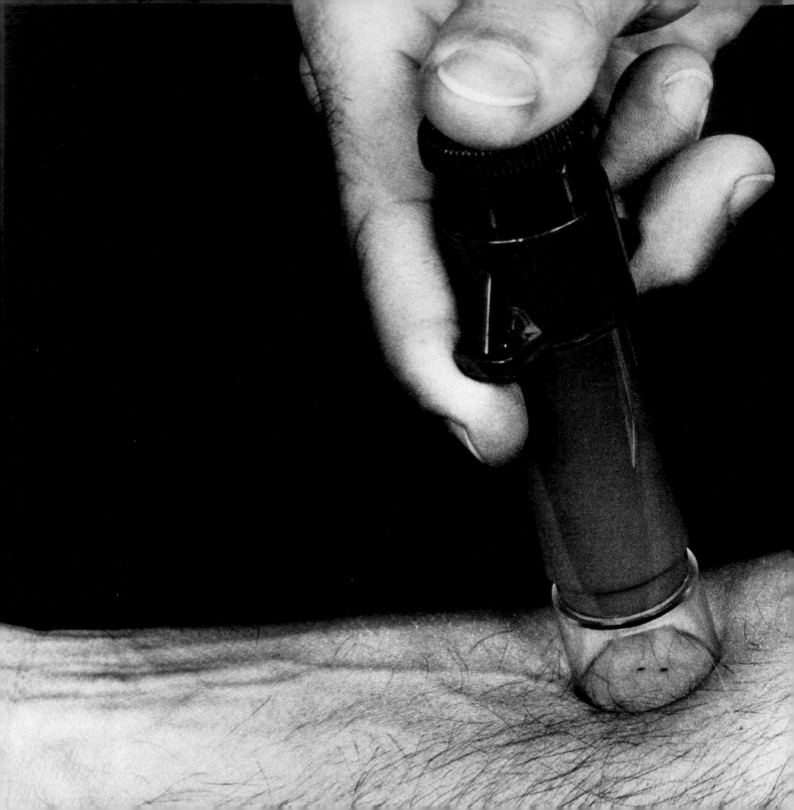

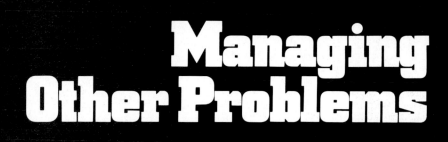

Managing
Other Problems

Systemic

Psychosocial

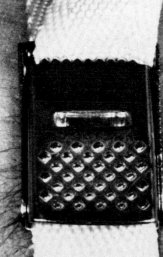

Systemic

In this sequence, you'll find information on how to manage problems that may affect your patient's entire body; for example, anaphylactic shock or a poisonous snakebite. Systemic problems challenge you to provide skilled nursing care on a moment's notice. Read on to learn more about your role in caring for a patient with systemic problems.

Learning about anaphylaxis

Consider anaphylaxis a life-threatening emergency situation. It occurs when a patient ingests or is exposed to a drug or other substance that causes a sensitivity reaction. Such substances include serums (usually horse serum), vaccines, hormones, local anesthetics, penicillin (most common cause) and other antibiotics, foods (nuts, berries, and seafood), and insect venom (from honeybees, wasps, or specific types of spiders).

Anaphylaxis can take place after a single exposure to an antigen or after repeated exposures. Generally, a reaction immediately after antigen exposure is more severe than a reaction that occurs later.

Initial signs and symptoms of anaphylaxis usually appear within minutes (usually no longer than 45 minutes after substance exposure). Insect venom reaction may take longer. These signs and symptoms include a sense of impending doom, weakness, sweating, sneezing, shortness of breath, nasal pruritus, urticaria, and angioedema. They may be followed rapidly by hypotension, shock, and cardiac dysrhythmias; nasal mucosal edema, profuse watery rhinorrhea, itching, nasal congestion, and severe sneezing attacks, possibly leading to pharyngeal and laryngeal obstruction (early signs of acute respiratory failure); and severe stomach cramps, nausea, diarrhea, and urinary urgency and incontinence.

To care for a patient with anaphylaxis, immediately administer 0.1 to 0.5 ml of epinephrine 1:1,000 aqueous solution. Repeat the dose every 5 to 20 minutes, as necessary. If your patient's conscious, you can administer epinephrine intramuscularly or subcutaneously. To speed absorption, massage the injection site after administering the drug.

If your patient has a severe reaction and loses consciousness, administer epinephrine intravenously. In addition, keep your patient's airway open. If you detect early signs of laryngeal edema, such as stridor, hoarseness, and dyspnea, administer oxygen. Also monitor your patient's vital signs, and watch for signs and symptoms of shock, such as low blood pressure; cold, clammy skin; rapid, shallow respirations; and tachycardia, with weak, rapid pulse. If he suffers cardiac arrest, initiate cardiopulmonary resuscitation measures. Finally, get your patient to the emergency department as soon as possible.

To help prevent anaphylaxis, teach the patient to avoid any substances that may cause him to have an allergic reaction. For example, a patient who's allergic to insect venom should avoid grassy or wooded areas and should carry an anaphylaxis kit whenever he goes outdoors.

Note: The following photostory shows the proper method for using an anaphylaxis kit.

Teaching a patient to use an anaphylaxis kit

Joan Simmons, a 42-year-old printer's assistant, is allergic to wasp stings. Because the doctor's instructed Ms. Simmons to carry an emergency anaphylaxis kit whenever she goes outdoors, he's referred her to you for instructions on the use of the kit. Complete your teaching. Then, watch her perform the technique without your assistance.

In this photostory, the patient is using the Emergency Anakit®, which contains a 1-cc syringe of epinephrine 1:1,000, two sterile alcohol wipes, one tourniquet, and four Chlo-Amine (antihistamine) tablets.

After being stung by a wasp, Ms. Simmons' first step is to ask someone to immediately contact the doctor. Then, she'll try to remove the stinger. Warn her that pinching, pushing, or squeezing the stinger may force it further into her skin. Remind her to go on to the next step if she can't remove the stinger quickly.

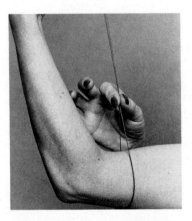

1 If Ms. Simmons is stung on the arm or leg, she'll apply a tourniquet between the sting site and her heart. Have her tighten the tourniquet by pushing down on the metal ring, as shown here. (Remind her to release the tourniquet after 10 minutes by pulling the metal ring.) After applying the tourniquet, she'll use an alcohol swab to clean a 4″ (10-cm) area of skin above it.

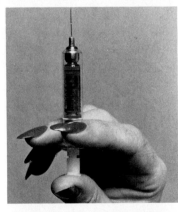

2 Now, she'll remove the needle cover from the syringe. Then, holding the syringe, with the needle upward, have her push the plunger to expel trapped air.

Next, your patient will insert the entire needle into her skin and pull back slightly on the plunger to check for blood. If she notices any, she'll withdraw the needle and reinsert it. If she doesn't, she'll push down on the plunger and inject the epinephrine.

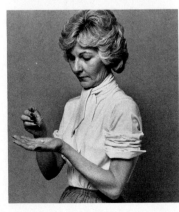

3 After withdrawing the needle, your patient will chew and swallow the four Chlo-Amine tablets. Tell her to apply an ice pack to the affected area to relieve pain and reduce swelling. Urge her to avoid exertion, keep warm, and notify the doctor if she hasn't already done so. If she doesn't notice an improvement in her condition after 10 minutes, encourage your patient to give herself another dose of epinephrine following the same procedure.

Tourniquet: When to use it

How often have you used a tourniquet? If your answer is "rarely," you've probably learned the first rule of safe use: Use a tourniquet only as a last resort. Why? Because improper use can cut off blood supply to the affected arm or leg, causing severe tissue destruction and necessitating amputation. Also, the tourniquet itself may cut into or further injure the skin and underlying tissue.

Use a tourniquet only when direct pressure, elevation of the extremity, pressure points, and pressure dressings aren't effective in controlling life-threatening bleeding.

If one's available, you can apply a ready-made, standard tourniquet to a patient. Or, you may improvise a tourniquet, using a belt, handkerchief, towel, necktie, cravat bandage, or other suitable material. To distribute pressure over tissues correctly, the tourniquet you choose should be 3″ to 4″ (7.6 to 10 cm) wide to avoid cutting your patient's skin.

Important: Never use wire or cord as a tourniquet. It may cut into your patient's flesh.

When using a tourniquet, keep these guidelines in mind:
• Apply the tourniquet proximal to the injury site, between the wound and the heart.
• Apply the tourniquet tightly enough to stop the bleeding but not so tightly that nerves and blood vessels are damaged by compression. Remember, however, that a loose tourniquet restricts blood flow in the veins but not the arteries; this results in the patient losing more blood than he would without a tourniquet, because the arteries conduct blood to the injured area, but the veins can't return it to the heart.
• When you've applied the tourniquet, don't loosen it unless directed to do so by a doctor. Loosening the tourniquet may dislodge blood clots or cause bleeding to resume, resulting in shock.
• Make sure the patient's transported to the emergency department immediately, so the doctor can remove the tourniquet as quickly as possible. Gangrene may develop if the tourniquet's left in place too long.

Learning about poisonous snakebite

Like anaphylaxis, a poisonous snakebite requires emergency intervention. If poisonous snake venom enters your patient's bloodstream, it may cause life-threatening complications. Therefore, you'll need to act quickly.

Snakebites are most common on the arms and legs, below the elbows and knees. But any bite into a blood vessel's dangerous, regardless of location.

Signs and symptoms of poisonous snakebite include local and facial numbness and tingling, convulsions, extreme anxiety, difficulty in speaking, fainting, weakness, dizziness, diaphoresis, mild to severe respiratory distress, headache, blurred vision, marked thirst, nausea, vomiting, diarrhea, tachycardia, hypotension, and shock.

Treatment of a snakebite victim usually involves transporting him to the emergency department as soon as possible, for the administration of antivenin. The following measures should be taken, however, before the patient's transported.
• Try to establish the type of snake.
• Apply a slightly constrictive tourniquet 2″ to 4″ (5 to 10 cm) above the bite. Don't apply the tourniquet, however, if more than 30 minutes have elapsed since the bite occurred.
• Never give the victim alcoholic drinks or stimulants.
• Never apply ice to a snakebite.

Using a snakebite kit

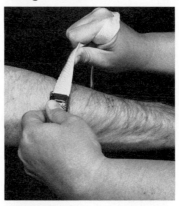

1 Suppose you encounter a person who has been bitten by a poisonous snake. Would you know what to do? If you're unsure, follow these steps.

First, remove the tourniquet from the Norton Snake Bite Kit® and apply it 2″ to 4″ (5 to 10 cm) above the bite. The tourniquet should be snug enough to prevent the return flow of blood to the heart but loose enough to allow you to slip a finger under it.

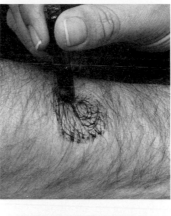

2 Remove the sterile swab from its wrapper. Break the plastic seal containing the povidone-iodine solution to moisten the end of the swab. Then, use the swab to clean the wound site.

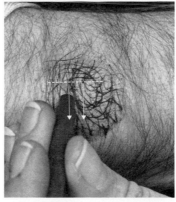

3 Remove the protective cover from the lancet blade. With the blade, make an incision about ½″ (1.3 cm) long and ⅛″ (3 mm) deep in your patient's skin at each fang mark. To locate the appropriate sites for the incisions, imagine a line connecting the fang marks. Then, begin the incision at each fang mark, perpendicular to the imaginary line, as shown here. Continue each incision slightly below the fang mark, where the venom's deposited.

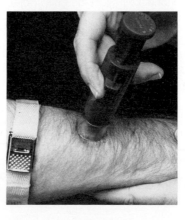

4 Attach the adapter to the suction device and place the device over the incisions you've made. To increase suction, pump the plunger two or three times. Release the plunger. When the plastic adapter cup fills with fluid, remove and empty it. Then, reapply it and continue with suction for about 30 minutes. Afterward, apply an adhesive bandage over the wound site. Send your patient to the hospital immediately.

Psychosocial

You know that ambulatory-care nursing puts you in close contact with your patients. While this situation affords you some special rewards, it also presents special challenges. For example, your familiarity with a patient's day-to-day activities may help you identify a psychosocial problem, such as insomnia or depression. Or, you may recognize a patient with a drug dependency.

For help in managing these problems, read the following pages. In them, you'll find information on:
• taking your patient's psychosocial history.
• caring for a patient with a sexually transmitted disease, such as genital herpes.
• detecting a patient who is abusing alcohol or drugs.

Taking your patient's psychosocial history

As an ambulatory-care nurse, you evaluate and manage your patient's emotional and psychological makeup as well as his physical condition. As you know, total patient care isn't easy. Your patient may be reluctant to talk about certain things. And, of course, you can't force him to do so. In such a situation, you'll have to call on your observation and assessment skills to detect a problem.

Try to develop a rapport with your patient. This'll help your psychosocial assessment. He'll trust you and will feel at ease talking with you. If you have frequent contact with your patient and have cared for him in the past—whether in the community, on the job, or at school—you'll be better able to determine changes in his behavior that may signal an underlying problem. Knowing his family, friends, or employer will also help.

For example, take the case of Bob Hilliard, a 39-year-old carpenter, with a wife and two daughters. He comes to your clinic complaining of fatigue and loss of appetite. From previous visits, you know Mr. Hilliard's usually cheerful and friendly. But you notice that now he appears depressed. You also note that he is unkempt, a change from his normally tidy appearance. In addition, you've learned that Mr. Hilliard hasn't been showing up for jobs or has been delaying them.

Now that you suspect a problem from your observations of Mr. Hilliard, you'll have to tactfully ask him some questions to confirm your suspicion and discover the problem's source. To help him relax, you need to be open and friendly and gain his trust. Begin by asking broad, nonthreatening questions, such as "How has work been going lately?" If he replies, "Not so good," you can guide him in a direction that provides you with the necessary information by saying, "What seems to be the problem?"

Of course, you're careful not to press Mr. Hilliard too hard for an answer. You encourage him to talk freely, asking him more pointed questions as he becomes more comfortable. Eventually, you learn that his wife left him recently and took their two daughters with her. The breakup has upset Mr. Hilliard so much that he isn't eating or sleeping properly.

As you can see, taking a patient's psychosocial history can be challenging. As an ambulatory-care nurse, you're in a unique position to help uncover his emotional or psychological problems. And when you do discover these problems, you can refer him to the appropriate agencies for additional assistance.

To help your assessment, consider gathering answers to these questions when taking your patient's history:
• Are your patient's clothes neat and clean? Are they appropriate to place, age, and weather conditions? Does he have an odor? Does he keep himself clean? If your patient's female, is her makeup appropriate?
• What's your patient's posture? Does he stand erect or slumped over? Does he pace or move about restlessly? Are his movements slow, or sudden or jerky?

• Are your patient's facial expressions appropriate to his comments? Does his face lack expression?
• Does your patient seem uncomfortable talking about his problems? Does he have trouble expressing his feelings? Does he speak loudly or softly?
• Does your patient appear anxious? Can he describe the feeling? When does he usually feel this way?
• What type of mood does your patient feel he's usually in?
• Does he get along well with other people? Does he seem to enjoy relationships with people?
• Has your patient recently been separated from someone he loves?
• Does he appear to have emotional support from his family and friends?
• Does he avoid involvement with other people?
• Is your patient worried about his financial situation? Why? Does he often talk about money? Does he have a steady job? Does he miss work frequently? Is he often late for work? Is he afraid of losing his job? Who manages his finances?
• Can he afford to buy necessary items, such as food?
• Does your patient appear to have trouble concentrating or thinking logically? Is his thought process slow or rapid?
• Does your patient seem preoccupied with a particular subject, always returning to it?
• Does your patient understand your questions? Can he provide the answers to easy questions? For example, can he name the four seasons of the year?
• To test your patient's judgmental ability, ask him what he would do if he lost something he borrowed from a friend?
• What eating pattern does your patient follow? Has he lost or gained weight recently? Does he follow any special diet? Where does he eat his meals?
• What life-style does your patient lead? Does it change frequently?
• Does your patient have a stable and comfortable home environment? Does he live with someone or alone?
• Is your patient often fatigued?
• Does your patient have trouble falling asleep? Does he need anything to help him sleep?
• Can he walk? Does he use any ambulatory aids, such as a cane or walker?
• Is his house neat and clean?
• Does your patient often feel under stress? What's his idea of a stressful situation? How does he think he handles stress? What does he usually do to relax?
• Does your patient have problems that are affecting the responsibilities of other family members? How does he feel about this?
• Has anyone in your patient's family had a stress-related disorder, such as coronary artery disease or a peptic ulcer? Has anyone had a psychiatric disorder?
• Is your patient satisfied with his sex life? Has it changed recently? Does your patient call attention to his or her own sexuality; for example, by wearing tight, seductive clothing?

Nurses' guide to sexually transmitted diseases

Because patients with sexually transmitted diseases usually seek treatment in a community setting, you can expect to encounter this type of problem frequently.

To refresh your memory of these diseases, review the following chart:

Gonorrhea
Cause
- *Neisseria gonorrhoeae*

Incubation period
- 3 to 6 days

Signs and symptoms
In males:
- Urethritis, with purulent urethral discharge and dysuria
- Redness and swelling at infection site
- Some infected males may be asymptomatic.

In females:
- Patient is usually asymptomatic.
- Green-yellow cervical discharge (most common)
- Dysuria
- Urinary frequency and incontinence
- Itchy, red, edematous urethral or vaginal opening
- Occasional itching, burning, and pain in vulva caused by exudate from adjacent infected area
- Severe pelvic and lower abdominal pain; muscular rigidity and tenderness
- As infection spreads, nausea, vomiting, fever, tachycardia in patients with salpingitis or pelvic inflammatory disease (PID)

Other possible signs and symptoms:
- Abdominal pain in upper right quadrant in patients with perihepatitis
- Pharyngitis and tonsillitis
- Rectal burning and itching
- Bloody, mucopurulent discharge

Nursing intervention
- Collect a specimen for culture from infection site.
- Dispose of all contaminated equipment according to your working protocol.
- Before treatment, establish whether the patient has any drug hypersensitivities. Observe patient closely for drug reactions during therapy.
- If gonorrhea's uncomplicated by any other disease, administer 1 g of probenecid (Benemid*) P.O., followed in 30 minutes by 4.8 million units of penicillin G procaine (Wycillin*) I.M. injected at two separate sites into large muscle mass, as ordered. Or, therapy may consist of 3.5 g of ampicillin (Amcill*) P.O. and 1 g of probenecid P.O., given

*Available in both the United States and Canada

together.
- If patient's allergic to penicillin, give tetracycline hydrochloride (Tetracyn*), unless patient is pregnant, or spectinomycin dihydrochloride (Trobicin*) I.M., as ordered.
- For outpatient therapy of gonorrheal PID, give tetracycline hydrochloride or penicillin G procaine I.M. each with 1 g probenecid P.O., followed by continuous antibiotic therapy for 10 days, as ordered.
- Advise patient that a follow-up culture from infection site should be performed 7 to 14 days after treatment is completed and again in 6 months.
- Tell an infected pregnant patient that she'll need a culture before delivery.
- Warn your patient that until culture results are negative, he's still infectious and can transmit gonococcal infection. Urge patient to avoid sexual activity.
- Instruct patient and family how to prevent spread of infection; for example, not sharing washcloths.
- Urge patient to inform all sexual contacts of his infection so they can seek treatment.
- Report all cases of gonorrhea to public health officials.

Lymphogranuloma venereum (LGV)
Cause
- *Chlamydia trachomatis*

Incubation period
- 1 to 3 weeks

Signs and symptoms
- Painless lesion on the glans penis or coronal sulcus in males; lesion may appear on the fourchette, urethral meatus, or medial surface of the labia in females; may range from a slight erosion to a small macule or papule; usually heals spontaneously within a few days; often goes undetected because of location
- Two weeks after lesion heals, inguinal lymph nodes swell, possibly becoming fluctuant, tender masses (especially in males)
- Possibly regional node enlargement, appearing as unilateral or bilateral buboes
- Thick, yellow, granular discharge from ruptured, untreated buboes; may result in formation of scar or indurated, inguinal mass
- Possibly iliac and sacral lymphatic obstruction in females; may also develop genitoanorectal syndrome (mucopurulent rectal discharge, bloody diarrhea, pararectal abscess formation)
- After initial lesion heals, myalgia,

headache, fever, chills, malaise, backache, and weight loss

Nursing intervention
- Collect blood samples and drainage specimens for culture.
- Administer tetracycline, oxytetracycline, or chlortetracycline P.O. for 14 to 28 days or sulfadiazine P.O. for 14 days to relieve systemic symptoms (enlarged, inflamed lymph nodes in groin area)
- Aspirate fluctuant buboes to decrease swelling and pain, according to working protocol. Such complications as strictures or fistulas may necessitate surgery.
- To cleanse affected area and reduce discomfort, tell patient to take warm sitz baths three or four times daily.
- Have patient cover ruptured buboes with nonadhesive dressings.
- Encourage patient to avoid using lotions, creams, sprays, and ointments on affected area.
- Advise patient to avoid all sexual contact during the infectious period—3 weeks for males and up to several months for females.
- Stress to female patients the need for biannual pelvic examinations.

Nonspecific genitourinary infections
Causes
- *Corynebacterium vaginale*, staphylococcus, diphtheroids, coliform, and, in males, *Chlamydia trachomatis* or *Ureaplasma urealyticum*

Incubation period
- 1 week to 1 month after coitus

Signs and symptoms
- Both males and females may be asymptomatic.

In males:
- Scant or moderate mucopurulent urethral discharge
- Variable dysuria
- Occasional hematuria
- If untreated, may lead to acute epididymitis

In females:
- Persistent vaginal discharge
- Acute or recurrent cystitis without specific cause
- Cervicitis with inflammatory erosion

Nursing intervention
- Collect specimen of prostatic, urethral, or cervical secretions for culture.
- Administer oral tetracycline, erythromycin, or streptomycin, followed by a sulfonamide, as ordered.
- Instruct female patient on use of sulfa vaginal cream, if ordered. Tell her to cleanse her pubic area

before applying the medication and to avoid using tampons during treatment.
- To help prevent nonspecific genitourinary infections, tell patient to refrain from sexual contact with infected partner, to use condoms during sexual activity, and to urinate before and after intercourse.
- Instruct patient to increase and maintain fluid intake.
- Advise female patient not to use douches and hygiene sprays or to wear tight-fitting pants or panty hose.
- Urge patient to inform all sexual contacts of his infection, so they can seek treatment.

Syphilis
Cause
- Spirochete *Treponema pallidum*

Incubation period
- *Primary syphilis:* up to 3 weeks
- *Secondary syphilis:* several days to 8 weeks after appearance of primary chancre (small, fluid-filled lesion, with indurated, raised edges and clear bases)
- *Latent syphilis:* from initial infection throughout life
- *Late syphilis:* 1 to 10 years after chancre appears

Signs and symptoms
- *Primary syphilis:* one or more chancres, usually on genitalia; may also be on the breasts, cervix, and vaginal wall in females and on the fingertips, anus, tonsils, or eyelids in both sexes; chancres usually disappear in 3 to 6 weeks.
- *Secondary syphilis:* rash with mucocutaneous lesions and general lymphadenopathy; rash can be macular, papular, pustular, or nodular; lesions are uniform, well defined, and generalized; usually appears in warm, moist areas, such as the perineum, scrotum, and vulva, and between rolls of fat; lesions enlarge, erode, and produce highly contagious pink or gray lesions (condylomata lata)

These signs and symptoms accompany secondary syphilis: headache, malaise, anorexia, weight loss, nausea, vomiting, sore throat, brittle or pitted nails, and slight fever. Alopecia may occur with or without treatment and is usually temporary.
- *Latent syphilis:* absence of clinical symptoms but a reactive serologic test for syphilis
- *Late (noninfectious) syphilis,* consisting of one or more subtypes: *Late benign*—chronic superficial nodules or deep, granulomatous lesions (which are usually painless,

Psychosocial

Nurses' guide to sexually transmitted diseases continued

solitary, indurated, and asymmetric) appear on bones or organs; may affect various body systems, causing epigastric pain, tenderness, enlarged spleen, and anemia (if liver's involved); perforation of the nasal septum or the palate (if respiratory system's involved). *Cardiovascular syphilis*—fibrosis of aorta's elastic tissue, leading to aortitis, usually in ascending and transverse sections of the aortic arch. *Neurosyphilis*—meningitis and widespread central nervous system damage, such as general paresis, personality changes, and arm and leg weakness.

Nursing intervention
• Collect blood sample for the fluorescent treponemal antibody absorption (FTA-ABS) test, the Venereal Disease Research Laboratory (VDRL) slide test, and the rapid plasma reagin (RPR) test to help confirm diagnosis.
• Check history of drug hypersensitivity before administering first treatment dose.
• If patient has early syphilis, administer 2.4 million units of penicillin G benzathine (Bicillin L-A*) I.M. as a single dose; or 600,000 units/day of penicillin G procaine (Wycillin*) I.M. for 8 days; or penicillin G procaine in oil with 2% aluminum monostearate (initially, 2.4 million units/dose for two subsequent doses given 3 days apart), as ordered.
• If patient has had syphilis for longer than 1 year, give penicillin G benzathine I.M. (2.4 million units/week for 3 weeks) or penicillin G procaine I.M. (600,000 units/day for 15 days).
• If patient's allergic to penicillin, administer tetracycline hydrochloride (Tetracyn*), as ordered, or erythromycin base, estolate, or stearate 500 mg P.O. four times a day for 15 days for primary or secondary syphilis or 30 days for late infection. (Tetracycline hydrochloride is contraindicated if patient's pregnant.)
• Make sure patient understands dosage schedule and precautions for medications.
• Promote rest and adequate nutrition.
• In secondary syphilis, teach patient to keep lesions clean and dry. Instruct patient how to dispose of contaminated material.
• Instruct patient to repeat VDRL test after 1, 3, 9, and 12 months to detect possible relapse. In latent or late syphilis, tell patient to have a blood study at 6-month intervals for 2 years.
• Warn patient to avoid becoming pregnant during treatment of

active disease because syphilis can cross the placental barrier and infect the fetus.
• Urge patient to notify all sexual partners of the infection, so they can seek treatment.
• Report all cases of syphilis to public health officials.

Trichomoniasis
Cause
• *Trichomonas vaginalis*
Incubation period
• Varies
Signs and symptoms
• Most patients are asymptomatic.
In males:
• Mild to severe transient urethritis, possibly accompanied by dysuria and frequency; may also affect the prostate gland, seminal vesicles, and the epididymis
In females:
• Gray or green-yellow, possibly profuse and frothy, malodorous vaginal discharge
• Severe itching, redness, swelling and tenderness in vagina and urethra; may also affect endocervix, Bartholin's glands, Skene's glands, and bladder
• Dyspareunia
• Dysuria
• Urinary frequency
• Occasional postcoital spotting, menorrhagia, or dysmenorrhea
• Signs and symptoms may persist for a week to several months and may be more pronounced just after menstruation or during pregnancy.
Nursing intervention
• Collect vaginal or seminal discharge specimen to identify causative organism.
• Administer metronidazole (Flagyl*) to patient and sexual partner. Give in small doses for 7 days or in a single, large dose, as ordered.
• After treatment, remind patient and sexual partner that they'll need a follow-up examination to check for residual signs of infection.
• Warn your patient to abstain from alcoholic beverages while taking metronidazole, because alcohol consumption may provoke a disulfiramlike reaction.
• Warn patient that metronidazole may cause his urine to turn dark brown.
• Instruct female patient to douche with a vinegar and water solution to relieve itching and pain.
• Caution female patient not to use over-the-counter douches and vaginal sprays.
• To help prevent reinfection during treatment, urge abstinence from intercourse or encourage patient to use a condom.

*Available in both the United States and Canada

How to culture a penile discharge

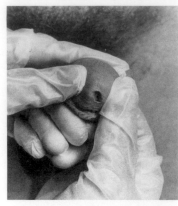

1 Let's say you're examining your patient's penis. While inspecting the urethral opening, as the nurse is doing here, you notice discharge. Do you know what to do? First, note the amount, color, consistency, and odor of the discharge. Then, check for bacterial growth by collecting two separate specimens for cultures. To proceed, follow these steps.

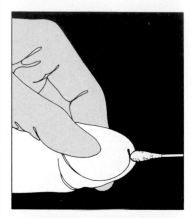

2 Remove the sterile cotton-tipped swab from a Culturette™ tube. Roll the swab in the discharge.

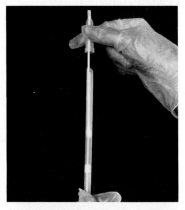

3 Next, return the swab to its tube, as shown here. Make sure you don't touch the outside of the tube with the swab. Then, squeeze the end of the tube containing the culture preservation medium. Make sure the swab's completely immersed in the medium.

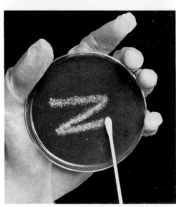

4 Obtain a second sterile cotton-tipped swab and roll it in the discharge. Using the swab, smear the specimen over a Thayer-Martin plate in a Z-pattern, as shown here. Then, immediately cross-streak the plate with the swab, unless this step is performed by the laboratory. Label both specimens and send them to the lab for analysis.

Genital herpes: Know the facts

"I just haven't felt like myself lately," Fran Rowland tells you in the clinic's waiting room. "I feel dragged out and have a headache, and when I urinate, it hurts."

When you start assessing Ms. Rowland's condition, you discover additional signs that warrant attention. For example, Ms. Rowland has a heavy vaginal discharge, and she says she has a dull ache in the entire genital area. Your vaginal exam reveals blisters on the vaginal wall and cervix. You document these and other findings in detail, so you can incorporate them into your patient's care plan.

Does Ms. Rowland have genital herpes? What do her signs and symptoms suggest? Among other things, possibly genital herpes. To ensure accurate diagnosis, you'll need to collect a specimen of tissue for culture or of secretions for a smear. Remember, genital herpes has been mistaken for venereal warts, syphilis, and nongonococcal urethritis.

Laboratory tests to identify and diagnose herpes include cytologic smear (Papanicolaou test), viral culture, and blood studies (antibody titers). Be aware that none of these tests detects the differences between herpes simplex virus type 1 (HSV-1) and herpes simplex virus type 2 (HSV-2). Tests that differentiate between these viruses are expensive and usually only performed in life-threatening situations, such as herpes infections in newborns.

How did Ms. Rowland contract herpes? Genital herpes is spread through skin-to-skin contact with any open lesion; for example, during sexual intercourse. It may also be spread by sharing contaminated items, such as a towel, or from an infected toilet seat or a bath tub. In addition, a patient with genital herpes may transfer contagious secretions from an infected area during masturbation, genital washing, or self-examination. And after the initial genital herpes infection, various

types of stress—menstruation, tension, pregnancy, or poor physical condition—may cause lesions to recur.

As you probably know, the incubation period for genital herpes can last from 2 to 20 days; the average period is 6 days. For most patients, active infection lasts about 3 weeks, with symptoms peaking at 10 to 14 days. Keep in mind that a patient is contagious from the time the lesions appear to the time they heal. But even when the lesions heal, the virus still remains in the patient's nerve cells. When infection recurs, the attacks are usually milder and of shorter duration than the initial one. In most cases, each successive attack of herpes heals faster and the time between attacks lengthens. As mentioned earlier, two types of herpes simplex virus exist. HSV-1, on the one hand, causes fever blisters on the lips, mouth, and face. On the other hand, HSV-2 causes lesions in the genital area. And although fever blisters and genital lesions are caused by two different viruses of the same family, a small number of genital lesions may be caused by HSV-1 and a few cases of fever blisters may be caused by HSV-2.

Tracking down signs and symptoms

Signs and symptoms of genital herpes vary from patient to patient. Some patients are asymptomatic whereas others experience symptoms with the initial herpes attack and subsequent recurrences.

In most cases, the first noticeable symptom is itching or irritation, accompanied by redness in the genital area. Later, a lesion (which may be wet and ulcerous) appears. Women are less likely to develop visible lesions. Other signs and symptoms may include burning during urination; hematuria; dysuria; increased vaginal discharge; fatigue; aching or tingling of legs, buttocks, or lower back; fever; chills; headache; nausea; vomiting; fever; and, in women, leukorrhea.

Herpes: Helping your patient adjust

Let's say the diagnostic tests show that Ms. Rowland has herpes simplex virus type 2 (HSV-2), also known as genital herpes. No doubt she'll express fears about how this disease will affect her life.

Thoroughly explain genital herpes to her, advising her to have frequent gynecologic exams. Remember to tell her that a possible link exists between herpes and cervical cancer. Although no conclusive evidence connecting herpes and cervical cancer is available, women with genital herpes are four to six times more prone to cervical abnormalities than those without herpes.

Listen to her fears and encourage her to ask questions. Be informative and honest. Even though you can't promise she won't have another attack, you can instill confidence in her ability to cope with the disease. Inform her that no effective treatment for herpes has been found; acyclovir (Zovirax), a new antiviral agent, is being tested. This drug doesn't kill the herpesvirus, but it prevents further virus production. Be sure to tell Ms. Rowland that the drug may help minimize her symptoms if she has another attack and may prevent a recurrence.

When you talk to your patient, review these important points:
• To prevent recurrences, advise her to minimize stress and tension as much as possible. Tell her to try to determine what triggers an attack—for example, working overtime—and then avoid it.
• Advise your patient to keep her towel, washcloth, toothbrush, toothpaste, and bathroom cup in her bedroom. This way family members will be less likely to use these personal items.
• Recommend that she wear cotton underwear to decrease irritation and promote lesion healing.
• Emphasize the importance of telling her current or future sex partners about her herpes history.
• Suggest that she routinely check her genital area for swollen, reddened areas and excessive vaginal discharge.
• Tell her to abstain from sexual activity during active infection, to protect her partner from infection. If they choose to have sexual intercourse during this time, urge her to have her partner use a condom. Make sure she understands that a condom may not protect her partner from the infection.

Note: If your male patient has genital herpes and chooses to have sexual intercourse, advise him to use a condom.

Psychosocial

Identifying substance abusers

Substance abusers cross all barriers—social, occupational, racial, and gender. They are as common in rural areas as in large cities. As an ambulatory-care nurse, you may be the first health-care professional to encounter such a person.

People abuse substances for various reasons. Some want to escape problems they can't deal with; others are looking for a way to stimulate their senses. Some people abuse substances to defy their parents, teachers, or other authoritative figures or to be accepted into their peer group. Others do it to relieve physical symptoms—real or imagined. And still others become addicted inadvertently, when they take prescribed drugs for an illness.

If you suspect your patient may be abusing drugs, alcohol, or inhalants, follow these guidelines:
• Don't jump to conclusions. Try not to make decisions about substance abuse based on your patient's appearance, your detection of substance odor, or the kind of companions he's with.
• Don't pass judgment or impose your values on the patient. If you feel hostility toward him or are contemptuous of him, he'll sense it and become defensive or withdrawn. Then your chances for developing rapport are remote.
• Don't let the patient or his family manipulate you.
• Be honest with him. You're more likely to gain his trust by being concerned and frank.
• Protect yourself legally by documenting your suspicions and confirmed reports of illegal drug use.
• Ask a co-worker who has encountered a similar situation for help or suggestions.
• Don't feel guilty that you can't cure your patient of his problem.
• If you're caring for a patient who is suspected of taking an overdose, monitor him carefully until an ambulance arrives. Your patient may be conscious one moment and lapse into unconsciousness the next.

Identifying abused substances

Although identifying substance abusers isn't easy, you can detect specific signs of addiction and abuse, such as euphoria, dilated pupils, and slurred speech. Take care, however, not to base an identification only on physical signs or abnormal behavior. For one thing, most symptoms suggesting substance abuse are common to various diseases. Study the chart below for more details.

Stimulants
• amphetamines (Biphetamine, Dexedrine*)
• methylphenidate (Ritalin*)
• cocaine
Street names
• For amphetamines: speed, uppers, bennies, pep pills
• For methylphenidate: fast freddies, crank
• For cocaine: coke, flake, dust
Duration of effect
• For amphetamines: 2 to 12 hours
• For methylphenidate: 2 to 4 hours
• For cocaine: 1 to 2 hours
Possible psychological effects
• Euphoria, insomnia, agitation, confusion, hallucinations, paranoia, talkativeness, tremors, delirium, violent outbursts, giggling, rapid speech, dependence
Possible physical findings
• Lip licking, excessive nose rubbing, skin picking, worn-down teeth from grinding while intoxicated, needle marks, skin abscesses, nasal abnormalities from sniffing, increased blood pressure, tachycardia, arrhythmias, headache, angina, increased respiratory rate, anorexia, dry mouth, vomiting, weight loss, dilated pupils in overdose, hyperactivity, hyperreflexia

Depressants
• chloral hydrate (Noctec*, Somnos)
• barbiturates (Nembutal, Phenobarbital, Seconal, Amytal*, Butisol)
• glutethimide (Doriden*)
• methaqualone (Quaalude, Optimil, Parest, Sopor)
• benzodiazepines (Ativan*, Valium*, Dalmane*, Librium*, Serax*, Tranxene*)
Street names
• For chloral hydrate: knock-out drops, joy juice, Peter, Mickey Finn (when mixed with alcohol)
• For barbiturates: downers, yellow jackets, barbs, blue devils, redbirds, blue heavens, peanuts, rainbows
• For glutethimide: downers
• For methaqualone: quads, ludes, soapers, sopes, Qs
• For benzodiazepines: lemons, downers
Duration of effect
• For chloral hydrate: 5 to 8 hours
• For barbiturates: 1 to 16 hours
• For glutethimide: 4 to 8 hours
• For methaqualone: 4 to 8 hours
• For benzodiazepines: 4 to 8 hours
Possible psychological effects
• Drowsiness, confusion, irritability, poor

memory, drunken appearance, depression, slowed comprehension, argumentativeness, somber appearance, stupor, dependence
Possible physical findings
• Clammy skin, abdominal cramps, gastric distress (nausea, vomiting, diarrhea), dizziness, headache, nystagmus, ataxia, varied pupillary reactions, slurred speech, decreased tendon and pain reflexes, shallow and slow breathing, decreased blood pressure and pulse rate

Alcohol
Street names
• Hooch, booze, brew, grog, spirits, firewater
Duration of effect
• Depends on body weight and chemistry, speed of consumption, previous dietary intake, alcoholic content of beverage consumed, and patient history
Possible psychological effects
• Depression, mood swings, guilt, self-destruction tendencies, lack of self-esteem, easy frustration, dependence
Possible physical findings
• Alcoholic breath odor, facial edema, poor coordination, slurred speech, broad-based footdrop, slapping walk, visual disturbances (such as blurred vision), bloodshot eyes, blackouts, nausea, vomiting, anorexia, diarrhea, insomnia, liver damage

Narcotics
• opium (Paregoric*, Dover's Powder)
• morphine sulfate*
• heroin (diacetylmorphine)
• methadone (Dolophine)
Street names
• For opium: poppies, schoolboys
• For morphine: Miss Emmas, first lines, mud, morf, white stuff
• For heroin: big H, horse, powder, smack, scag, stuff, seat, snow, Harry, joy powder
• For methadone: meth
Duration of effect
• For opium: 3 to 6 hours
• For morphine: 3 to 6 hours
• For heroin: 3 to 6 hours
• For methadone: 12 to 14 hours (after cumulative use)
Possible psychological effects
• Euphoria, lethargy, apathy, slow comprehension, stupor, inattentiveness, dependence
Possible physical findings
• Watery eyes, loss of appetite, cool and clammy skin, nausea, vomiting, constipation, cramps during withdrawal, constricted pupils with negative reaction to light and poor accommodation, convulsions, shallow and slow breathing, urine retention, increased pigmentation over veins, thrombosed veins, skin lesions or abscesses, swollen nasal mucosa, needle marks, decreased blood pressure

Hallucinogens
• Lysergic acid diethylamide (LSD)
• mescaline, peyote
• phencyclidine

*Available in both the United States and Canada

Street names
- *For LSD:* acid, microdots, California sunshine, sugar, cubes, trips, big D
- *For mescaline, peyote:* mesc, cactus, buttons, moon
- *For phencyclidine:* PCP, hog, angel dust, killer weed (when combined with marijuana)

Duration of effect
- *For LSD:* 8 to 12 hours
- *For mescaline, peyote:* 8 to 12 hours
- *For phencyclidine:* varies

Possible psychological effects
- Euphoria; delusions; hallucinations; poor perception of time and distance; distortion of sight, hearing, touch, and body image; excitation; psychoses; sudden behavioral changes; blank stare; suicidal or homicidal tendencies; mood swings; dependence

Possible physical findings
- Cold, sweaty hands and feet; chills; incoherent speech; palpitations; abdominal cramps; dry mouth; vomiting; nausea; anorexia; diarrhea; dizziness; dilated pupils in overdose but constricted in intoxication; muscle aches; irregular respiratory rates; increased blood pressure, pulse, and temperature

Marijuana derivative

Street names
- Pot, hash, THC, joints, Acapulco gold, tie sticks, reefers, locoweed, giggle smoke, Mary Jane

Duration of effect
- 2 to 4 hours

Possible psychological effects
- Euphoria; paranoia; psychosis; hyperactivity; relaxed inhibitions; distorted time and sense of perception; delusions; hallucinations; mild levels of suspiciousness, confusion, disorientation, and panic with toxic dose; dependence

Possible physical findings
- Talkativeness, dilated pupils, craving for sweets, tremors, decreased motor coordination and muscle strength, nystagmus, headache, dry mouth, increased respiratory rate, decreased blood pressure, tachycardia, decreased testosterone, male impotence

Inhalants
- Cleaning fluid
- Model airplane glue
- Lighter fluid
- Gasoline
- Paint thinner

Street names
- None

Duration of effects
- Varies with body weight and chemistry

Possible psychological effects
- Delirium, hallucinations, lethargy, restlessness, disorientation, violent behavior, dependence

Possible physical findings
- Runny nose, watery eyes, poor muscle coordination, drunken behavior without odor of alcohol, odor of fluids or other solvents, mucous membrane irritation, vomiting, bloody diarrhea, coughing, gagging, dyspnea, cyanosis, rales

We'd like to thank the following people and their companies for their help with this PHOTOBOOK:

ABBEY MEDICAL
(formerly Accurate Medical Service)
Willow Grove, Pa.
Chuck Hepler, Manager

©AMERICAN ACADEMY OF DERMATOLOGY
Evanston, Ill.

AMERICAN LUNG ASSOCIATION OF PHILADELPHIA AND MONTGOMERY COUNTY
Norristown, Pa.

AMERICAN MEDICAL INSTRUMENT CORPORATION
Subsidiary of Vernitron Corporation
Flushing, N.Y.
Grace Giordano, General Manager

BARNES-HIND PHARMACEUTICALS, INC.
A Division of Revlon Health Care Group
Sunnyvale, Calif.

W.A. BAUM CO. INC.
Copiague, N.Y.

BILSOM INTERNATIONAL, INC.
Reston, Va.

THE BURDICK CORPORATION
Hackensack, N.J.
Jules Pitsker, District Manager

CENTERS FOR DISEASE CONTROL
Atlanta, Ga.

CONNEY SAFETY PRODUCTS
Madison, Wis.

THE DEVILBISS COMPANY
Health Care Division
Somerset, Pa.

ENVIRONMENTAL TECHNOLOGY CORPORATION
Cleveland, Ohio

JOHNSON & JOHNSON PRODUCTS INC.
Patient Care Division
New Brunswick, N.J.

MEDTEK CORPORATION
Princeton, N.J.

MEDTRONIC INC.
Minneapolis, Minn.

NATIONAL HEALTH INFORMATION CLEARING HOUSE
Rosslyn, Va.

NATIONAL HEART, LUNG AND BLOOD INSTITUTE
Bethesda, Md.

NATIONAL HIGH BLOOD PRESSURE EDUCATION PROGRAM
Bethesda, Md.

NORCLIFF THAYER INC.
Tarrytown, N.Y.

NORTON COMPANY
Safety Products Division
Rockford, Ill.

ONOX INC.
Palo Alto, Calif.

PURITAN-BENNETT CORPORATION
Bellmawr, N.J.

J. SKLAR MFG. CO., INC.
Long Island City, N.Y.

SMITHKLINE DIAGNOSTICS
Sunnyvale, Calif.

SYBRON CORPORATION
Medical Products Division
Rochester, N.Y.

TELEDYNE WATER PIK
Fort Collins, Colo.

TERUMO CORPORATION
Piscataway, N.J.

Berks County Office of the Aging
Reading, Pa.

Eleanor M. Brower, RN
Clyde L. Nash, Jr., MD
St. Luke's Hospital
Cleveland, Ohio

William P. Bunnell, MD
Director of Orthopedics
Alfred I. DuPont Institute
Wilmington, Del.

Casa Colina Hospital
Pomona, Calif.

Commonwealth of Pennsylvania
Department of Health
   Donald Mixon
   Public Health Advisor
   Immunization Program
   Norristown, Pa.
   Elizabeth Powers, RN
   Community Health Nurse Supervisor
   West Reading, Pa.

Maureen Hamilton, RN
Staff Development Coordinator
Chestnut Hill Hospital
Philadelphia, Pa.

Clem J. Hill, DMD
Professor, Pediatric Dentistry
University of Florida
Gainesville, Fla.

Mark Lapayowker, MD
Professor, Radiology
Radiology Department
Temple University
Philadelphia, Pa.

Joan Reilly, RN, PNP
North Penn School District
Lansdale, Pa.

Sister St. Gregory, BS
St. Joseph's Villa
Flourtown, Pa.

Also the staffs of:

BERKS VISITING NURSE HOME HEALTH AGENCY
Reading, Pa.

CHESTNUT HILL HOSPITAL
Philadelphia, Pa.

COMMUNITY GENERAL HOSPITAL
Reading, Pa.

THE FRANKLIN MINT
Franklin Center, Pa.

UNIVERSITY OF MICHIGAN
Ambulatory Nursing Department
Ann Arbor, Mich.

VISITING NURSE ASSOCIATION OF EASTERN MONTGOMERY COUNTY INC.
Abington, Pa.

Selected references

Books

Alexander, Mary M., and Marie S. Brown. PEDIATRIC HISTORY TAKING AND PHYSICAL DIAGNOSIS FOR NURSES, 2nd ed. New York: McGraw-Hill Book Co., 1979.

American Heart Association. HEART FACTS 1982: A PSYCHOPHYSIOLOGIC APPROACH. Dallas: American Heart Assoc., 1982.

Arndt, Kenneth A. MANUAL OF DERMATOLOGIC THERAPEUTICS, 2nd ed. Boston: Little, Brown & Co., 1980.

ASSESSING YOUR PATIENTS. Nursing Photobook Series. Springhouse, Pa.: Springhouse Corp., 1980.

ASSESSMENT. Nurse's Reference Library. Springhouse, Pa.: Springhouse Corp., 1982.

Bates, Barbara. A GUIDE TO PHYSICAL EXAMINATION, 2nd ed. Philadelphia: J.B. Lippincott Co., 1979.

Benson, Evelyn R., and Joan Q. McDevitt. COMMUNITY HEALTH AND NURSING PRACTICE, 2nd ed. Englewood Cliffs, N.J.: Prentice-Hall, Inc., 1980.

Brown, Marie S., and Mary A. Murphy. AMBULATORY PEDIATRICS FOR NURSES, 2nd ed. New York: McGraw-Hill Book Co., 1980.

Brunner, Lillian S. THE LIPPINCOTT MANUAL OF NURSING PRACTICE, 3rd ed. Philadelphia: J.B. Lippincott Co., 1982.

Budassi, Susan A., and Janet Barber. EMERGENCY NURSING: PRINCIPLES AND PRACTICE. St. Louis: C.V. Mosby Co., 1980.

Burkhalter, Pamela K. NURSING CARE OF THE ALCOHOLIC AND DRUG ABUSER. New York: McGraw-Hill Book Co., 1975.

Capell, Peter T., and David B. Case. AMBULATORY CARE MANUAL FOR NURSE PRACTITIONERS. Philadelphia: J.B. Lippincott Co., 1976.

Conway, Barbara L. CARINI AND OWENS' NEUROLOGICAL AND NEUROSURGICAL NURSING, 7th ed. St. Louis: C.V. Mosby Co., 1978.

Cosgritt, James H. AN ATLAS OF DIAGNOSTIC AND THERAPEUTIC PROCEDURES FOR EMERGENCY PERSONNEL. Philadelphia: J.B. Lippincott Co., 1978.

DEALING WITH EMERGENCIES. Nursing Photobook Series. Springhouse, Pa.: Springhouse Corp., 1980.

DeJong, Russell N. THE NEUROLOGICAL EXAMINATION, 4th ed. New York: Harper & Row, 1979.

DIAGNOSTICS. Nurse's Reference Library. Springhouse, Pa.: Springhouse Corp., 1982.

DISEASES. Nurse's Reference Library. Springhouse, Pa.: Springhouse Corp., 1981.

ENSURING INTENSIVE CARE. Nursing Photobook Series. Springhouse, Pa.: Springhouse Corp., 1981.

Estes, Nada J., et al. NURSING DIAGNOSIS OF THE ALCOHOLIC PERSON. St. Louis: C.V. Mosby Co., 1980.

GIVING CARDIAC CARE. Nursing Photobook Series. Springhouse, Pa.: Springhouse Corp., 1981.

Jarvis, Linda L. COMMUNITY HEALTH NURSING: KEEPING THE PUBLIC HEALTHY. Philadelphia: F.A. Davis Co., 1981.

Leitch, Cynthia J., and Richard V. Tinker. PRIMARY CARE. Philadelphia: F.A. Davis Co., 1978.

Mann, James K., and Annalee R. Oates, eds. CRITICAL CARE NURSING OF THE MULTI-INJURED PATIENT. American Association of Critical Care Nurses. Philadelphia: W.B. Saunders Co., 1980.

Pierce, Donald S., and Vernon H. Nickel, eds. THE TOTAL CARE OF SPINAL CORD INJURIES. Boston: Little, Brown & Co., 1977.

Sanderson, Richard G., ed. CARDIAC PATIENT: A COMPREHENSIVE APPROACH. Philadelphia: W.B. Saunders Co., 1972.

Sokolow, Maurice, and Malcolm B. McIlroy. CLINICAL CARDIOLOGY, 2nd ed. Los Altos, Calif.: Lange Medical Publications, 1979.

Spradley, Barbara Walton. COMMUNITY HEALTH NURSING CONCEPTS AND PRACTICE. Boston: Little, Brown & Co., 1981.

Swift, Nancy, and Robert M. Mabel. MANUAL OF NEUROLOGICAL NURSING. Boston: Little, Brown & Co., 1978.

Tackett, Jo J., and Mabel Hunsberger. FAMILY-CENTERED CARE OF CHILDREN AND ADOLESCENTS. Philadelphia: W.B. Saunders Co., 1981.

Turek, Samuel L. ORTHOPAEDICS: PRINCIPLES AND THEIR APPLICATION, 3rd ed. Philadelphia: J.B. Lippincott Co., 1977.

Whaley, Lucille F., and Donna Wong. NURSING CARE OF INFANTS AND CHILDREN. St. Louis: C.V. Mosby Co., 1979.

Zenz, Carl, ed. DEVELOPMENTS IN OCCUPATIONAL MEDICINE. Chicago: Year Book Medical Publishers, 1980.

Periodicals

American Heart Association Subcommittee on Emergency Cardiac Care. *CPR and Emergency Cardiac Care: New Standards and Guidelines,* EMERGENCY MEDICINE, 12:65-77, August 15, 1980.

Amilar, R.N., and L. Dubin. *Sexual Response to Disease Process,* JOURNAL OF SEX RESEARCH, 4:257-264, November 1968.

Batterman, B., et al. *Hypertension: Treatment and Nursing Responsibilities,* CARDIOVASCULAR NURSING, 11:41-44, September-October 1975.

Brown, Margie E. *Introduction to Assessment of the Skin,* OCCUPATIONAL HEALTH NURSING, 28:8-121, August 1980.

Boyd-Monk, Heather. *Practical Methods of How to Examine the External Eye,* OCCUPATIONAL HEALTH NURSING, 29:10-14, June 1981.

Clark, N., et al. *Developing Education for Children with Asthma Through Study of Self-management Behavior,* HEALTH EDUCATION QUARTERLY, 7:278-297, Winter 1980.

Dupont, Jeanne. *EENT Emergencies,* NURSING79, 9:65-70, November 1979.

Fleming, J.W. *Common Dermatologic Conditions in Children,* AMERICAN JOURNAL OF MATERNAL CHILD NURSING, 6:346-354, September-October 1981.

Gaston, Susan F., and Lorna Lou Schuman. *Inhalation Injury: Smoke Inhalation,* AMERICAN JOURNAL OF NURSING, 80:94-97, January 1980.

Janz, Nancy, and Richard M. Lampman. *Coaching Your Cardiac Patient Along the Path to Recovery,* NURSING81, 12:36-41, December 1981.

Joseph, L. *Self-care of the Nursing Process,* NURSING CLINICS OF NORTH AMERICA, 15:1, March 1980.

Linde, B.J., and N.M. Janz. *Effect of a Teaching Program on Knowledge and Compliance of Cardiac Patients,* NURSING RESEARCH, 28:282-286, September-October 1979.

Mills, J. *The Common Cold: Nuisance or Serious Problem?* JOURNAL OF RESPIRATORY DISEASES, 9:16-27, September 1981.

Pleuss, J., and M.S. Kochar. *Dietary Considerations in Hypertension,* POSTGRADUATE MEDICINE, June 1981.

Potter, M., et al. *Is Your Patient Also an Alcoholic?* JOURNAL OF PRACTICAL NURSING, 30:17, May 1980.

Rogers, Terry. *Clinical Problems in the Adult with Asthma,* NURSING CLINICS OF NORTH AMERICA, 16:293-298, June 1981.

Smith, C.R. *Patient Education in Ambulatory Care,* NURSING CLINICS OF NORTH AMERICA, 12:595-608, December 1977.

Turner, R., and J.O. Hendley. *How Colds Spread: Surprising New Data,* JOURNAL OF RESPIRATORY DISEASES, 3:97-106, January 1982.

Webster, Katherine P. *Planning and Implementing Health Screening Programs,* JOURNAL OF SCHOOL HEALTH, 50:493-495, November 1980.

Wise, Thomas. *Sexuality Counseling,* MEDICAL ASPECTS OF HUMAN SEXUALITY, March 1978, pp. 93-107.

Woodbery, Patricia Moran, and Ann B. Hamric. *Emergency Exercise,* NURSING81, 12:32-34, December 1981.

Index

Index

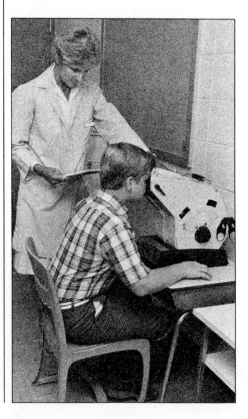